GW00656575

Sky Wards

Sky Wards

A History of the
Princess Mary's
Royal Air Force Nursing
Service

MARY MACKIE

Foreword by HRH The Princess Alexandra
Patron of the PMRAFNS

ROBERT HALE · LONDON

© Mary Mackie 2001
First published in Great Britain 2001

ISBN 0 7090 6976 6

Robert Hale Limited
Clerkenwell House
Clerkenwell Green
London EC1R 0HT

The right of Mary Mackie to be identified as
author of this work has been asserted by her in accordance with the
Copyright, Designs and Patents Act 1988

A catalogue record for this book is available from the British Library

2 4 6 8 10 9 7 5 3 1

Set in Sabon by
Derek Doyle & Associates, Liverpool.
Printed by
St Edmundsbury Press Limited, Bury St Edmunds
and bound by
Woolnough Bookbinding Limited, Irthlingborough.

CONTENTS

ACKNOWLEDGEMENTS

This book could not have been written without the help and support of many people. I should like to express my unbounded gratitude and appreciation to all of them, in particular:

To Air Commodore Robert H. Williams, RRC QHNS, Director of Nursing Services and first male Matron-in-Chief of the PMRAFNS, for his determination to have a history of the Service brought to print; for allowing me the privilege of being the one to do it; and for his unswerving support and assistance during the many months of work involved in bringing the project to completion.

To you, Bob, this book is dedicated.

To Group Captain Annie Reid, OBE ARRC, Matron-in-Chief from March 2001, for her kindness in providing me with much help and useful information; to my tireless ally and research assistant Wing Commander (Rtd) Angela Scofield, ARRC, who spied out the land at the museums, did some of the interviews, provided stories and pictures, and helped to set me right on technical details; to Air Commodore (Rtd) Valerie Hand, RRC, for her own stories and her eagle eye for factual and grammatical accuracy; and, not least, to Mrs Marion Donaldson (PMRAFNS Rtd) for her personal support and encouragement and, in her role as editor of the *PMRAFNS Magazine*, source of invaluable information and assistance.

To all members of the PMRAFNS, past and present, who allowed me and my husband, or Anji Scofield, into their homes where they recounted their own amazing stories. They are all named in the

Appendix. However, I must add a special thank you to Group Captain (Rtd) Liz Sandison, RRC, for being such a wonderful hostess over the two days when a squadron of PMs gathered at her home to talk with us and share their experiences. The welcome could not have been warmer. Thank you, Liz.

To the many, many other PMs, and their husbands and families, RAF doctors, patients, WAAFs, medics – everyone who has so willingly responded to my appeals for information and bombarded me with photographs, cartoons, maps, menus and wonderful stories that have made me laugh out loud or brought a lump to my throat – sometimes both. Some of you have swiftly answered my follow-up queries and in some cases put up with phone calls to check yet more final details. Thank you all for your kindness and your good wishes. I'm only sorry that lack of space has forced me to leave out much that I had hoped to include. However, as you know, everything you sent will be added to the records and preserved for the future. Some day there may be another book.

To all at the RAF Museum at Hendon, especially to Peter Elliott, Senior Keeper, and Andrew Cormack (Uniforms), and to the cheerful, friendly staff in the Wings Café – couldn't have done without you!; to Jean Buckberry, College Librarian at RAF Cranwell; to Sandy Gilbert-Wykes, Community Relations Officer at RAF Coningsby; to Mr Stankus at the Royal Signals Museum, Blandford; to all at Air Historical Branch, London, and Personnel Records, Innsworth; and to the staff of the Imperial War Museum and the Public Record Office (PRO). My work at the latter was immensely aided by a list of relevant files kindly sent by Enid Zaig, to whom special thanks for saving me so much time. And to Jean Holmes, for sharing with me her research into the youngest VC, RAF Sergeant John Hannah.

Finally, to Chris, my long-suffering husband and unpaid assistant, for help too varied to detail, for being a strong shoulder when the going got tough, and such a supportive cook and bottle washer over eighteen months when my word processor saw more of me than he did!

Thank you, all.

Foreword

As Patron, I am delighted to welcome the publication of this long-awaited history of the Princess Mary's Royal Air Force Nursing Service. It is an extraordinary story of dedication, professionalism, courage and humour, set against a backdrop of eighty eventful years of world history, illustrated by many personal stories of past and present members of the Service. It also shows the development of medical and nursing practice over the last century, and the vital role the Royal Air Force has played in those advances.

I am pleased to add my personal tribute to all members, past and present, of the PMRAFNS.

Alexandra

HRH The Princess Alexandra
Patron of the PMRAFNS

ILLUSTRATIONS

Between pages 32 and 33

Between pages 64 and 65

Between pages 96 and 97

9

Illustration Credits

INTRODUCTION

A history of the Princess Mary's Royal Air Force Nursing Service (PMRAFNS) was first envisioned seventy years ago, in 1930, when the first Matron-in-Chief began to gather anecdotal material. Her rough jottings, plus letters from early sisters telling their own stories, waited in the archive like diamonds for me to mine. Other researchers, over the years, have gathered bits and pieces of material which I have gratefully incorporated in this present book. Meanwhile, time has been galloping on and every year adds yet more stories. The present book must be somewhat longer than the one originally planned.

As I've discovered, even in books which purport to cover the whole RAF, little or no mention is made of the PMRAFNS. Huge and busy hospitals fail to merit so much as a footnote in tomes giving minute details of airfield squadrons, and even the *History of the RAF Medical Service for World War Two* – three huge volumes – gives the PMs only ten pages. One history of RAF Halton, whose hospital is regarded as the well-spring of both the medical and the nursing services, adds insult to injury by mentioning the hospital in passing but getting its name wrong. Its author calls it 'Queen Mary's RAF Hospital' instead of 'Princess Mary's' – an entirely different lady!

I was, therefore, delighted to be asked to set matters right and produce a book telling the story of the RAF's nursing service, not as a dry and dusty record of facts and figures alone but as a human tale with plenty of lively personal anecdotes. I must admit that when I accepted the task I was not fully aware of the mountain I had to climb (not quite Everest, but approaching K2!); however, despite the hard work and moments of hair-tearing, it has been a journey of discovery, full of interest, excitement and entertainment. It has also made me aware of the courage of the thousands of women and, latterly, men who across eighty years have been proud to call themselves 'PMs'. I hope that the result will please all members, whether retired, currently serving, or prospective. I also trust it will provide 'a good read' for anyone interested in nursing, or in the air force, or simply in a rattling good story of human beings with all their virtues, faults and foibles, and their wonderful sense of humour.

A word about the style of the book

A professional writer I am, but on the subject of this book I started out with (almost) a blank sheet. Perhaps that was a good thing: I've been able to research it from scratch and write it for a wide audience, trying to avoid nursing or service jargon which might make some readers feel excluded. Clinical purists please forgive me, but 'fainting fit', for instance, is understood by all, whereas 'vasovagal attack' would send most people rushing not for smelling salts but for a dictionary. In most cases I've settled for plain English.

The book is broken up into sections covering sweeps of history and the chapters too are divided into segments, with side headings, for those who like to dip in and out. Or the book can be read from beginning to end as a flowing story.

I needed to establish a consistent and logical way of referring to the people who, via their letters and interviews, have helped me to tell this story. To this end, contributors other than PMs are fully identified within the text: 'Jimmy Brown, RAF Sgt' or 'Cpl WAAF Polly Perkins', or 'patient Mrs Johnson' speak for themselves. Any name without such explanation is, or has been, a serving member of the PMRAFNS. To avoid complications caused by changes of rank and, in the case of the ladies, by maiden and married names, I've settled for the simple approach, referring to nearly every lady by her maiden name, adding her married name, as appropriate, in brackets. So someone identified as 'Joan Smith (Mrs Bloggs)' will mostly remain Joan Smith, or simply Joan, during the rest of that segment. If we meet her again in a later chapter she will be re-identified as 'Joan Smith (Mrs Bloggs)' for clarity. The style of the book generally lets the writers speak as they were when they had these experiences, so this way of identifying them seemed logical to me. The men, too, you'll generally find as 'Sam Jones' or simply 'Sam', whether they were Aircraftman or Group Captain. Occasionally, for variety and flavour, I've slipped in a 'Sister Joan Smith' or 'PM Sally Spigot' or 'Flight Lieutenant Sam Jones'. For anyone interested in discovering more about these contributors – when they served, what rank they held and where I gleaned their stories – an appendix details all PMs actually quoted in the text. I have not included awards and honours against these names: there being no time to check every single one, rather than risk making a mistake and causing offence, I've compromised by leaving them out. In fact, very many PMs have been awarded such honours as the Royal Red Cross or the Order of St John of Jerusalem, as is made clear in the main text.

When it comes to capital letters I've followed current practice for minimizing them. It's correct to write 'the prince visited the coalmine' without a capital letter for prince, though when using full name and title the capital is employed: 'Prince William visited the coal mine'; so this book refers to the 'sisters' mess' and the 'commanding officer', not to the 'Sisters' Mess' and the 'Commanding Officer', though in direct quotes I've left the capitals as the writers preferred them. This usage, I hope, makes the book more reader-friendly.

Another problem in a book of this kind is the use of initialisms and acronyms: everyone knows what RAF stands for but other terms such as NBC and MDHU are less familiar and may have different meanings in different contexts. I've endeavoured to keep them to a minimum or, where necessary, to write the words in full; if anyone gets really lost, one of the appendices has an alphabetical list.

Other appendices give the main dates and details of all RAF hospitals, one list for the UK, the other for overseas. This is the first time such lists have been compiled. In one or two instances, exact opening and closing dates of these units have eluded me; some details seem impossible to pin down without spending months poring over daily records, and in some cases the records no longer exist. Spellings of foreign place-names provide another area for error – where there's an anomaly unsolved by recourse to atlases and libraries, I've settled for the most widely-used spelling.

Writing a book of this kind, one is faced by a minefield of possible misinformation. In addition to my own double-checking, members of the PMRAFNS have provided invaluable technical help and my copy-editor has ironed out a few of the remaining unforced errors. Any mistakes that remain are my own and I take full responsibility for them. In spite of them, I hope you will enjoy reading this celebration of the Princess Mary's Royal Air Force Nursing Service.

Mary Mackie
March 2001

PART I

'Nothing shall deter us'

'*Nec aspera terrent*'
Motto of the PMRAFNS

ONE

Hurricane Hattie

1961 . . . Yuri Gagarin rides through space. Teenagers gyrate to a
new dance called the twist. The Beatles are still unknowns and
Coronation Street has been on British screens for just a year. In
Russia, Nikita Khrushchev holds the reins of power, while over in
Washington DC the charismatic young president, John F. Kennedy,
is newly settled in the White House. Political tensions keep armed
forces alert, ready to respond at the first sign of aggression.

Britain's Royal Air Force patrols the skies from airfields across
Europe, the Middle East and the Far East. And, equally far-flung,
members of Princess Mary's Royal Air Force Nursing Service carry
out their daily duties: in the Mediterranean, Flight Officer Joy
Harris is enjoying 'trooping' aboard *Devonshire*; and Flight Officer
Jane Stott is in Singapore, at RAF Hospital Changi. Not so very
long ago, Changi endured horrors during Japanese occupation;
now, when a Royal Navy vessel passes, merry midwives wave
nappies in greeting from louvred windows. At home, at RAF
Hospital Cosford, Shropshire, Flying Officer Eileen Smith is beginning a romance with Flying Officer David Dodds. The same unit
welcomes young Bob Williams, a boy entrant to the Medical
Branch, to begin eighteen months' training as a nursing attendant;
he will emerge, in due time, as Warrant Officer Boy Entrant and
Head Boy of the School, ready for the next stage in his Royal Air
Force career.

On 30 October of that same year, the latest Russian atom-bomb
test explodes a massive sixty megatons, provoking world-wide
protest. And the following day . . .

17

On 31 October 1961, Flight Officer Dorothy 'Hutch' Hutchins was in a cinema enjoying a film when a message flashed up on the screen summoning her back to her unit immediately. A stir of curiosity rippled through the cinema as she hurried out. Arriving at RAF Hospital Wroughton, she found that she and her colleague Flying Officer Iris Rawlings – both on call for aeromedical evacuation duties – were ordered to RAF Lyneham. They and the rest of the aeromed team were to gather their equipment and prepare to fly to the Caribbean, where Hurricane Hattie had devastated British Honduras, flattening its capital, Belize.

Iris Rawlings (Mrs Kerse) takes up the story:

> Within a couple of hours we were at RAF Lyneham meeting the rest of the team and being issued with what was to be our uniform for the next two weeks – men's khaki drill shirts and trousers. The rest of the team consisted of a medical officer, about a dozen technicians, and an adjutant, Flight Lieutenant Pinks – 'Pinkie' – whose home was in Belize and who was to prove invaluable to us.

The team boarded a Britannia and flew 6,000 miles across the Atlantic, to find the town of Belize wrecked and the airfield flooded. Their landing was tricky, on an airstrip marked out by lamps.

> HMS *Trowbridge*, a RN vessel, had been first on the scene. We were met at the airport by some of her crew and guided, through knee-high water, to the town library, which they had made their Mess. They gave us a meal and afterwards, since we had brought stretchers and blankets, we were invited to choose our bed space. We elected to sleep beneath a sign saying 'Unusual Hobbies'.

Next morning, borrowing wellington boots from the Navy, Iris and Hutch went out to survey the damage.

> The shore was only about a foot above sea level and the tidal waves had removed the roofs from all the houses and completely wrecked the less substantial ones (the majority).

The church, one of the few brick buildings, had been used as a refuge and its subsequent collapse had resulted in the highest death toll – running into hundreds.

It was decided that we should rehouse and tend the patients from the local hospital, which had been totally demolished. We commandeered the remains of the house of a local dignitary. This was the largest house in the area and, having been two-storeyed, still had one floor with a ceiling . . .

Once the patients were comfortably installed (two to a bed!), we had to prepare the upper floor for our occupation. The technicians fitted a tarpaulin roof, we unpacked the stretchers and blankets, and there was our 'home'.

Dorothy Hutchins recalls:

Sanitary arrangements consisted of a bucket which, for lack of other means of disposal, had to be emptied into the sea. There was a nightly curfew because of escaped prisoners and looting, a fire watch duty because of hurricane lamps . . . and the US Air Force dropped emergency food packs and tinned goods – including tinned bread, tinned butter, even tinned Smarties . . .

Unexpected horrors imprinted themselves on Iris Rawlings' memory:

Next to the hospital there was a water storage tank, where people would queue with their receptacles. Hutch and I would sometimes go out on what remained of the verandah and watch. One day we were told that a body had risen to the top of the tank . . .

One of our patients died and an army truck came round to collect the body. I talked to one of the soldiers, who couldn't have been more than eighteen years old. It seemed their daily task was to go round collecting bodies and taking them for cremation on pyres by the sea shore. The ground was too flooded for burial – sheer volume of bodies apart – and the bodies could not be kept. I asked the young soldier how they coped and he said they were given a bottle of whisky each day to see them through. I imagine the memory must haunt him for life – it does me, and I only heard about it.

Eventually it was decided that we had done all we could and it was time to leave. We were to spend a day or two in Jamaica, as guests of the QAs [Queen Alexandra's Royal Army Nursing Corps]. Imagine our joy when we were met at the aircraft by their Matron and told she had made hairdressing appointments for us that afternoon. Only a woman would think of that! We were also told that no female help was being allowed into Belize – we had rather jumped the gun. How glad I am that we did because it was an adventure I wouldn't have missed for anything.

As a result of this 'adventure', Dorothy Hutchins was made an Associate of the Royal Red Cross (ARRC) and Iris Rawlings received a Commendation from the Air Officer Commanding-in-Chief (AOC-in-C) – just two of the many awards earned over the years by members of the PMRAFNS.

TWO

Introducing the PMs

Once, long ago, arrow, sword and shot sufficed to despatch an enemy. The twentieth century added the sophisticated niceties of mustard gas, the fighter plane, the doodlebug, the nuclear bomb, napalm, the 'smart' bomb, chemical and biological weapons . . . All of these enable us to wage more impersonal war, with human targets obscured by distance and technology. Fortunately, our capacity for inflicting pain and death has obliged us also to learn better ways of soothing and healing, not only the wounds caused by our warfare but also illnesses which have plagued humankind for generations. Many of these medical advances have been pioneered and perfected with the help of the Royal Air Force Medical Service (RAFMS) and its twin sibling the Princess Mary's Royal Air Force Nursing Service (PMRAFNS). Members of this latter Service refer to themselves affectionately as 'PMs'.

The story of this elite and specialized group of women and men mirrors the political, military and medical story of the twentieth century. Born out of the horrors of the Great War, 1914-18, in the following two decades the Service spread to aerodromes across Britain and put down roots in the turbulent Middle East. As another world war shattered yet more bodies and minds, its supportive tendrils reached across three continents, from Iceland to Japan. It held steady as Korea erupted, as Cyprus revolted, and as hurricanes howled. Through the Falklands conflict, in the Gulf, in the Balkans, and during thousand upon thousand of individual dramas in between, PMs have answered the call for nursing aid.

Their main claim to uniqueness lies in their mobility. Wherever

21

an emergency arises, even halfway across the world, specially trained aeromedical teams can fly to the scene within hours, using the most up-to-date planes and carrying the latest equipment. Their expertise in in-flight nursing has been honed and perfected over eight eventful decades.

Those years have seen many changes in the service. Nurses are no longer simply ministering angels, offering little beyond soap and water, tender smiles and the touch of a soft feminine hand. PMs enter the third millennium as highly qualified, multi-skilled professionals, male and female, officers, warrant officers, NCOs and students. They work closely alongside naval and army nurses, as part of the Defence Medical Services. But they proudly continue to proclaim and defend their identity as members of the PMRAFNS.

The legacy of Florence Nightingale

The history of nursing, both civil and military, has been chronicled in detail elsewhere. Suffice it here to say that until comparatively recent times nursing was the province of amateurs and/or ill-paid incompetents. In warfare, while steel and shot killed a good many fighting men, far more died of wounds gone rotten through well-meaning ignorance and lack of hygiene. Not until the mid-nineteenth century did nursing become first a respectable occupation and eventually a fully trained profession, thanks largely to the efforts of Florence Nightingale.

By the time Miss Nightingale died in 1910, she had established the basis of a system of nurse-training that was to be adopted throughout the world. Its military ethos spawned all those terrifying sergeant-major-style matrons who have been parodied down the years. But out of those schools came the women who were to form the nursing services of Britain, the various civilian branches as well as those of the three armed forces: the Royal Navy, the Army and – as the early years of the twentieth century drew half the world into war – the Royal Air Force.

Genesis

In 1900 powered flight was in its infancy. Few people imagined that those first flimsy aircraft and the daredevils who piloted them would ever prove as effective in war as a cavalry charge or bombardment from a battleship. But some visionaries thought the possibilities worth exploring. An Air Battalion of the Royal Engineers came into being on 1 April 1911. It comprised two companies, one working with balloons and airships, the other with aircraft. In May of the following year, this battalion became a corps – the Royal Flying Corps (RFC), divided into a military wing and a naval wing later to be titled the Royal Naval Air Service (RNAS). With the arrival of 1914, intrepid young pilots swiftly improvised new techniques for waging aerial war.

In those early days, medical and nursing care for members of the RFC and RNAS came from whatever source lay closest. Sick or injured flyers, treated initially by unit medical officers and orderlies of the Royal Army Medical Corps, were passed on, as necessary, to the nearest military or naval hospital and the care of doctors and nurses of the army or navy. However, this state of affairs rapidly proved impracticable, mainly because flying stations (as they were then called) had to be situated on level uplands, with ample room for take-off and landing. Most of the airfields which sprang up during the Great War lay deep in the countryside, well away from large concentrations of population and established hospitals, whether army, navy or civilian. Clearly, special medical arrangements must be made to serve the needs of flying stations.

A sick bay for flyers of aeroplanes, airships and balloons was opened at the RNAS training station at Cranwell, Lincolnshire, in 1916. Around the same time, a fund was launched to establish a hospital for flying officers of the Royal Flying Corps; the unit opened that same year at Bryanston Square, London, with twenty available beds. Shortly afterwards, thanks to the generosity of voluntary contributors, the fund was sufficient to open a larger unit at Eaton Square. A third RFC hospital, at Mount Vernon, appointed its first medical specialist – a bacteriologist – on 11 October 1917, and soon a convalescent home was established in a large hotel with 200 acres of grounds at Shirley Park, Croydon. These facilities were staffed by nurses 'borrowed' from either the army – the Queen Alexandra's Imperial Military Nursing Service (QAIMNS), as it was then called; or the navy – the Queen Alexandra's Royal Naval Nursing Service (QARNNS). As yet, the embryo flying services had no separate medical or nursing branch of their own.

On 1 April 1918, under the command of Major General Sir (later Lord) Hugh Montague Trenchard, the two wings of the RFC merged, assuming their new and enduring title of The Royal Air Force. Just three weeks later the new service won its first famous victory when one of its pilots shot down and killed the top-scoring German fighter ace, Rittmeister Manfred Freiherr von Richthofen, the 'Red Baron'.

On 1 June that same year, the fledgling Royal Air Force acquired its own (temporary) nursing service. Qualified civilian nurses might apply, and army and naval nurses could elect to leave QAIMNS or QARNNS and become members of the Royal Air Force Nursing Service (RAFNS), for the duration of the war at least.

Four Women

Looking back at those days of early 1918, we find a world in turmoil. At the front, young men were still fighting and dying, knee-deep in mud; at sea, U-boats menaced great iron-clad warships, while in the skies fragile flying machines augmented the forces of land and sea. And all the while, in the background, millions of people toiled in support. They included many women – girls who turned their soft hands to painting and doping, to carting artillery shells, butchering meat rations or, in the more traditional way of women through the ages, tending the hurts of those who returned from the front. Among those carers were four particular women – Margaret, Kate, Marion and Mary.

Differences of age and rank separated them, not to mention geography, but each of the four was involved, in her own way, in the war effort and in nursing. Three were well-experienced nurses: Margaret was based in India, Kate in London, Marion close to the front in France, and Mary, the youngest of the four at only twenty, had for some time been deeply involved with volunteer war work in England. None of them had met any of the others, nor did they suspect the roles that awaited them. Their only connection, back then in early 1918, was the vocation that had called them.

Joanna Margaret Cruickshank, known to her family as Margaret, was born on 28 November 1875, the second child of William Cruickshank. Her father, a Scotsman from Aberdeen, ventured out as a young man, first to try life in Australia and later to settle in

India. His five children were all born in India and grew up as part of the Raj, in an era when the British Empire was still a powerful force in the world.

It is thought that Joanna Margaret's interest in nursing began in India, perhaps through work with Lady Minto's Indian Nursing Association (INA). She eventually returned to the UK to take professional qualifications, starting as a probationer nurse at Guy's Hospital in 1907 at the somewhat advanced age of thirty-one. After completing a general nursing course she gained extra diplomas in massage and midwifery and, around 1912, she travelled back to the east to rejoin her family and become a sister with Lady Minto's INA. In 1917 she joined Queen Alexandra's Imperial Military Nursing Service.

The Great War was at its height. In the mountains and deserts of the North-West Frontier and the Middle East, Indian soldiers fought beside their British comrades. Margaret Cruickshank was one of the army nurses who cared for them amid the heat and the dust – and the mosquitoes. In common with many of her patients, she contracted a malignant form of malaria. Stricken by recurring fevers which depleted her strength and left her unable to work, she sought relief in the Punjabi hills, whose cooler air might restore her health. Sadly, it failed to do so and in March 1918 she was invalided home to the more temperate climate of Britain.

The journey proved an eventful one, especially for a sick woman of forty-two. Interviewed later by the press, she described her voyage from India as being fraught with 'delay, difficulties and dangers'.

The culminating point was when the ship was torpedoed in the Mediterranean: we had, of course, been aware of the danger, but none of us realised just what it would feel like. Even now . . . that moment when the ship was struck is as vivid in my memory as when it happened. We had to take to the open boats and after a few hours at sea we were picked up by a Q-boat and sent home overland through Spain. We expected at any time to be detained as prisoners of war.

Fortunately, she arrived home safely.

*

During July 1918 the Air Ministry had launched its nursing service by advertising in the nursing press for a matron-in-chief and four matrons, plus forty sisters and staff nurses. The first quota was filled mainly by army and navy nurses, but some civilians also applied. When the first Director of Medical Services (DMS) for the RAF, Lieutenant-General (later Sir) Matthew Fell, asked the authorities at Guy's Hospital, London, to recommend suitable candidates for his new service, among the names put forward was that of Kate New.

Kate had done her general nursing and midwifery training at Guy's Hospital, beginning in 1908 at the age of twenty-five. Once qualified, she stayed on at the same hospital. She had volunteered to join the forces as soon as war was declared, but had been persuaded that her talents were more urgently needed at Guy's. However, in October 1918, when the air force nursing service offered her a post, she readily accepted.

Another early recruit to the new service was Marion Welch, who celebrated her thirtieth birthday in January 1918. Trained at Huddersfield, where she won a Gold Medal, she too became a qualified midwife, with an extra diploma in dispensing from Apothecaries Hall. She worked at hospitals in England and later served in France with the British Red Cross Society, in a tented unit not far from the battlefield. In the year before she applied to join the RAFNS, she had been nursing at the War Hospital in Chichester.

As for young Mary, on her twenty-first birthday, 25 April 1918, her parents agreed to allow her to apply to one of the London hospitals to become a probationer nurse. Persuading them to grant her this dearest wish can have been no easy task. Girls of her station did not, as a rule, take up a profession of any kind. But the war had changed many things. When Victoria Alexandra Alice Mary Saxe-Coburg Gotha – simply 'Mary' to her family and friends – became a trainee at the Hospital for Sick Children in Great Ormond Street, the matron was advised that her new recruit was to be 'treated as one of the nurses under all circumstances'. The order came from Buckingham Palace. The new probationer was the only daughter of King George V.

First members

If His Majesty had no objections to his daughter's working as a nurse, he did have reservations about allowing her to be named as

Royal Patron of the newest nursing service. The Air Ministry considered her the perfect candidate, young and fresh, modern and caring, the personification of the RAFNS itself. But when her father was approached, as early as October 1918, with requests that his daughter's name might be linked with the RAFNS, he chose to withhold his consent until the service was 'thoroughly constituted and working on a sound and efficient basis' – probably a wise decision, as it turned out.

Even in this first inchoate 'temporary' incarnation, the new service took time to organize. To begin with, an acting principal matron had to be appointed. The successful applicant was Miss L.E. Jolley, another product of Guy's Hospital. She had lately been a matron at the Royal Southern Hospital in Liverpool and then a sister/acting matron in the QAIMNS Reserve. Being forty-eight at the time of her appointment to the air force nursing service, she was already well over the upper age limit for military nurses, which owing to the urgent needs of 1914-18 had been raised to forty-five; but the matter of age was waived in her case. Her officially stated role was to act as adviser in the formation of the new service, with a salary of £300 per annum but with 'no guarantee of permanence in the post'. In common with all other members of the early RAFNS, Miss Jolley was appointed for the duration of the war only. On those terms, she began work at the Air Ministry in July 1918.

Later that month, the Assistant Medical Administrator (AMA), Lieutenant-Colonel Heald, asked her to draft a document setting out conditions of service for the RAFNS. He added: 'This will be very simple as it is merely a question of putting down the pay and conditions of service of the QAIMNS.'

On 4 September Miss Jolley wrote a rather testy memo (on economical brown Air Ministry paper, in a flourishing script and flamboyant blue-green ink!): 'Can I be informed, please, as to what units are likely to be opened and when, also of any vacancies to be filled by nurses, as I want to give applicants some idea when their services will be required.' The answer came: 'Matlock may be ready within 2 or 3 weeks – an asst matron, 2 sisters and 3 nurses, with 1 masseuse, will be required'. Another two weeks later, the AMA advised Miss Jolley not to engage more nurses than they were likely to need, but 'the three nurses for whom you have no immediate billets . . . can be absorbed on to the Matlock establishment'.

As summer turned to autumn, air force sisters and staff nurses replaced army and navy nurses at the small hospital units in London and at Cranwell; others went to Women's Royal Air Force depots at Glasgow, Birmingham and Sheffield; to the convalescent centres at Matlock, in Derbyshire, and at Hastings; and to station sick quarters at the recruit training camps around Salisbury Plain. With them went members of the equally new RAF Medical Service, whose personnel included male and female doctors and dentists, with male nurses and medical orderlies. Women of the Voluntary Aid Detachment (VADs, trained in first aid and home nursing) acted as ward orderlies, cooks and general assistants. Later, in October 1918 and January 1919, air force personnel replaced army staff at existing hospitals in Blandford and Hampstead. From 1919 these places begin to appear in the records as RAF hospitals.

First uniforms

Inevitably, in those first few months the various branches of the new air force comprised a merry mix of army and navy flyers and ancillary personnel, plus a few former civilians. A month after the air force had been formed, the authorities decreed that khaki should be worn as service dress during the war; when peace came a new light blue uniform would be introduced as standard. However, while war lasted, this new light blue could be worn as mess dress if desired. Most air force personnel continued to wear versions of their old army and navy uniforms, but a few invested in the new light blue. A letter in the archive, from Mary Edwards (Mrs Sellors) recalls: 'Those officers who had been in the Army wore their khaki uniform until they got the pale blue uniform of the RAF. This uniform had gold rank markings. I only saw one Sqn Ldr wearing this uniform, and I thought it most unserviceable and rather theatrical.' This 'theatrical' pale blue was, presumably, the same as the 'light blue colour adopted for the RAF' which is specified in an order for '3000 yards of blue whipcord' to make uniforms for the RAFNS in October 1918. Little hard evidence remains of this early colour, but later files mention a 'new' air force blue introduced around October 1919, so one may guess that the pale blue was swiftly superseded by the more practical and now-familiar blue-grey. Thousands of RAF personnel down the years must have been grateful for the change of mind!

The black 'Dick'

One aspect of uniform (one that holds memories for every nursing officer who ever wore it) made its debut very early on. For some it was the bane of their lives, for others a dear friend, but to all it became a close companion. This item was, and still is, the formal black highwayman-style headgear worn by female nursing officers with their blue-grey outdoor uniform and fondly referred to as a 'Dick' (as in Turpin). Its distinctive quatrecorn shape came into being in September 1918.

An early proposal that the new service should adopt a black *tricorn* head-dress raised alarums in the Women's Royal Naval Service (WRNS), whose Deputy Director, Miss Crowdy, wrote to protest. She had been asked by the Director of WRNS to say that 'since officers of the WRNS have already adopted such hats, the (D)WRNS deprecates this shape being used by another service.' In a memo, the Medical Administrator (RAF), Major-General R.C. Munday, noted: 'It is considered desirable to avoid any ill-feeling with the WRNS and I therefore propose adopting a four-cornered hat for the RAF Nursing Service . . . The Matron in Chief is in favour of the four-cornered hat.'

All subsequent PMs who had problems with that darned hat now know who to blame! Still, it was to be some time before the exact shape and style were agreed, and even then the hat continued to evolve over the years, sometimes officially, by order of Matron-in-Chief, sometimes by individual and less orthodox methods, as we shall discover.

While outdoor uniform was, as yet, a type of military motley, for members of the RAFNS indoor ward dress was simple: light blue ankle-length cotton dresses, white caps and long white aprons, with black shoes and stockings. In winter, as one sister remembers, some added Burberrys and gumboots.

Conditions which demanded such practical clothing were to arrive, along with the killer flu, later that first year.

First hospitals

Some postings led nurses to comfortable billets in picturesque areas. Others, as Marion Welch later observed, 'worked under greater hardship and difficulties than many on active service during war'.

One of the more desirable postings was Matlock, the spa resort in the Derbyshire hills of central England, which became the site of the RAF's No. 1 Health Centre. Before 1914 the building, set on a steep hillside with terraced gardens, had been the luxurious Rockside Health Hydro; it would become so again once the war ended. But now it was turned into a convalescent hospital for air force officers. Its matron, Miss W. Charlesworth, left a report which paints a happy picture.

> Most of the Hydro furniture was removed and stored in a building at the bottom of the hill and was replaced by barrack and hospital equipment. The patients admitted were all walking cases and usually required treatment such as massage and medicated baths. The Hydro contained a small swimming pool where the patients used to take a cold plunge before breakfast. There were also most types of medicated baths. A PT instructor used to give exercises and games to the patients in the ballroom. There was a tennis court attached to the Hydro and the golf links were quite handy.
>
> The Hydro had one of the best ballrooms in Matlock and many a gay evening was spent there by the patients as they were allowed to hold a dance there about once a fortnight. The civilians had a hospital at the Royal Scotch Matlock Bath and the civilian Sisters were always invited to the patients' dances at Rockside. In those days the RAF Nursing Staff were not allowed to dance with the patients so they had to be onlookers.
>
> The Rockside Café adjacent was a popular rendezvous for the patients as delicious home-made cakes were served there.
>
> There was quite a lot of talent among the patients and one or two very successful concerts were given . . . We were asked to give this concert and play at the civilian hospital (which contained quite a lot of Tommies) a few days later and Sister Rees and I had a very nice box of chocolates each, presented to us by one of the Tommies.

In Hastings, on the south coast, however, things were not quite so rosy. One of the early sisters, recalling her experiences, wrote to her matron-in-chief:

We arrived at Hastings on a cold winter afternoon, and went straight to the hospital, the Hermitage. We were met by a very worried CO: 'So sorry, Sister, no accommodation for you. Hospital not opened yet, or equipped. No room for you at all.'

But, having received a wire that afternoon announcing our impending arrival, he had gone over the road to a YWCA Hostel, and they would put us up. Like shop-girls we shared cubicles in a large dormitory; but for the Matron, Miss Nicholson, we managed to get a tiny room, so small that when she pulled her trunk from under the bed the door wouldn't open! It was bitterly cold . . . Most days we spent there were meatless . . .

This same sister (whose name, alas, is not recorded, though her writing tells vivid tales) soon moved along the south coast from Hastings to Dorset, to a place known as Blandford Camp.

Then I was posted to Blandford . . . colder than ever . . . camp about four miles from the town. When we took over the hospital from the Army, conditions were really awful . . . where we slept at night, by day became the operating theatre. They got us billets in Blandford, and about 7 a.m. daily we were taken for the day to the camp by ambulance or lorry (most of them on their last legs – or wheels!). We always took with us a huge churn of milk, and where the road was very rough it would splash over us in spite of the lid . . . We had to balance it most carefully when we went in one old ambulance that was so decrepit that we all had to sit on one side or it would have collapsed. The churn seemed to take up all the room.

Night duty in those days was eventful – it always seemed pitchy dark and we had to walk endless distances to our hutted wards, over rough tracks and duckboards (mostly missing) – and mud – with rats running everywhere . . . Sisters going round two- or four-hourly to do their treatments by the light of hurricane lamps. And the gales! One night I was hopelessly lost – lamp blown out – and suddenly out of the black darkness a voice: 'Halt! Who goes there?'

Knowing there was a bayonet not far away, I gasped,
'Sister!'

'Pass, Sister!' and the sentry re-lighted my lamp for me.

Then the disused railway cutting! If one missed it and
slipped over, one could get a nasty fall . . .

Blandford Camp, Dorset

Blandford Down, outside the town of Blandford Forum, plays a
brief but interesting role in the history of air force nurses. Located
on open uplands rising out of pleasant green woods, the area had
been used by the military for two hundred years.

The first winter of the Great War saw a vast hutted camp of the
Royal Naval Division spread across the downs, wooden billets,
ablutions huts and stores all linked with duckboard walkways to
save the boots of thousands of recruits from miring in the mud.
Other huts held a YMCA, a Methodist mission, a Church of
England church, a post office with telegraph facility, canteens for
the men, wardrooms for petty officers and messes for officers. The
camp also boasted a divisional medical area, with a hutted hospital
unit not far away – a hospital that was to become very familiar to
members of the RAFNS. From this sprawling base on the
windswept Dorset Downs, men went out to the trenches of Belgium
and the carnage of Gallipoli. Among them was the young Sub-
Lieutenant Rupert Brooke.

By 1916 Blandford Camp had expanded further with the opening of two separate detention centres for German prisoners of war.
These men might be employed on duties within the camp or hired
out to local farmers. They were not allowed to sit idle.

As the war ground on, the huge training camp was adapted for
use by the RFC, which in April 1918 became the RAF. That
summer, Blandford Camp became an RAF recruits wing. A three-
mile extension of the railway link with Blandford Forum boasted a
platform 200 yards long. In September the RAF Record Office came
to the camp, followed in November by Women's Royal Air Force
(WRAF) Records. Blandford developed into a huge hutted city,
where recruits and other personnel of both the RAF and the WRAF
rubbed shoulders with German PoWs going about their chores. The
hospital was busy, army nurses soon giving place to new arrivals

Portrait of Joanna M. Cruickshank,
first Matron-in-Chief of the
PMRAFNS 1918–30

HRH The Princess Mary in
Red Cross uniform, 1920
(by kind permission of
The Earl and Countess of
Harewood and the Trustees
of Harewood House)

HRH The Princess Mary and Matron-in-Chief, Joanna Cruickshank,
visit Central RAFH Finchley, 1922 (© British Crown Copyright/MOD)

The first sisters to be posted overseas, pictured aboard the troopship
Braemar Castle, September 1922 (© British Crown Copyright/MOD)

RAF Hospital, Hinaidi, Iraq (© British Crown Copyright/MOD)

Sister Kathleen Sweeny, 1920s

from the air force. They coped with the usual crop of illnesses and accidents, plus a bad bout of summer flu which no one realized was a mere foretaste of things to come.

Members of the WRAF at Blandford turned their hands to whatever work arose. A WRAF butcher, who had been a milliner in civilian life, handled huge carcasses which supplied meat rations to the troops. WRAF electricians worked two shifts in the power house, which supplied all the power for the great camp and brought light to the busy hutted hospital. Going to and from work on wintry nights, nurses of the RAFNS and members of the WRAF trekked across the downs through wind, hail and snow, with wet skirts swishing about their ankles and hurricane lamps swinging.

That November, when peace was finally declared on the eleventh hour of the eleventh day of the eleventh month, Blandford became a repatriation camp. Personnel came there from overseas to wait to be demobilized, many of them shattered both mentally and physically. A line from one of Marion Welch's letters strikes a chill down the spine: 'That suicide wood at the back of the hospital lines was a grim reality and *not* a piece of newspaper fiction exploited by "John Bull".'

As winter set in, with rain and freezing winds, hospital staff had their hands full. Reporting to her matron-in-chief ten years after the events, Marion Welch recalls:

The winter was a severe one . . . Much of the camp was under canvas and the war huts set aside for the hospital wards were far from weatherproof, and a considerable distance apart. So limited was the accommodation available for sisters' quarters that several had to sleep in the operating theatre at night, and day and night staff had to use the same quarters. After the first couple of months, billets were found in the old market town of Blandford, some five miles from the camp. A great debt of gratitude is owing to some 6 or 8 residents for their unfailing care and kindness to those Sisters of the RAF who were privileged to live in their homes.

[But] the really interesting tales could never be published in the press. Who would credit the fact that we had to nurse men on stretchers in empty huts without any hospital equipment? The weather was so appallingly wet that even though we kept in gumboots and Burberry coats we were drenched going from hut to hut and constantly held up by armed sentries when on night duty.

On occasion, these night-duty excursions had hilarious consequences. The unnamed sister quoted earlier says:

When the ambulance deposited us at the camp we had quite a walk along the disused railway line to our night quarters and tiny duty room – which we often saw little of on busy nights. There were three or four of us walking along the line one night, and I was carrying the PUDDING – Matron had an idea we didn't need any food at night (we often used to buy food for ourselves) but as a concession we had been allowed to make the rice pudding! In the dark I caught my foot on a railway sleeper, and down I came! Away went the pudding, but so solid was it, it just hopped out of its dish whole! By the light of a lamp we found it. It had lost nothing, but gained a good quantity of coal- (and other) dust. We put it back carefully in its enamel pie dish. Cook (we had a good cook for the patients) washed it – it made three puddings! But it was the last time I was allowed to carry 'the pudding'.

Then came the awful pneumonia and flu . . .

Spanish flu, 1918-19

In June and July, that summer of 1918, a brief outbreak of flu had claimed the lives of two young RAF recruits at Blandford. Now, as autumn became winter, a great pandemic swept across the world.

At the time, viruses were beginning to be recognized as such, but nothing could counter the strain of Spanish flu which struck in the winter of 1918/19. In particular it attacked healthy young people such as the thousands of recruits and repatriates who crowded the camp at Blandford. Victims died within two or three days, with haemorrhage and fluid on their lungs: unable to breathe, they drowned in their own bodily fluids. Some sources suggest that this particular virus came from birds, transmitted direct from avian to human. World-wide, it claimed even more lives than had the recently ended war.

From the Air Ministry, Medical Administrator R.C. Munday reported in October to the Secretary of State: 'In order to cope with the urgent needs at Blandford, rendered still more serious by reason of the recent influenza outbreak, the immediate taking-over of the Workhouse has been effected . . . and the cleaning and equipment of five huts as an hospital extension. A statistical report on the epidemic is in course of preparation.'

Kate New, recently recruited to the RAFNS, was appointed matron of the 200 bed auxiliary hospital in the old workhouse at Blandford. Pausing only to collect her uniform from an outfitters in Westminster, Kate caught a train to Blandford Camp. She found the old workhouse under-staffed, ill-equipped, and filthy. She and her assistants – a handful of male nursing orderlies and general-duty bods – had only ten days in which to turn the place into a hospital. They set to and started scrubbing, exterminating weevils from the walls and evicting mice from every nook and cranny. The mice were especially well-settled in the old cheese store, which was to be Kate's office and bedroom.

Just as the first patients arrived, reinforcements appeared in the shape of three trained nurses; then five more arrived. Soon there were fourteen members of the RAFNS working at Blandford's old workhouse. They were badly needed. In this second flu outbreak, between September and December 1918, twenty-four RAF men died, mostly youngsters from the recruits wing, along with six German prisoners of war. The anonymous sister adds:

Many of the patients died after but a few days' illness. The old workhouse in Blandford had been taken over, but its accommodation – or lack of it – was even worse. [We were] under-staffed – patients pouring in, lying on the floor on mattresses and stretchers – not enough of anything with which to cope. Fifty SI [seriously ill] or even DI [dangerously ill] patients to one Sister, and one orderly between two Sisters. When I took over from a Night Sister, she pointed to the [duty] bed and said, 'I found those sheets left by the last Sister, 'fraid you'll have to use them, there aren't any more.' Any that could possibly be used had to go to the patients. We were short of hypodermics, utensils, everything.

Amid the grimness, however, lighter moments did occur. As matron at the auxiliary hospital, Kate New was responsible for the catering for her nurses. The RAF cook objected to being told how to do his job by a 'mere nurse' and refused to speak to her for ten days after she suggested he might bake the sausages rather than serve up what she describes as 'nasty grey things boiled in water'. Another airman cook had learned his trade 'by watching his wife, miss'.

Rations of bread and meat were doled out by the RAF – 'You took what you were given and were grateful for it,' says Kate New – but other items of food had to be bought by Matron, with a daily cash allowance of 2s 6d (12½p) for each nurse. Even in 1919 this called for frugal and ingenious shopping.

Blandford has one final claim to fame in the annals of RAF history – its personnel formed one of the early RAF bands. Kate New well remembered hearing, over and over again, the new march that was to develop into the famous, stirring, tingle-down-the-spine theme known to all as the 'Royal Air Force March Past'.

The anonymous sister says:

> Those early days are hard to describe, now. All was terrible and difficult. But when I left Blandford some months later, it was with sadness. There were many happy times, and as things improved we were able to look after the patients better. Transport back to billets often there was none, but it was a lovely walk if the weather was good . . .

The emergency auxiliary hospital at Blandford closed in 1919 and Kate New went as matron to the hospital at RAF Old Sarum (Salisbury). Slowly the whole huge camp on the Dorset Downs wound down, soon to be demolished and revert to downland and arable, until needed again for military purposes in 1939. It is now the home of the Royal Corps of Signals.

Last to leave in early 1920 were four members of the WRAF. The main hospital had closed. The recruits had all gone home. RAF Records had moved on. Auditors had drawn a final line under WRAF Records – indeed, the entire Women's Royal Air Force had been found surplus to requirements and was ordered to disband: the service officially ended on 1 April 1920, having been in existence for just two years. (Like Blandford Camp itself, the women's branch of the air force was to rise again in 1939, metamorphosed into the wartime WAAF.)

In the rationalization of affairs after the Great War, the future of the Royal Air Force itself was in question. What hope of continuation had the temporary, wartime-only Royal Air Force Nursing Service?

THREE

Trenchard

After 1919 British military planning worked on the premise that there could not possibly be another major war for at least ten years. Britain's most powerful enemies had been silenced and the few remaining problems in the Middle East and Bengal were minor skirmishes by comparison. What was more, the struggle against Germany had left the country in turmoil and in debt. Her people, weary of war, wished only for life to return to normal.

A regime of steady demobilization returned men and women of the reserves to their thankful families. Men gladly rejoined factories and mines; most women turned with relief to hearth and home. They were happy to believe that the recent conflict had indeed been 'the war to end all wars'. That being so, what purpose could be served by maintaining a separate air force? Better to save money by reabsorbing it into the two established services.

This idea pleased both the Navy and the Army. The Admiralty urged the return of its flying wing: it was planning to build more ships capable of carrying and launching aeroplanes; naturally it wanted the whole operation under its sole control. For its part, the War Office knew itself to be perfectly capable of organizing its own air battalions; they were, after all, only glamorous and rather showy extras, playing a supportive role to real fighting men – so the army chiefs of the day reasoned.

Taking the opposing view, Sir Hugh Trenchard, who had once led the RFC and was now Chief of the Air Staff (CAS), strongly argued air power as the key to future military greatness. The air force must be nurtured as an independent entity and allowed to

38

develop its full potential, with the highest standards demanded of all its personnel: *Per ardua ad astra* (through adversity to the stars). That ideal was, is and always will be the goal of every branch of the RAF.

The effectiveness of air power was soon to be demonstrated. In 1920, a single squadron of DH9s quelled uprisings in Somaliland, largely by swooping over the heads of the so-called Mad Mullah's riders and carrying out bombing raids on pre-warned and therefore empty villages. Later, on the north-west frontier of India and in Mesopotamia (soon to be Iraq), the RAF flew effective sorties in support of army operations. These successful 'side-shows' proved far less costly, in terms of both money and casualties, than long, arduous ground campaigns. The voices raised against the air force grew fewer. Trenchard was vindicated. He held his appointment as CAS for ten years, during which time the RAF flew many more successful campaigns. And, despite his professed dislike of the tag, he is still best remembered as the 'Father of the Royal Air Force'.

But, if the RAF itself had established its right to exist, in Whitehall the question of its maintaining separate medical and nursing services continued to create controversy.

Arguments for a separate Medical Service

During the war, medical problems peculiar to the flying service had revealed themselves. Aerial activity posed new problems for the human body and mind: improved artillery defences forced planes to fly higher, where lack of oxygen caused what was then called 'mountain sickness'; higher speeds brought increased stresses on bone and muscle and nerve; and spending hours alone in a cockpit could do strange things to a man's mind. A report from the Medical Administrator to the Secretary of State, dated November 1918, notes that seaplane pilots require especially strong nerves: '. . . the long, lonely patrols over the sea are not to be entrusted safely to a man with an imagination.' Aircrew selection committees, and medical officers responsible for the health of airmen, were obliged to develop new methods to cope with these new challenges. They would obviously require the support of a specialist medical and nursing service. As an Air Ministry memo sharply observed:

It appears to be quite illogical that the air force should have no medical service of its own while not only the Navy and Army but the Indian Army, the Prison Service, the Police Service, the Post Office, the Home Office, the Local Government Board, the Board of Education and every other Government Department each has its own medical service . . .

Memos flew back and forth between the War Office, the Air Ministry and the Secretary of State for War and Air (whose name was Winston S. Churchill). The Army Council, foreshadowing events eighty years in the future, took the view that an effort should be made to 'initiate an Imperial Medical Service providing jointly for the needs of the Navy, Army and Air Services'. The Director General of Army Medical Services asserted: 'We can supply all that is required . . . As regards nurses, QAIMNS can be used in the Hospitals where Air Service Officers and men are admitted . . .' His Quartermaster-General added waspishly, 'In war . . . when the Air Force comes down out of the sky, [it] must clearly have its territorial requirements provided for by the Army.'

In response, the Chief of the Air Staff wrote that the War Office seemed to assume that the air force existed solely to co-operate with the army. His lengthy and impassioned memo sums up by saying:

I strongly deprecate the continuous efforts . . . of the War Office to say what services ought to run for the benefit of the Air . . . the Army Medical Service know nothing about the diseases of the Air, or the peculiarities of the Air from a Medical point of view . . . If this goes on, I cannot see why we should not state that it would be better and more convenient for the Air Service to run the Army Tanks . . .

Miss Joanna Margaret Cruickshank joins the fray

The original acting principal matron of the RAFNS, Miss Jolley, resigned after only six months in office. She had been appointed in an advisory capacity, for the duration of the war only, and she was no longer a young woman. Given the contentious atmosphere that swirled about Whitehall in the wake of the war, she may have been glad to retreat. The RAFNS appeared in danger of being swallowed whole by the much larger and older army nursing service. If it were to survive, it obviously required a leader of strong mettle and feisty character.

Fortunately, just such a woman waited not far away.

We have met her before: Joanna Margaret Cruickshank, who earlier that year had enjoyed an adventurous voyage home from India while suffering from malignant malaria. She joined the RAFNS in October 1918 as a matron attached to Miss Jolley's staff at the Air Ministry, and she became acting matron-in-chief on 25 November, just three days before her forty-third birthday. Her nieces and nephews remember her as 'Aunt Margaret', but to her nursing colleagues she is best known by her first Christian name and her later title: Dame Joanna Cruickshank.

Whatever the history books may say, it can be argued that the defining moment for the RAFNS – the moment when the bedraggled fledgling first stretched its wings, stuck out its scrawny neck and pecked those who threatened it – came on Friday, 5 July 1919. On that day the redoubtable Miss Cruickshank, matron-in-chief of (temporary) air force nurses, came face to face with the equally formidable matron-in-chief of (long-established) army nurses. They were members of a committee of ten, comprising five representatives of the army medical and nursing services, three from the Air Ministry (including the then Brigadier-General Sir Matthew Fell, Director of Medical Services for the RAF), and two senior matrons from civilian hospitals in London. On that fateful Friday the committee convened 'to consider the administration of the RAF Nursing Service as a branch of QAIMNS'.

Asked to state his views, Sir Matthew Fell said that the Air Ministry would prefer the two services to remain 'entirely distinct', with members of QAIMNS seconded to the RAFNS for a period of three years.

That, said the army, would cause problems with promotion, and what about the expense of providing a second uniform? Also . . . and, moreover . . . and what of . . . ?

The crunch came when the lady who ruled army nurses learned that nursing sisters of the Royal Air Force would be stationed not only at the main hospitals but at station sick quarters on many airfields across the land. Indeed, some were already working at these scattered units, as far afield as the wild reaches of Salisbury Plain.

'But who is in charge of them?' cried she, appalled by the idea of young women working so far from the supervisory eye of an older matron.

Miss Cruickshank replied crisply, 'They're grown women. They don't need a nanny.' Or words to that effect. As she later observed, in her opinion the nurses she led were 'of discretionary age and . . . quite capable of looking after themselves'. Women had grown beyond the need for chaperonage: she herself was ample proof of that.

The head nurse from the War Office vehemently objected. She would never allow any of *her* ladies to work under such conditions. Good heavens, the very idea!

It was a moment Joanna Cruickshank never forgot. As her writings reveal, she decided then and there that air force nurses could not and would not return to the old-fashioned, matriarchal regime that governed the army fold.

Something of the acerbity of the discussion lingers between the lines of the draft minute of that July meeting. Setting out army objections to the proposal, it notes that nurses would 'have to serve in sick quarters, RAF hospitals and in WRAF hostels, under conditions possibly at variance with the Matron-in-Chief of the War Office's views [!] and under officers not under the control of the Army Council'. What was more, 'Matron-in-Chief of the War Office could no longer control the posting and movements of the nurses.' Interestingly, these phrases are omitted from the more formal draft of the report.

As ever was and is with government policy, the question of finance formed one of the main arguments for amalgamation. It soon became evident that no appreciable saving would result. Indeed, given the strong opposition, and the unique medical needs of the air force, a move to enforce a merger might cause actual harm. As Joanna Cruickshank (quoting W.S. Gilbert) charmingly phrases it, the representatives from the Air Ministry ' "took heart of grace", and decided, come what may, to go for a Nursing Service of their own'.

Consolidation

In view of the cut-backs in the post-war RAF (a total of over 180 operational squadrons had dwindled to a mere twenty-five by March 1920), the Air Ministry and the War Office agreed that hospital accommodation and treatment for air force personnel in most areas should be provided, *pro tem*, by existing army establishments. Exceptions were RAF Halton, home of the Aircraft Apprentice School; RAF Cranwell, where the Royal Air Force College was being established; and the RAF's Central Hospital, then located in Finchley, Middlesex. These three centres, already established, should continue. Overseas, too, the army foresaw no medical difficulty except possibly in Egypt, Palestine and Mesopotamia, where special arrangements might be necessary. Given these parameters, the RAFNS could now decide how many nurses it needed.

Official figures for membership of the RAFNS at this period differ wildly: for 1920 alone, one authoritative source quotes forty, another seventy-eight, another a hundred and one. Some figures include VAD nurses, others are vague about exactly who they include. Evidently great fluctuations occurred, month by month, as the Service settled down in the wake of the war years. However, order was about to be restored.

Royal approval

The first official Terms and Conditions of Service were presented to Buckingham Palace in January 1921. On the 21st of that month, King George V granted the RAF Nursing Service a Royal Charter and established it by Royal Warrant as a permanent branch of the RAF.

Candidates for membership were required to be twenty-five to thirty-four years of age, and to have completed at least three years' training in a large civil hospital. On entry they became staff nurses with the princely annual salary of £60 and faced six months' probation before their appointment could be confirmed. Promotion was by recommendation. They wore a prescribed uniform but remained civilians, and though they enjoyed officer status they did not hold military rank – they were addressed by their professional titles: Staff Nurse, Sister, Matron.

Dame Joanna Cruickshank, writing after the Second World War, explains the problem of status more fully:

Should nurses rank as officers? – this question arose early. Though nurses in the British Services did not hold commissioned rank, it was already common form in both the Army and the Navy that they should be accorded the respect and obedience due to officers. Should they become officers in fact and in law?

This question had been raised before and was revived by the arrival in this country of USA Army nurses during the 1914-18 war. Australian Nursing Sisters, too, throughout the war, had worn on their shoulder straps the same stars or crowns as the men. But, despite this precedent, after the war the proposal for officer-status of British Forces Nurses was not accepted . . . in 1919 the Services were not ready for such a change – and most members of the Nursing Services felt that their old titles of Matron, Sister and Staff Nurse (the last since done away with) conferred all the authority they needed. In fact . . . the majority felt that the granting of military rank might take away rather than strengthen their status as women devoted to selfless vocation.

This situation obtained until another world war demanded changes, but that time lay in the unguessed future.

By 1921, many military nurses had retired or returned to civilian hospitals; some who now wished to join the permanent service found themselves well over the required upper age limit of thirty-four years. Indeed, Joanna Cruickshank herself would have been excluded had the new parameters been strictly applied. She pleaded the cause of her older nurses, pointing out their excellent record, their loyal and satisfactory service and their valuable experience. As a result, in certain cases the appointment board agreed to waive the age limit rule.

Matron Kate New was one of the older nurses. Since the three remaining RAF hospitals already had matrons established, the only post available to Miss New was as a senior sister at the isolation hospital at Halton. Feeling that the RAF no longer offered a real career, she chose to return to civilian nursing. She became one of the first district nurses, a vocation in which she continued until she retired at the age of sixty-five.

Meanwhile, with the RAFNS now 'thoroughly constituted and working on a sound and efficient basis', as His Majesty had once desired, when the Air Ministry approached him again the King agreed that his daughter might be formally associated with the new Service.

The original PM

We left Her Royal Highness the Princess Mary beginning as a probationer nurse at the Great Ormond Street Hospital for Sick Children in spring 1918, when she was twenty-one years old. But her interest in caring for others began long before that.

Born on 25 April 1897, at York House, Sandringham, amid the woods and fields of Norfolk, Mary was the third child and only daughter of parents who were then the Duke and Duchess of York. Her great-grandmother, the Queen Empress Victoria, still ruled a vast empire, and for paternal grandparents the little princess had the flamboyant Bertie, Prince of Wales (soon to be Edward VII), and his beautiful, long-suffering wife, Alexandra of Denmark.

When Edward VII died in 1910, Mary's father succeeded to the throne as King George V; her mother became Queen Mary. As for her two older brothers, familiarly called David and Bertie, the first is better known to history as the romantic figure who gave up a throne for love – the uncrowned Edward VIII, Duke of Windsor – and the second as the self-effacing George VI, reluctantly obliged to take the throne in his older brother's stead. Three younger brothers completed Mary's family: Henry, Duke of Gloucester, survived into his seventies; George, Duke of Kent, was killed in an air crash while serving with the RAF in 1942; and the youngest, John, born in 1905 and afflicted with epilepsy, lived to be only fourteen.

All four of her surviving brothers, as they grew to manhood, learned how to fly aeroplanes. So it was hardly surprising that, when the chance came, Mary eagerly associated herself with the newest of the armed services.

When war broke out in 1914, the Royal Family responded with vigour. King George and Queen Mary raised morale by showing themselves in support of their people: they attended parades; they visited hospitals, mines and factories; and as food and goods grew scarcer, owing to German attacks on sea-borne supply convoys, the King introduced strict rationing into his own household, ignoring the occasional grumbling of his royal offspring. His two oldest sons actively participated in the conflict: young Bertie was already in the navy despite his poor health, while David, Prince of Wales and heir to the throne, insisted on going out to the front to see for himself the horrors that faced the boys of the British Expeditionary Force. For her part, the King's only daughter plunged into the war effort with dauntless spirit. She accompanied her mother on visits to factories, hospitals and children's homes, and in spare moments she knitted for the mud-bound troops such invaluable comforts as socks, scarves and balaclava helmets. Her handiwork added to the tens of thousands of warm garments which went out to the fighting front via the collecting point at St James's Palace.

Not content with these efforts, the seventeen-year-old princess conceived a scheme whereby she might send a personal Christmas gift to every British soldier and sailor. When advised that her own allowance would not stretch to this, she launched a fund which, aiming to raise £100,000, exceeded itself magnificently and, by the time it closed, totalled £162,000 – a massive sum in those days. She succeeded in sending to each of over 500,000 fighting men a small brass box embossed with her portrait. Each box contained a card, inscribed 'From Princess Mary and friends at home, With best wishes for a Happy Christmas and a Victorious New Year,' and a gift of smoking materials – cigarettes or a pipe and tobacco, with a flint lighter. Non-smokers received chocolates or sweets. The young princess's thoughtfulness touched many hearts. It was a sign to 'the boys over there' in that bitter winter of 1914 that they had not been forgotten, and many an old soldier kept his 'Princess Mary' tin long after the contents had been put to good use.

Across Britain, voices had hopefully declared that the trouble would 'all be over by Christmas', but despite a brief truce between front-line soldiers on Christmas Day the war dragged on, and on.

Women began to clamour for something useful to do in support of their courageous menfolk and, in response, Queen Mary founded her 'Work for Women' Fund. Across the country, women of all ages, from terraced backstreet or country mansion, earned calluses and cuts by turning their hands to manual labour, from chopping down trees to loading barges to toiling in salvage depots or driving horses to plough fields.

The teenage princess joined her mother in the fund-raising effort. Journeys to inspect and bring heart to troops provided interludes in a diary filled with visits to hospitals, soup kitchens and munitions factories. On one occasion, watching her chat with soldiers about to embark for France, Lord Kitchener remarked to General Haig that the princess's example 'has done more than anything to rally the women of England to the colours'. She became a member of the VAD, attended a course of first aid lectures at Buckingham Palace and sat the required exams. She served meals to workers in a munitions factory canteen, or sorted reports and files at Devonshire House. She worked with the Girl Guides, the Women's Land Army, the Needlework Guild and the Red Cross.

As we have seen, on her twenty-first birthday, rather than indulging in the customary 'coming out' ball, which might have been thought frivolous in those austere times, she chose to begin work as a children's nurse. Granted her royal sire's permission, she earned the respect and affection of other staff for her willingness to roll up her sleeves and set to, however menial and messy the chore. Bed-making, nappy-changing, bottle-feeding, applying poultices, feeding by nasal tubes and bathing by water, vapour or hot air failed to daunt her. Having mastered the basics of the medical wards, she went on to offer tender loving care to young surgical patients.

Perhaps her brother David had told her of the makeshift hospitals and first aid tents he had seen on his visits to Belgium and France. There, VADs with only minimal training served as assistants to the more professional sisters of QAIMNS, while women of the First Aid Nursing Yeomanry (fondly known as FANYs) emulated the legendary Valkyries by riding on horseback into inaccessible spots to bring back the wounded. Where sailors needed nursing care, QARNNS sisters leapt into action, and locally the Territorial Army Nursing Service gave help.

As hostilities lessened, Princess Mary visited the front lines in person, taking 'a message from the Queen' to all women serving in France. She saw how nurses shared the privations – wet, muddy conditions with few comforts; basic food, and not much of that; water that had to be boiled before it was fit to drink; beds of straw, in draughty wooden huts, where one slept fully clothed both for warmth and for decency. All of this the nurses endured while caring for men badly wounded by battle or simply made sick by conditions. Soldiers living in trenches, up to their shins in freezing muddy water, suffered horribly from trench foot and frostbite. Diphtheria, and secondary infections such as tetanus and septicaemia added to the toll of misery. Of the nurses she encountered, the princess later commented, 'I am glad to know how the girls really lived. I used so often to think of them and wish I could have joined them earlier in the war.'

After the war, the King decided to allow his children to seek marriage partners among the British aristocracy. Many eligible suitors flocked round his only daughter, but it was Viscount Lascelles, heir to the Earl of Harewood and fourteen years her senior, who won her heart. They were married on 28 February 1922, and a year later the Princess Mary, Viscountess Lascelles, bore her first son, George.

In response to the request that she might consider lending her name to the RAFNS, Her Royal Highness expressed her pride and pleasure in 'being associated with such a magnificent Service as the Air Force'. On 14 June 1923 she became President of what was proudly renamed in her honour the Princess Mary's Royal Air Force Nursing Service.

So began the fully-fledged PMRAFNS, as an all-female branch of qualified nurses. Members worked beside doctors and male nurses of the RAF Medical Service, which also supplied nursing orderlies, nursing attendants and theatre assistants, all male until the WRAF reformed in 1939. Together, these personnel staffed sick quarters on flying stations scattered across the south and east of Britain. And in larger numbers they worked at the first three permanent RAF hospitals – Finchley in Middlesex, Cranwell in Lincolnshire, and Halton Park in Buckinghamshire, all of which had their origins in the very early days of military flying.

Central Hospital, Finchley

The first small scattered hospitals of the RFC, RAF and WRAF which existed in the London area between 1917 and 1920 had mostly been sited in individual houses (see Appendix II). Among them was an officers' convalescent hospital at Avenue Road,

Finchley. As the Service consolidated, these units all merged into one Central Hospital at East End Road in Finchley, not far from RAF Hendon (scene of the first RAF Tournament in July 1920 and now the home of the RAF Museum). What was then a pleasant semi-rural location with room for a grassy airfield is now lost amid the sprawl of Greater London.

Finchley was the smallest of the three post-war RAF hospitals, employing a matron and seven RAFNS sisters. Opened in 1919, it was the first RAF hospital graced by an official visit, in April 1924, from Princess Mary, the new President of the PMRAFNS. But it was also the shortest-lived of the original hospitals – it closed in June 1925, when its function moved to Uxbridge and it became the RAF Officers' Hospital.

Cranwell

RAF Cranwell lies five miles from the market town of Sleaford, in Lincolnshire. Well known as the home of the RAF College and Basic Flying Training School, it can claim to be one of the very first flying stations. As early as 1915 the site was chosen by the RNAS as a training centre for officers and men destined to serve in and with aeroplanes, balloons, airships and kites.

Princess Mary's second brother, 'Bertie' (later George VI), had been stationed at Cranwell as officer-in-charge of one of the navy squadrons. When the RNAS dispersed into the RAF, the prince transferred with it. Four years later authority designated Cranwell as one of the three main RAF hospitals.

In common with most of the hastily erected units flung up during the Great War, early Cranwell was a sprawl of wooden huts connected by duckboard walks. The RAF College officially opened in February 1920. Its cadets endured a regime that was strict, spartan and physically demanding, but after two years they emerged fully equipped to be officers of the RAF. Amid a landscape of rolling fields and wide, windswept skies, each man learned how to fly his aircraft to its limits – and how to recover it if he stretched it beyond those limits. Between 1920 and 1925 only two men died in air accidents at Cranwell, which says much for the skill of the young pilots and their instructors.

Staff at the hutted hospital coped with all injuries sustained by

Cranwell personnel, whether from flying or some more mundane cause. Led by a matron and ten other members of the RAFNS, they also dealt with the usual illnesses prevalent among young men, and cared for pregnant RAF wives.

Princess Mary paid her first official visit to Cranwell aerodrome in April 1925, to see both the RAF hospital and the cadet college. She was greeted by Matron-in-Chief Miss Joanna Cruickshank, among others, and after inspecting a guard of honour formed by cadets she went straight to the hospital where some of the nurses were presented. The *Daily Telegraph* noted that she spoke to almost every one of the eighty patients in the hospital, but spent most time in the female ward, 'where she stopped by the bedside of the wife of an RAF man at Cranwell, and chatted with her about her baby boy, born only six days ago'.

The same article later tells of emergency procedures for accidents on the nearby aerodrome: 'An officer of the watch is always on duty, and at the least accident he gives telephonic warning to the hospital, when motor ambulances, and a motor fire engine to cope with any outbreak of fire that may occur, are rushed to the ground, while beds in the special accident ward are, at the same time, instantly warmed by electricity . . . ' The report reminds us how new and exciting it all was then – an aerodrome, with aeroplanes overhead, and on the ground motor vehicles, telephones, and electricity!

One of the sisters who worked at Cranwell in those days remembered that Princess Mary also paid less formal visits, when she ate lunch in the sisters' mess.

> On these visits, Princess Mary thought of herself as one of us . . . when seated at a table she would kick off her shoes . . . When taking coffee, she filled her cup with sugar crystals and these she ate with a spoon. On one occasion she produced a cigarette case – this was handed round, one noticed, with a rather mischievous smile: smoking at this time was allowed, but not approved . . . The conversation was about members, and especially those serving overseas; Princess Mary knew all members personally. We numbered 105 . . .

So wrote Louise Hardy, who was there.

Halton Park

Set amid the rolling hills and woods of beautiful Buckinghamshire, RAF Halton has glamorous origins. The estate was owned by the super-rich de Rothschild family, and during Victorian and Edwardian days the big house – which was to become (and still is) the officers' mess – saw its share of gaiety.

In the early days of the First World War, the bachelor Alfred Charles de Rothschild offered the use of his estate to the army, which cleared vast areas of timber and erected hundreds of tents for recruits summoned by the sternly pointing finger of Lord Kitchener: 'Your Country Needs You' boomed the posters. Then in 1917 the RFC took over and opened its Boys' Training School, where apprentice fitters and riggers, known as 'Trenchard's Brats', learned their trade – most of the wooden workshops of the Aircraft Apprentice School were built by German PoWs in the latter years of the Great War.

In January 1919 the RAF Medical School opened at Halton. More wooden huts, set on a hillside, contained the new hospital. Long wooden corridors connected the huts, with the wards set in pairs either side – medical and surgical wards, a theatre and all facilities, plus a separate isolation wing. They had beds for officers, for families and for maternity cases, but with a thousand young apprentices on the camp, prey to accident and illness, the boys' ward was busiest of all. By the end of 1920, male nurses and orderlies (many of whom had served through the late war) tended their patients with the help of thirty-five sisters and staff nurses of the RAFNS, all under the guiding eye of an experienced matron.

Halton Park quickly established a reputation as the main RAF medical centre. The Central Pathological Laboratory set up its business there; the first pathologist transferred from the earlier RFC Hospital at Hampstead and his particular interest, in tropical diseases, led to the development of the famous Institute of Pathology and Tropical Medicine. The medical school became the RAF Medical Training Depot (later the Medical Training Establishment and Depot), which produced orderlies, medics, theatre assistants, laboratory technicians and other allied trades.

Of the three early hospitals, only Halton survived in its original location. It grew from strength to strength, pioneering a wide range of medical and surgical techniques. It also provided an introduction to service life for generations of PMs. Many of them still regard Halton as their Service's true home.

Early privations

Life in those early wooden huts was often hard, especially during the winter when Britain's climate turned the ground into either deep squelching mud or frozen ruts. Nurses trudged from ward to hutted ward on rotting duckboards, clutching their great-coat collars about their throats, trying to keep their long skirts from trailing in the wet, and lofting their feeble lamps to guide their way through storm and sleet. Little wonder that some, like Kate New, retreated to more civilized conditions.

Younger and more hardy souls stayed on, among them Marion Welch, who reports a moment of black farce: 'Shall I ever forget the night when that mad orderly Jones tried three times to set fire to the camp and hospital. The AOC's car dashing up at 2.30 a.m. and cutting the only decent length of fire hose we possessed . . . '

She adds:

Halton's early days were rather grim – huts that let in all the weather. I have seen patients pulling wool from their dressings and stuffing it into holes in the boards to keep out the draughts. One might have to hoist an umbrella over one's bed in heavy rain, and I used to be fascinated watching the snowflakes coming [between] the boards of my bedroom to form a lovely little heap on the floor. We had a bathroom to each hut, the stove of which we often had to stoke ourselves.

Two lines of the hutted wards were joined by an open passage [which] we called the 'dark hole of Calcutta'. It was floored with cinder dust. Later it was roofed in and properly floored, but for months it was a horrible alleyway. The wards were all old Army huts which had had their day, but they served their purpose, they lasted on, and stood many years of patching up.

One or two of the older matrons had also 'had their day but lasted on'. Mary Edwards (Mrs Sellors) remembers a certain Miss Cameron:

... matron of Halton when I went there in 1922 before going abroad [Mary was posted to Basra, Iraq]. She was most particular that our rooms were tidy, so much so that she threw out [a box containing] a white hat which had been specially made for a sister going abroad as she had a very small head!

[Miss Cameron] was to be matron of Baghdad hospital. We were in huts then and she met me on the duckboards and asked me if I wouldn't prefer to go to Baghdad with her. It was rather difficult for me to say, 'No, thank you,' but I did.

She rather annoyed us by calling us by our surnames . . .

Over the years to come, more than one matron acquired the habit of addressing juniors by surname alone. As a result, through the Second World War and beyond, sisters themselves hardly knew one another's forenames: Sister Higgins became eternally 'Higgie'; Sister Thomas became 'Tommy' – at reunions one still hears these affectionate nicknames on many lips as old friends meet. And the story goes that one formidable senior matron so far forgot herself that she addressed a surgeon by roaring his surname down the ward: 'Jones!' Stung, he turned and bawled back, 'What do you want, SMITH?!'

Dame Joanna Cruickshank summed up the early days:

The new Service came to birth in critical times, when neither was the 1914-18 war ended nor victory assured. Under the forced incubation of hard struggles that lay ahead, its growth was rapid, though the new Service was soon to experience the pangs of under nourishment when the aftermath of war brought the campaign for economy and the committee known as the 'Geddes Axe'.

PMRAFNS, as it is now termed, is unique in that it was born and grew up with its parent Air Force as one of the family – cherished, but not spoiled – and, as the story of its work will show, it has never failed its parent, working hand in hand with the Medical Branch – for doctors and nurses own the same calling . . .

The oft-repeated tradition of 'sixty original sisters' is difficult to pin down to an exact date. As we have seen, recorded numbers vary bewilderingly. By August 1923, according to official files in the Public Record Office, the PMRAFNS counted 101 permanently appointed members. It would continue to do so, with minor fluctuations and a slight but steady overall increase, until 1937, when the war reserve began to form. However, in 1923 there were indeed about sixty sisters on duty at home in Britain. By that time, the other two fifths of the total hundred-odd had been posted overseas.

They had gone out to the mysterious Middle East – to Mesopotamia.

PART II

The Wide Blue Yonder

ONE

Mespot

The land of Mesopotamia – nicknamed 'Mespot' by British troops
– encompassed parts of Persia (Iran) and much of present-day Iraq.
Watered by the ancient rivers Tigris and Euphrates, and peopled by
various tribes and itinerant desert peoples, it once formed part of
the mighty Ottoman (Turkish) Empire. Britain's interests in the area
had increased with the opening, in 1869, of the Suez Canal, which
made the trading route through the Red Sea to India so much
shorter. It was important to keep the canal and its environs in
friendly hands.

Since the Turks had allied themselves with Kaiser Wilhelm
during the Great War, in 1918 they shared his defeat. Their empire
crumbled, leaving the Middle East in danger of descending into
chaos, with tribal factions fighting each other for supremacy. As a
preventive interim measure, the League of Nations decided to
govern the area by mandate – that is, they gave control of the ex-
Turkish territories to the European allies, each country to adminis-
ter its given areas, to the benefit of the inhabitants, until the emer-
gent nations grew stable enough to govern themselves. Britain's
particular areas of responsibility were Mesopotamia, Palestine and
Transjordan; she already had a colony at Aden and protectorates
along the south-east coasts of Arabia. She administered these territories as part of the Indian Empire, garrisoning them with British
and Indian troops to safeguard trade routes with the Far East.

Humiliated by their defeat in the war, the Turks encouraged
unrest among the area's tribes, some of whose leaders resented the

imposition of foreign rule. Tribal clashes and anti-British uprisings caused nearly 3,000 British casualties by the end of 1920. In the following year, the League of Nations created an Iraqi kingdom whose first monarch, Faisal I, had been an ally of Lawrence of Arabia.

To allow Faisal time to establish his authority, his country remained under British mandate, in conditions of political ferment and unrest. RAF squadrons went out to support the peace-keeping efforts of British and Indian troops. Often the mere sight of an aircraft swooping over the desert was enough to give rebels pause, though some of the warriors became deadly accurate using rifle-fire against the airborne enemy. But to friendly tribes RAF crews proved to be helpful allies; on occasion their aeroplanes flew seriously ill Bedouin sheikhs to British service hospitals for emergency treatment.

Such mercy flights did much to increase the friendship between Britain and the people of Mespot. They also added to the RAF's ever-widening expertise in evacuating casualties. Indeed, the RAF's first major 'casevac' was to take place in Mesopotamia before long. Fortunately, by that time a brand new RAF hospital, staffed by members of the PMRAFNS, had been established beside the River Tigris, at Hinaidi.

The interrupted voyage of the Braemar Castle

With trouble escalating in Mesopotamia and more squadrons being posted there for duty, the RAF's Director of Medical Services proposed that some of his nursing sisters should take over from army nurses already established in desert areas. These first overseas postings took ten PMs to Iraq.

On 13 September 1922, a matron and nine sisters sailed aboard the troopship *Braemar Castle*. Among them was Mary Edwards (Mrs Sellors), bound with one or two others for Basra while the rest were posted to Baghdad. The voyage was not to be a pleasure cruise; as their ship sailed towards Gibraltar, trouble brewed at the far end of the Mediterranean.

For some time, Turkish forces under the leadership of Mustapha Kemal Bey (Ataturk) had been threatening the peace of the mandated territories. In mid-September 1922 they arrived at the neutral zone surrounding Gallipoli and set up camp outside the town of Chanak (Cannakale), whose fortifications commanded the narrows of the Dardanelles straits. They seemed intent on shattering all peace treaties and sweeping aside the European forces who barred their way to Constantinople. As the crisis deepened, the French and Italians withdrew, but British Prime Minister Lloyd George resolved to hold Chanak. Britain and Turkey stood on the verge of war.

In response to the crisis, the *Braemar Castle* diverted to the area and anchored outside Constantinople. The PMs remained on board, but the RAF contingent went ashore to join the defending troops. The seaplane carrier HMS *Pegasus* sailed closer to add its weight to the argument, and more RAF squadrons set out from the UK. However, with the onset of winter floods and frost the tension ended and a peace pact was drawn up.

Hinaidi Hospital, Baghdad

After ten days' delay, the PMs' long voyage continued, through the Suez Canal and the Great Bitter Lake, down the Red Sea, round via Aden and the Arabian peninsula and up the Persian Gulf. Mary Edwards remembers transferring to a British Indian ship in the Shatt-al-Arab (the confluence of the Tigris and Euphrates) for the last few miles up to Basra. But at Basra the army hospital was not ready to receive air force nurses, so all the PMs went on to Baghdad. There they took over at No. 23 British Combined Services Hospital.

Within weeks, Mary Edwards was sent to work at the Indian sick quarters at nearby Karradah. She did not take up her originally intended post, at Basra, until the following year, when the RAF opened the Combined British and Indian Hospital in that city.

Soon, other PMs joined those first few. Twenty sailed for Mespot around the turn of the year and by midsummer 1923 another nine had arrived in Palestine. Early that same year, the staff at the old army hospital in Baghdad moved to a splendid new purpose-built RAF British General Hospital at Hinaidi, on the banks of the Tigris, some eight miles outside Baghdad.

As described by Marion Welch, who was twice matron there, the hospital at Hinaidi comprised seven or eight large buildings

containing wards with high, cool ceilings and wide verandahs to
alleviate the heat, with space for 500 patients of both the air force
and the army benefiting from all the latest (1920s) equipment.

Louise Hardy, posted there in 1926, remembers, 'a superb building, the wards named after the Air Aces of the 1914 war . . . Our
Mess and living quarters were also on the grand scale, and the ante-
room [was] very attractive and comfortable, the floor covered with
beautiful Persian carpets. Our bedrooms were very large, each with
its own bathroom. On the flat roof above was a second bedstead
where one could sleep in the hot weather.'

Over fourteen eventful years, Hinaidi was to be the home of
many PMs. They enjoyed the services of a domestic staff of Assyrian
bearers, hospital assistants both Iraqi and Indian, and leisure facilities including two fine tennis courts and stabling for fourteen horses
– 'It was customary to ride in the early morning before breakfast,'
writes Louise Hardy. 'In accordance with the social etiquette of
those days, we had to pay calls and receive callers. We were also
elected to membership of the British Club . . . the centre of social
life for the British Community.'

Despite these apparent luxuries, it was not an easy life. Nurses
and troops alike endured the heat, the dust and the flies for what
was then an overseas tour of a full five years, far from home and,
for most of the men, far from wives and families, too – only a few
privileged officers had their wives with them.

1923 saw eight RAF squadrons based in Iraq – three at Hinaidi, two
at Baghdad West, one at Shaibah and two further north among the
hills at Mosul. Aircrew continued very active, flying sorties against
rebellious tribes and Turkish forces. Death and injury stalked every
flight over craggy gorges, inhospitable mountains and baking
deserts, in climate and conditions never foreseen by the manufac-
turers of those early 'string-and-sealing wax' aircraft. Since ageing
planes often obliged their crews to make a forced landing in hostile
territory, the aircraft usually flew in pairs, so that the second one
could land nearby and lift the stricken crew to safety, often under
attack from tribesmen intent on mutilation, murder and pillage.
Parachutes were not a regular part of equipment until the late twen-
ties and few accurate maps existed.

With the practice of tropical medicine still in its early stages, endemic diseases also took their toll, and the climate added its own punishment – men could die of simple heatstroke. Nor were recommended precautions always effective: regulations obliged the wearing of a 'spine-pad', a four-inch wide pad of felt which hung down the back suspended from a cord round the throat; this item of equipment was deemed necessary to protect a man's spine from the 'deleterious rays of the sun'!

The then-commander of Hinaidi-based 45 Squadron, later Sir Arthur 'Bomber' Harris of Second World War fame, wrote in his book *Bomber Offensive* that he would 'never forget the appalling climate, the filthy food, and the ghastly lack of every sort of amenity that our unfortunate men were compelled to put up with in "peace time" '.

The first major 'casevac' by air

Aerial evacuation of casualties began, so history tells us, in 1870, when during the siege of Paris 160 patients were successfully lifted away from danger, courtesy of a hot-air balloon. For the RAF, involvement with casualty evacuation – 'casevac', as it became known – began in 1918, when at Helwan in Egypt a patient strapped firmly to a stretcher and swathed like a mummy against the dust was loaded into a cut-out section of the fuselage of a De Havilland 6 'Dung Hunter' for the fifteen-mile hop to the Stationary Hospital at Cairo. A couple of years later, during the war with the Mad Mullah, three patients on stretchers fixed inside the fuselage of a DH9 were flown 175 miles to hospital.

At RAF Halton in England, the first air ambulance service, using specially fitted aircraft, began and ended in the mid-twenties. A similar service lasted longer in the Middle East. However, purpose-built air ambulances proved unnecessary since most troop-carrying planes could easily be converted to carry casualties, and in real emergencies almost any aircraft could make shift as an ambulance.

In Mespot at this time, rebel Turkish leaders Kemal Ataturk and Sheikh Mahmud had vowed to reclaim large areas of upper Iraq, including Kurdistan. This northernmost part of Britain's mandated territories was, like the Persian Gulf, blessed with 'black gold', which made it contentious ground. The Turks, with their eyes on the oil, claimed that the Kurdish people were actually Turkish nationals, who must be protected from exploitation by the British. The Kurds (then as now) regarded themselves as an independent people with a right to self-determination.

In February 1923 British Intelligence discovered that Sheikh Mahmud planned to spark a general uprising in northern Iraq. In response, RAF detachments flew to Kirkuk, Mosul and Erbil, to reconnoitre and make bombing sorties in support of the ground troops. They also supplied rations and other necessaries to inaccessible areas; and, as had become a regular habit, they evacuated sick or wounded troops back to the hospitals and sick quarters.

However, casevac skills were put to their first real test when a severe outbreak of dysentery struck in the remote, arid mountains of Kurdistan. Original plans for evacuation had involved the use of river rafts, but the stricken troops had penetrated far into the mountains, beyond the river's navigable limits. The only available means of ground transport were mules and donkeys, an impossible method with life-threatening disease felling scores of men. Back in Baghdad, emergency plans swung into operation and soon the largest casevac yet seen was under way.

Over four days, using twelve aircraft and covering a total flying distance of nearly 10,000 miles, the RAF conveyed a total of 359 patients some 200 miles to the splendid new hospital at Hinaidi and the tender loving care of PMRAFNS sisters. Without this prompt air action, many lives would inevitably have been lost. The operation conclusively proved the vital role which the RAF could play in the future transport of sick and wounded personnel.

Social life

But work, war, danger and disease provided only part of the picture. Mespot had its fair share of social life, too, most of it centred on the capital, Baghdad, where the large British community, which included many civilians, enjoyed cricket matches, dances and teas, church outings, film shows and horse races. Romance also blossomed in a community where single men far outnumbered the few marriageable women. Inevitably, several members of the PMRAFNS joined the ranks of blushing Baghdad brides.

Sister Kathleen Isobel Sweeny, for instance, met her future husband in Mesopotamia. He was Flight Lieutenant Fairweather of

No. 30(B) Squadron, RAF Kirkuk. The wedding took place at RAF Kirkuk, in the north of Iraq.

Their son, John Fairweather, says that his mother was known fondly as 'Sister Sunshine' because she was 'not at her best first thing in the morning'. Being a fever-trained nurse and the only one in Mespot with such qualifications, she had found herself in charge of the fever ward at Hinaidi. There she came up against a formidable matron who insisted on pristine neatness and cleanliness on the ward, particularly in areas behind the bedhead, and who had been known 'to go on her knees and personally check these areas with her white gloves'. One day just before Matron's rounds, the ward admitted a new patient who needed an injection, administered by Sister Sweeny. When Matron arrived to find the bedside locker still littered with kidney bowl, hypodermic etc., she declared it 'a disgustingly filthy ward almost unfit for human habitation. She then went on her knees to check the skirting behind the bedhead and, being of ample proportions, displayed a rather large and well-corsetted posterior. A soldier in the next bed, who had "taken a bit of a shine" to Sister Sunshine . . . leaned over, grabbed the syringe and jabbed it straight into Matron's derrière.' Mr Fairweather adds that his mother, 'swore that Matron's shrieks would be heard three wards away and her false teeth were picked up three beds further down!'

The soldier, it seems, was put on a charge and sentenced to detention. 'The Doctors however, considered him unfit to undergo punishment, so he served his sentence in my mother's ward in the company of a Military Policeman . . . the Doctors discharged him as fit for duty coincidentally on the day he completed his sentence!'

Kathleen Sweeny resigned her appointment with the PMRAFNS when she married her dashing aircrew officer. Married women were not allowed to remain in the Service in those days.

Mary Edwards tells of her friend Miss Oliver, who 'was matron at Finchley when I was there and was posted to Basra':

She married out there: one Colin Macpherson. I was her bridesmaid.

Before she married, I went to Baghdad with her in an oil tanker which tied up at the Maud Bridge. One night I was awakened by a coolie who came into my bunk. I dashed up and caught hold of his coat, but he wriggled away from me. I got such a fright that I went to Miss Oliver's cabin and told her. She was most sympathetic and told me she had never seen me so frightened before.

Occasionally, naivety caused even more hair-raising incidents. Louise Hardy and a friend, having just completed a three-month stint of night duty, with no time off to keep in touch with local affairs, went into Baghdad to buy film for their cameras. Unaware that it was the final week of the Muslim festival of Ramadan, they were persuaded to go in a taxi to see an interesting mosque in a nearby town – 'the third holy city of Moslems'. The mosque had a courtyard paved with blue and white mosaic glimpsed through gateways, but 'across these were heavy golden chains. Fortunately we only wished to see and not go in . . . We saw pilgrims praying, kneeling on glorious Persian rugs . . . We walked round to look through several gates . . . We were very impressed and realised fully that it was a very holy place to the Muslims following us.'

Evidently they didn't realize quite fully enough. As the growing crowds around them began to talk ever more loudly and heatedly, a man drew the two women aside and warned them in English that they must leave at once. He told them to have money ready to throw into the crowd, to distract them while the nurses gained the safety of their taxi, which by this time was 'covered with Arabs sitting on the roof and the bonnet . . . the driver slumped over the wheel quivering with fear.' They threw the money, the men leapt down to squabble over it, and the taxi shot off: 'He drove like a maniac. We bumped and rolled along until in sight of Baghdad. By this time the radiator was boiling and we were bruised from being thrown around . . .'

Later that week they heard that there had been a riot in the town they had visited, with 200 headless bodies found outside the walls. The problem seemed to have stemmed from anger roused by the visit of 'two Christian women earlier in the week'.

Louise and her friend confessed that they had been the two women involved, with the result that they were questioned by their matron, by the hospital CO and then by the British Chief of Police. Finally they were called before the Air Officer Commanding, who said that if they had read 'Daily Routine Orders' they would have

Outdoor uniform 1930s. Note large brims on quatrecorn hats (© British Crown Copyright/MOD)

Carol-singing at Cranwell, 1938 – last Christmas before the outbreak of war
(© British Crown Copyright/MOD)

Sister Elizabeth Smallwood with staff and patients, Ward 11,
Halton Hospital, Christmas 1941

RAFH Wroughton, 1945

PMRAFNS sisters with friends at Giza, 1945

'Les Girls' of 61 MFH India, 1944, with (*back row, second and third from right*) Jessie Higgins and 'Tommy' Thomas known that Baghdad and all other towns were out of bounds until the end of Ramadan.

Presumably the truth about this particular escapade did not reach the local press. Usually, news of the British community – details of cricket scores from the UK and reports of the social whirl of Mespot – appeared in at least two English-language newspapers. The *Iraq Times*, printed and published in Baghdad, vied with the *Times of Mesopotamia*, which in June 1924 claimed to be 'the oldest established British newspaper in Iraq'; it was printed in Basrah/Basra/Busrah/Busra – all four spellings are to be seen on the front page!

Marion Welch had been matron at Hinaidi for just over eighteen months when, in May 1926, she fell ill and had to be invalided home to England. She spent three weeks in hospital under observation and was then granted a week's sick leave before returning to duty as matron of the RAF Officers' Hospital at Uxbridge. In August, however, she was taken ill again and underwent a major operation. Happily, this time she made a good recovery.

Having been at Uxbridge for just over a year, she was given a plum appointment – first matron at the newly-built hospital at Halton. We shall join her there shortly.

Aden

Legend claims that the name Aden derives from 'Eden', that it is the place where Cain and Abel lie buried and also the site of the building of Noah's Ark. It lies in Yemen, clustered around the edges of a vast bay which came under British control from 1802. After the opening of the Suez Canal, trade expanded rapidly and Aden, strategically placed near the entrance to the Red Sea, became not only one of the largest ports in the world but an important stop for passenger ships sailing between Europe and the Orient. In the rocky, mountainous desert hinterland lay various small states known as the Aden Protectorate. Britain protected the local rulers and in return those rulers levied a quota of soldiers to help British forces keep the peace.

Turkish incursions into the area called for military vigilance, but RAF squadrons based in Aden also helped patrol other problem areas such as Sudan, Kenya and British Somaliland. The first squadron went out in February 1927, to a place named RAF Khormaksar, which in the men's eyes replaced Iraq as 'the pits', as far as postings went.

RAF Khormaksar lay on the northern, inland side of the port of Aden, flanked on the western promontory by army encampments and the oil refineries of Little Aden. To the east, RAF Command Headquarters at Steamer Point clustered on hilltops with the main town below. The narrow confines of the inhabited coastal strip are surrounded by the famous 'barren rocks of Aden'.

The hospital, high over the bay at Steamer Point, benefited from thick walls which minimized the heat. It was said to have originated as a Turkish prison. The RAF took it over from the army in April 1928, re-equipped the wards and built a new operating theatre. Five members of the PMRAFNS arrived there in June 1928 – a matron, two sisters and two staff nurses. Others were to follow.

Aden's climate made life particularly trying. The warm 'winter' was bad enough but during the high summer season, from May to September, temperatures rose to 100°F and more. The only air conditioning came via great wooden fans that merely circulated the hot air and stirred up the dust. With humidity at 80 per cent, sisters spent their days drenched in their own sweat, sometimes changing their ward dresses four or five times a day.

With no natural water available, only tepid water, piped in across the desert, could be had, and that needed boiling before they dared drink it. Vegetation – small gardens and patches of lawn – had to be watered every day, otherwise it withered and died, blending into the uniform sere dusty brown of the landscape. Rain was so rare that when it did come it sent people out fully dressed to enjoy a soaking; unfortunately it usually arrived in torrents that broke walls and washed roads away.

The nursing sisters' mess lay almost at the top of the hill, separated from the town by a tortuously winding road. Whitewashed walls edged rocky ridges where the hospital buildings perched, each one higher than the next. Near the top, a tall and airy building with verandahs shaded by slatted blinds remained much the same during the forty years it served as a mess for PMRAFNS sisters. It commanded magnificent views over the town to the vivid blue of the bay, where visiting ships lay at anchor – cruise liners, yachts and cargo vessels – with Little Aden on the further headland, below a horizon of misty mountains which on homesick days might resemble the Cuillins on Skye.

Spectacular as the setting may have been, the hospital at Steamer Point was no place for idle dreamers. Nursing sisters looked after cases of dengue fever, sandfly fever and malaria, skin conditions such as prickly heat and dhobi itch, and the slow healing of septic wounds got by all the usual causes plus sea urchin spines in swimmers' feet, and bites from such local inhabitants as ants, scorpions and tarantulas. There were sharks in the sea, too. Not surprisingly, Aden was classed as an 'unhealthy' posting.

Palestine and Egypt

Policing the struggle between Palestinians and Jews was, for Britain, a thankless task and difficult to perform in a relatively well-developed, well-populated country. Anti-Jewish riots began in earnest with massacres in 1920, after 40,000 young Zionists arrived and established *kibbutzim*, and Hebrew became the official language of Jews in Palestine.

As the bloodshed and unrest continued, RAF squadrons dropped supplies and flew reconnaissance missions. Operations included the first use of wireless/telegraph packs mounted on camels and, where aircraft might be ineffective, the RAF even used armoured cars. One of these, as reported by PM Mary Gall, had once belonged to a gangster and was, reputedly, both bullet-proof and mine-proof. Happily, the truth of this was never tested.

PMs first went out to Palestine in 1924, to take over the army hospital at Ludd (Lydda), which was replaced by a new hospital at RAF Sarafand, opened in 1926 and visited two years later by Princess Mary. Sarafand remained a posting for PMs until 1940.

Neighbouring Egypt had been under British control for many years; it was peaceful, regarded as a kind of 'Clapham Junction' of the air, within easy reach of probable centres of unrest both east and west, and therefore a good location for a small RAF force to train and wait in reserve. Since many army troops were stationed there, army hospitals provided care for most British personnel. (The same was true of the north-west frontier in India). Two PMRAFNS sisters did briefly staff a station sick quarters at RAF Aboukir, on the Egyptian coast, from September 1924, but riots forced the place to close in 1925 and the sisters were transferred to Palestine. PMs returned again from 1928 to 1931, but were withdrawn owing to lack of patients.

However, the Second World War would bring them back to the land of the Pharaohs.

TWO

The new Halton

The scheme for constructing a permanent hospital at Halton had been approved in 1923, but it took four years for the new brick buildings with their Nightingale wards (long, wide rooms with a row of beds on each side) to be completed. In 1927, vacation of the old wooden huts took place in stages. First the offices, X-ray unit, dispensary and ancillary departments moved to their new premises. Next the new kitchens were equipped and stood ready for use. Lastly came the transfer of the wards, accomplished in a single day. By that time most of the patients had been discharged or sent on sick leave; only a few remained, some still 'bed' cases, others 'up' and reasonably mobile.

Marjorie Ells, then sister-in-charge of the ear, nose and throat ward, remembers it well:

> The great move began with the surgical and medical wards the first to go, and the Huts began to feel strangely empty. None of us had seen the new hospital or the wards, so it was an exciting occasion. My ward was the last to go, at about 8 p.m. All my patients were mobile, fortunately, for on arrival, to our horror, we found bedsteads and mattresses awaiting making up and, in the middle of the ward, a pile of bricks and rubble left by the builders. I gathered the staff together with the patients and we all got together to remove the debris, find buckets and form a team to scrub the place out . . .

A later PM, Lesley Cornwall-Jones (Mrs Howat), was actually born in the old First World War huts at Halton. Her father Richard,

69

a member of the Works Directorate, was involved with the building of the new hospital.

> Father used to tell the tale that when the hospital was opened and the first patients were wheeled in on stretcher trolleys, they couldn't get into the lifts! Only the length of the stretchers had been calculated and not the longer stretcher poles. In the usual manner of the English, the problem was soon overcome, when the carpenters were sent for and round holes were cut in the wooden walls of the lifts, to accommodate the ends of the stretcher poles . . . They were [still] there in the 1950s.

Despite these problems – not unprecedented in dealing with builders – the new Princess Mary's Royal Air Force Hospital, Halton, and the new sisters' quarters, were officially opened on 31 October 1927 by the PMs' Royal Patron and President, Princess Mary. One may imagine the excitement of the young apprentices forming the guard of honour, with the band playing and several VIPs, including Matron-in-Chief Joanna M. Cruickshank, lined up to greet Her Royal Highness. Later, Matron Marion Welch conducted the princess around the new wards.

At this juncture an ambulance arrived outside. It contained Louise Hardy (she who had started that riot in Iraq!). She writes of being invalided home from overseas and rushed straight to Halton, arriving 'as Princess Mary was doing her inspection, and I had to wait outside until it was over. I had the distinction of being the first sick sister at Halton.'

A case of shingles

Though as yet PMs had no RAF rank, their professional status was declared by stripes set on braid on the shoulders of capes or at the wrists of jacket sleeves. Staff nurses wore plain dark blue braid, sisters the same but with a single pale-blue stripe; senior sisters and above had maroon braid with pale blue stripes as appropriate – wider stripe, higher status.

The old blue ward dresses had been replaced by white cotton, worn with white linen collars, cuffs and aprons, plus a yard-square traditional 'veil' of white lawn fashioned into a deep triangle down the back and wings framing the head. Black stockings and shoes continued for a while but they too were soon replaced by all-white. An RAF blue cape, with a medical badge at each front corner, covered the shoulders when appropriate.

For formal evening occasions in the mess an elegant long blue satin dress might be worn, if acquired at the wearer's expense. This mess dress had self-covered buttons down to the waist, with Swiss lace at wrist and collar and a matching satin shoulder cape. A delicate organdie veil with blue wings at the back corner adorned the sister's head.

A veil was worn also with the grey-blue dress and shoulder-cape which made another option for mess and fairly formal wear. Or nursing sisters could go out and about in grey-blue jacket and skirt, white shirt and black tie, black shoes and stockings. This uniform suit was worn either with a double-peaked storm-cap or the black quatrecorn 'Dick Turpin'.

That hat created problems for the more fashion-conscious sisters in those days of 'flappers' and dropped waists. At a meeting of the Medical Advisory Board in February 1928, Miss Joanna Cruickshank informed her colleagues that matron after matron had approached her, on behalf of their nursing staff, with a request for a change in the style of the uniform hat. The sisters complained that the present style could not be worn neatly, or comfortably, on a fashionably shingled head, with hair cut severely short at the back. The company which made the hats had 'recommended the re-blocking of the hat to a shape that would meet all objections'.

A sample of the new shape was shown, but the committee 'agreed that a change was undesirable. Matron-in-Chief undertook to see whether the firm supplying the hat could offer further suggestions about making the hat suitable with either type of head, without in any way taking from the distinct character of the hat.'

Happily, by the time the committee met again in June, the hatters had produced an 'altered hat which in no way alters its character'. A close call for the 'Dick'.

Miss Welch and Miss Watt

Marion Welch remained in post as Halton's first matron for only a few months. The following April saw her promoted to the Air

Ministry to work with her friend Miss Cruickshank. Her place as matron at Halton went to Katherine Christie Watt.

Kate Watt had begun her RAF career in 1919, nursing at WRAF hostels in Glasgow and then at Great Yarmouth; she had worked at various RAF hospitals in Britain, including Old Sarum, Halton and Finchley, where she had been acting matron. When Uxbridge first opened she filled in as matron there, too, until the appointment of Marion Welch. She had worked with Miss Cruickshank at the Air Ministry, and had then been sent to Baghdad to replace Miss Welch when the latter had to be invalided home.

In fact, Kate Watt and Marion Welch had danced an intricate *pas de deux* through most of the important postings in the Service, with Miss Watt just that small step behind all the time. By 1929 they were both highly experienced, well-respected senior matrons of the PMRAFNS. And, as everyone knew, Miss Cruickshank was nearing retirement age. A new matron-in-chief would be needed. Which one would it be? Miss Welch or Miss Watt?

Airships

Despite earlier disasters, trial flights with airships continued. One of them caused a commotion at Halton Hospital when most of the patients on the orthopaedic ward (the single exception was a poor chap in traction!) ran out to stand on the lawn and watch the R100 'floating gracefully across the sky'. Charles James was one of 'Trenchard's Brats' at the time, in hospital with a damaged spine, treatment for which called for him to lie supine with the small of his back supported by two sandbags. He associates the airship's arrival with the smell of Sunday breakfast kippers, and great excitement, until a loud voice from the doorway ordered, 'Get back to your beds!' It was Matron, 'a woman of considerable size and vast authority. She was not amused.'

In October that same year, news of the trial flights of the latest airship, the R101, reached even the high seas. Marion Welch, now aged forty-one, was in the Mediterranean on board the *Nevasa*, bound once more for Iraq and another stint as matron of Hinaidi. On notepaper headed 'British India Steam Navigation Co. Ltd', she penned a letter to her friend Miss Cruickshank:

The *Nevasa* is a terrible ship for rolling even in a moderate sea. We should reach Port Said on Friday and have to coal there, so most people will take the opportunity to go ashore for a few hours. I shall be very glad when we reach the end of our journey.

A day or so later, she adds:

Another storm last night and most people had a return of *mal-de-mer*. Hope we shall find it calmer in the Red Sea. Miss Hards lands at 8.30 a.m. tomorrow, Port Said. Only herself, 1 Medical and 1 Flying Officer and 47 men to disembark for Egypt. The MO does not know his destination in Egypt until he reports at Cairo. Must finish my mail. So glad to see by wireless news that the R101 trial flight was so successfully carried out. Did you get a view of the airship when it passed over London?

The 'Miss Hards' she mentions was another long-serving member of the PMRAFNS – one wonders how she must have felt at the prospect of disembarking, for destinations unknown, as the only woman with forty-nine men!

She flies through the air . . .

On a summer day in 1930, at Grosvenor House, Park Lane, Matron-in-Chief Joanna Cruickshank held an 'at home' attended by many leading members of the nursing and medical services of all three forces. Guest of honour was Princess Mary, Countess of Harewood. Of this charming social event the nursing press reports that attending PMs 'were daintily and tastefully attired in afternoon dress, and wore on the left shoulder, as a distinguishing mark, a badge in crêpe de chine resembling a flower in the three Royal Air Force colours'. Some guests had come from long distances, especially the matron of the Palestine hospital, who 'had actually travelled from the Holy Land – not, as the uninitiated might think, by air, for that species of locomotion is forbidden to RAF nurses when on duty, but by the ordinary route.' The 'ordinary route' was, of course, the sea.

Back in 1920, Kate New had tried flying. While nursing at Old Sarum she had her one and only 'flip' in an aeroplane, suitably attired in a pair of serge bloomers (as popularized by Mrs Amelia Bloomer, of New York, for use while bicycling). Kate New thought these garments more suitable than 'pretty panties' for clambering into the front of a two-seater Avro, but before they set off she admonished the pilot not to get up to 'any tricks like looping the loop'. Hearing of this escapade, the Director of Medical Services (DMS), Sir Matthew Fell, was not amused. He made a special trip to Old Sarum to advise Miss New that 'nurses did not fly in service aircraft'.

The intrepidity of these women is exemplified by Mary Edwards, who on her second tour in the Middle East, in 1929, found herself at Hinaidi, from where 'we were allowed to fly to Egypt in training flights . . . On the return journey – fortunately outside the hills of Amman – I noticed oil pouring out of the engine; so we came down in the desert in mid-July. There was another 'plane with spare parts following us. It came down beside us; so we transferred to it.'

Two years later:

> I was transferred to Sarafand to do matron's duties . . . I went by aeroplane in which was ex-King Ali – brother of King Faisal. We had a terrible journey. As I was sitting beside the King I thought it better to move down to the tail and put my head down. When we reached Amman King Ali waited for me and said to me, '*Vous étiez très malade, madame* [You have been very ill]'. He passed me a bottle during the journey. I opened and smelt it. It was ether! So with thanks I returned it.

Perhaps the Middle East allowed for a certain licence in such matters. At home, the combination of women and wings was still anathema.

Dame Joanna Cruickshank, in later life, pondered the question:

> Should nurses be allowed in the air? It seems odd, now, to think that though they were in a Flying Service, in those early days it was only in very exceptional circumstances that the nursing sisters were permitted to be passengers in official

aircraft on duty. It was argued that they were civilians, and they might be killed! Whether killed or injured, questions might be asked in the House – always a bugbear to Ministers and their Civil Service henchmen. And how about compensation, even though the victims should have signed a certificate that they took the air at their own risk?

Writing after the Second World War, she merrily admits to having defied the ban herself:

On one occasion, the RAF hospital at Cranwell was being inspected by the then so-called Director of Medical Services (since just before the last war, this title has been Director-General of RAF Medical Services.) . . . For obvious reasons, the Matron-in-Chief PMRAFNS, Miss (now Dame Joanna) Cruickshank, wished – indeed, was expected – to be there to meet him. Owing to some unforeseen combination of accidental circumstance, she found herself unable to reach Cranwell in time if she travelled by train. She determined to fly, and managed somehow or other – not without perseverance – to get round the official taboo. However, she did not arrive by air! After the second of two forced landings she would still have gone on, but her pilot thought that he would 'call it a day'. So Matron-in-Chief had to proceed – in the Services one does not 'go', one 'proceeds' – ignominiously by car! And late!

Now it is but a 'normal occasion' for Sisters to travel on duty in Service aircraft, and the day may not be far distant when a Matron-in-Chief pilots her own light aircraft on an inspection tour.

Fifty years after Dame Joanna scribbled this account of her own adventures, modern matrons-in-chief are still waiting for that day to arrive.

A successor for Miss Cruickshank

With Miss Cruickshank due to retire on reaching the age of fifty-five in November 1930, two candidates appeared eligible to succeed her – Miss Marion Welch and Miss Katherine Christie Watt. Miss Cruickshank wrote references for each of these ladies, including details of their training, careers and her own recommendations on their suitability.

> In addition to holding very good professional qualifications, Miss Welch possesses outstanding administrative and organizing abilities. She has the power of maintaining a high standard of efficiency, has a wide range of knowledge, general and professional, a generous outlook, possessed of sound common sense and a sympathetic understanding of human nature. I have no hesitation in recommending her as my immediate successor.

Of Miss Watt, she concludes: 'Miss Watt's professional, administrative and moral qualifications equal those of Miss Welch, but she has not Miss Welch's wide range of general knowledge and experience.'

The Air Ministry evidently agreed with these conclusions. In July 1930 they wrote to Miss Welch in Iraq to inform her that she had been selected to succeed Miss Cruickshank – on the understanding that she would retire in 1936 after completing twenty years' service (they did not want her to think she, too, could hang on until her fifty-fifth birthday, thirteen years on!).

What must have been their reaction when Miss Welch turned them down flat? She informed them that she was resigning the Service. She had communicated her reasons to Miss Cruickshank.

A clue to those reasons lies in a delightful letter written from Hinaidi and dated 21 November 1930:

> Writing this letter, the last to you as our Matron-in-Chief, is a very sad event . . . I hope and pray that the next part of the road may be even more interesting though less arduous to travel . . . Miss Watt takes over when most of the spadework is done, though there will be plenty of battles to be fought in the future . . .
>
> I look forward to seeing you when I come home next year. Have not made any final plans about the wedding yet, but expect to get married about March and spend the summer in Europe.

Romance had belatedly struck for Matron Miss Marion Welch, then aged forty-two.

This same letter gives some amusing sidelights into everyday life and attitudes in British Baghdad:

> The Bazaar last week in aid of the Civil Chaplaincy Fund was a great success . . . Mrs Ludlow-Hewitt gave her first dinner party last Tuesday and Miss Walker, Adamson and I were the only ladies invited. She had to give it in the AOC's Staff Mess as her domestic trials with servants at present are very acute . . .
>
> Last night we had several health films shown in the hospital, one on Malaria, another on Hookworm and 2 comics called 'Giro the Germ' issued by the National Health and Cleanliness Council in London. The portable cinema apparatus was lent to Mr Lampard by the Ford Motor Co. On Saturday we are to have the latest Ford films on production of cars and farming implements. The men are always so interested in anything mechanical . . .

Giro the Germ sounds fun. I'm not so sure about *Malaria* and *Hookworm*! The gentleman who operated the 'portable cinema apparatus' was her intended, Mr Lampard, resident in Baghdad as secretary of the Young Men's Christian Association. He and Miss Welch were married in the spring of 1931.

And so Miss Katherine C. Watt became the second matron-in-chief of the PMRAFNS. She remained in the post until 1938.

Sour grapes?

Prior to Miss Cruickshank's retirement, the Air Ministry requested that the Treasury might grant her a special rate of pension: 'Miss Cruickshank was the first Matron-in-Chief. To her fell the onerous task of building up the Royal Air Force Nursing Service from its beginning and the efficiency of the Service today is due in no small measure to the good work that she has done.'

The ensuing discussion is on file only in scribbled memos between two writers whose identity is not clear, but some of the comments are revealing. One of them says that Miss Cruickshank's efforts at setting up the RAFNS were rewarded by her getting the CBE; that, he implies, should be sufficient, without giving her extra retirement pay too. (One wonders how he felt when she received the DBE in 1931!)

Another minute adds a bracketed PS concerning another senior nurse (matron-in-chief of the Ministry of Pensions): 'She has been a bit 'troublesome' . . . in the last year or two, but I suppose most of them get a bit that way; Matrons-in-Chief are so used to being auto-crats with the staff they control.'

The other chap replies, 'Miss Cruickshank was no doubt glad to get such a post as MIC at an age seven years above the usual maxi-mum. One cannot expect to enter a Service late in life and derive the same benefits as regards pensions as if one entered at the normal age.' He seems to forget that during the First World War nurses were gladly accepted up to the age of forty-five.

Not surprisingly, in view of these hostile male witnesses, the appeal for a special rate of pension was turned down. However, minutes of a meeting of the Nursing Service Advisory Board record 'high appreciation of the way in which Dame Joanna Cruickshank has discharged the duties of Matron-in-Chief during her long tenure in office. She had the responsible task of creating the Nursing Service, and the Board consider that its present state of high efficiency is largely due to her ability, guidance and example.'

Nor was she about to sit with her feet up. As the Second World War began, Dame Joanna accepted the demanding post of Matron-in-Chief of the Joint War Organization of the British Red Cross and the Order of St John of Jerusalem. She designed a special cap for nurses, a simple shape over which a gas mask could be fitted with ease. But she was no longer a young woman and perhaps she had taken on too much – ill-health forced her to resign her position in 1940. That same year she assumed the duties of Commandant of the Alien Women's Internment Camp on the Isle of Man, but again her health obliged her to relinquish this work in 1941.

Now aged sixty-five, she at last contented herself with a back seat and, some years later, turned her mind to writing a new and more personal history of the PMRAFNS. It would, no doubt, have been a lively read, but sadly only a meagre twenty typed quarto pages of a first rough draft survive – some of the highlights have illuminated this present account. What else might she have written, memories that only she could have told? Lost forever, alas.

Until she died in August 1958, aged eighty-two, she maintained a keen interest in the nursing services to which she had been attached. She was particularly pleased to renew acquaintance with old friends of the PMRAFNS, at reunions and at the annual inter-hospital tennis tournament which is named after her. The Dame Joanna Cruickshank Tennis Tournament is still played today, a happy summertime occasion. The trophy is a fluted silver rose bowl presented to the PMs by their first matron-in-chief in 1930.

Days of sunlight

The early thirties brought tranquil times and an increase in social functions. In 1931 the PMRAFNS 'Dinner Club' held its first reunion dinner, and later an 'at home' reception took place in the ballroom at Claridge's. Then in the New Year's Honours for 1932, the Service's Royal Patron received a new title when her father, King George V, created her Princess Royal. This honorary title may be conferred only by the sovereign on his or her eldest daughter and its last holder before Princess Mary was her aunt, Princess Louise, Duchess of Fife, who died in 1931.

The RAF's new hospital at Halton flourished and new buildings for the RAF College Cranwell were soon to be opened by the Prince of Wales (later Edward VIII, then Duke of Windsor).

The third hospital, located at RAF Uxbridge, served a huge depot where adult recruits entered ground-support trades. In those days all RAF personnel worked closely with aircraft and, whatever his trade, in order to win his 'props' (leading aircraftman insignia) a man had to prove himself physically capable of turning a real aircraft propeller.

PMs employed at the RAF Hospital Uxbridge had at last vacated their old wartime quarters and set up home in a new sisters' mess, built along the same lines as those at Halton and Cranwell – centrally heated with a whole suite of rooms for the matron and for each sister a separate bedroom with hot and cold water on tap. These luxuries must have brought some comfort after an epidemic of cerebro-spinal meningitis (spotted fever) hit the depot. Two hundred patients were isolated, half the camp quarantined and special precautions, including armed guards on the gates, taken to prevent the disease from spreading to the nearby town. Even so, six recruits died, despite being rushed to Halton Isolation Hospital.

Elsewhere, other young patients had happier outcomes. In Ireland, the family of sixteen-year-old Aircraft Apprentice R.J. McQuigg received an alarming telegram informing them that their son was in PMRAFH Halton suffering from something called nasopharynxitis. They rushed to consult their GP, who assured them that this polysyllabic terror was nothing more than a feverish cold. Mr McQuigg says drily, 'Thanks to a week of care from Princess Mary's Nursing Sisters, and the strict discipline of Matron, I made a good recovery.'

Another young apprentice, Charlie Chapman, developed rheumatic fever and spent six months in a ward at Halton. He particularly remembers the kindness of the staff, and also 'an import of victims of the Quetta earthquake disaster'. Quetta, now in Pakistan, was then in British Beluchistan and had long been an army outpost. When the earthquake happened, on 6 May 1935, thirty thousand lives were lost. This was the first occasion when an entire medical unit moved by air, when a team of army doctors, nurses and equipment flew from Karachi to the scene of the disaster. Evidently some of the victims ended up in the care of PMs at Halton.

The RAF's medical and nursing services continued to thrive and grow, developing expertise in specialist fields, particularly aviation medicine. Flying remained a dangerous occupation. However, interesting statistics from 1932 reveal that for every man killed or injured by flying in that year, twenty-seven were injured whilst taking part (often compulsorily) in games or physical recreation! Hopefully none of the sisters entering for the Dame Joanna Cruickshank Cup had their names added to the list.

As reported in the nursing press, at this time the tennis tournament took place in 'the lovely gardens of the Officers' Mess at the RAF depot, Uxbridge.' It developed into 'a delightful social function as well as a reunion of members of a very scattered service. On every side one could hear such names as "Basra", "Baghdad" and "Karachi" mentioned as casually as one ordinarily hears "Hyde Park" or "Oxford Circus".'

On another occasion the Nursing Times reporter observed the presence of 'umpires perched on a chair set on a table, "ball-boys" stalwart hairy-legged Air Force lads, spectators nurses in mufti with friends and officers. The stage was set . . . for the semi-final and final singles match . . .' That year Miss Helen Cargill won the trophy with Miss Veronica Ashworth as runner-up (both went on to become matrons-in-chief after the Second World War). Naturally air force nurses had their share of admirers – the report adds in a bracketed aside, 'There is always a very masculine element about the RAF nurses' functions . . .'

After years of complaints of a general shortage of good nurses, August 1936 brought a rise in pay and allowances, with a chance for swifter promotion. A new member of the PMRAFNS, joining as a staff nurse, could now expect promotion to the rank of sister in one year rather than three. Maximum pay for a sister could be achieved, by annual increments, in nine years rather than seventeen as previously. Along with improved pay for special qualifications, an increase in allowances and a greater number of substantive appointments in the grades of matron and senior sister, the opportunity to travel and work abroad made the PMRAFNS an attractive career for an ambitious young woman. Entering at the minimum age of twenty-four, she could hope to be earning £125 a year by the time she was thirty-three – always supposing she did not succumb to the urge to get married. Marriage still meant enforced retirement for women in those pre-war days.

Coming events cast their shadows

In a cuttings book kept by Dame Joanna, alongside snippets about the tennis tournament, with teas and parasols and happy chatter amid glorious summer weather, there is a column clipped from the *Iraq Times*. It reports an incident at RAF Hinaidi when a British civilian engineer was shot dead by an infuriated Iraqi mechanic. On the back of this cutting, only the last part legible (the rest is glued down), is a piece which reports a military review in Germany, in the presence of 'the former "Corporal Hitler", now Supreme Commander of the German forces. Herr Hitler, alongside General von Blomberg, reviewed 6,000 troops at the Zeppelin Meadows. Over 60,000 political leaders, Storm Troops and Guards were ordered to attend the demonstration. Though only a small part of the army took part, the military technique was "a revelation".'

Meanwhile, in Mespot

In the Middle East the RAF and its hospitals continued to deal with victims of skirmish, disease and accident. Between 1919 and the end of 1938, 2,806 casualties were moved by air, across hundreds of miles of inhospitable desert and mountain.

On one flight, from Egypt to Iraq, PMs Hards and White were among the passengers on a Vickers Victoria aircraft when something forced their pilot to head for an emergency landing, in the middle of the desert, at night. According to service instructions, a certain door had to be opened on such occasions, but the airman who performed the duty slipped and fell from the plane, some 700 feet above ground. 'The machine landed safely, and the remainder of the party were rescued at dawn by a plane from Baghdad,' said the *Daily Telegraph*. The unfortunate airman was buried with full honours at Hinaidi.

In August 1931, cholera broke out among the population of southern Iraq and queues formed outside the dispensaries at Basra. According to the *Iraq Times*, 'Thousands of Arabs from the desert, marshes and river villages for miles around are swarming in for inoculation, the value of which they fully realise. When the dispensaries close, crowds patiently sit outside waiting through the night.' As the epidemic began to abate, 633 cases had been reported, with only 300 surviving. But many others had been prevented from catching the disease. A dispensary orderly held the men's record of 1,500 injections given in one day, but a 'British girl nurse' had established a record for women – in one day she inoculated no less than a thousand desert Arabs.

Habbaniya

Under an Anglo-Iraqi treaty of June 1930, the RAF agreed to withdraw from Hinaidi and Mosul within five years of Iraqi independence, which was due in September 1932. A reduced RAF force was to reside at Sin el Dhibban, sixty miles from Baghdad. Construction work for the new camp, named RAF Dhibban, began in 1934; flying squadrons were based there from 1936; Squadron HQ took up residence the following January; and the hospital completed its move from Hinaidi in December 1937.

The camp lay in the flood-plain of the Euphrates, only a few miles from a treeless plateau where Lake Habbaniya rippled on dusty, gypsum-saturated shores. A rest and leave centre grew up near the lake, and a yacht club flourished on waters where Empire flying boats landed. The big, airy RAF hospital had 500 beds, including some for the Iraqi levies – troops enlisted from local tribes to serve beside British forces in their area.

The unit was officially renamed RAF Habbaniya from 31 May 1938. Some pronounced it Hab*ban*iya, some Habban*ee*ya, some preferred the shortened 'Habb' and others went on calling it Dhibban. Most personnel loved it.

However, PMs in Iraq did not permanently sequester themselves within the safety of their hospitals and the comfort of their well-staffed messes, nor even within the confines of the camp and the British community. Throughout their long acquaintance with the country, from 1922 to 1958, nursing sisters often travelled long distances to treat tribesmen and their families in remote villages. They also accompanied RAF personnel to their summer 'rest and recreation' camp, high and remote in the cooler climate of the Kurdistan hills.

Ser Amadia

Initially a summer training camp for Iraqi levies, Ser Amadia opened each summer, from the early thirties to 1954, with a break during the war years. PMs sent to work there dispensed first aid from a makeshift, tented sick quarters to which tribesmen from miles around would flock. Some came from beyond the Turkish and Persian borders. These men and their families might travel for days in order to camp nearby and await medical attention from these much-admired ladies and the doctors and medics who worked with them.

Among the sisters involved was Louise Hardy, who explains that, 'each year in May an advance party . . . composed of officers, airmen and two nursing sisters . . . left Hinaidi with tents and other portable equipment. The only fixtures remaining [at Ser Amadia] from one year to the next were the rifle range and a fine swimming bath.'

The medical team left Baghdad at sunrise, flying in Vickers Victoria aircraft to a small village north of Mosul, where they landed in a bumpy field of grass. Lorries took the main party on but the adjutant brought his car to convey the sisters 'by a shorter but more precipitous route . . . a typical mountain road, very steep and with exciting hairpin bends which had to be negotiated with care for flocks of goats and groups of horsemen might be met around any corner. The horsemen were fierce-looking Kurds . . . each carried a rifle across his saddle bow.'

By early afternoon they had reached another mountain village where 'having changed from uniform to jodhpurs, we mounted mules for the final climb . . . no defined path, but the mules picked their way very cleverly over great boulders and up steep paths until suddenly the camp came into view.' It was seven o'clock in the evening. Tired and hungry, they were shown to their tents by a bearer who had gone ahead with the advance party. 'Our quarters were very comfortable, and we liked particularly the leafy hut known as a *caprana*, which had been erected at the entrance to the tent. It was a cool and pleasant place to sit and have one's meals.'

Official morning sick parade took little time, the men being generally fit, but afterwards the sisters and the medical officer, Flight Lieutenant Bellringer, would walk across to the camp of their Assyrian guards, 'where an Indian doctor prescribed for local people'.

[He] was grateful for our help with the women patients, and Flight-Lieutenant Bellringer, an experienced surgeon, performed remarkable operations, using only a set of ward instruments and a kitchen table . . . We could not send the very sick to their homes, so gradually a small tented hospital grew up around the sick quarters. These hardy, mountain people recovered quickly from conditions which in those days, without the use of penicillin, would have killed a European. Their material needs were cared for by their own relatives, and goats, being 'rations on the hoof', wandered around everywhere.

On one occasion Louise and another sister rode for four hours on mules to attend an Arab woman in difficult labour. Having overseen the delivery of a healthy boy, they set out for the four-hour ride back, escorted by the child's father and a party of other men, with a bright full moon silvering the mountains. When they passed other riders the new father would shout the news of his son and the men all fired their rifles in salute – 'which startled us a little the first time it happened,' Louise Hardy admits. She had many adventures in Iraq but she particularly recalls those 'exciting periods of beauty in Ser Amadia'.

Farewells

When Matron-in-Chief Katherine Watt retired in January 1938, the press announced her intention of going on a travel tour to visit, among other places, 'Iraq, where she hopes to see over the new Royal Air Force Hospital, opened last December, at Dhibban.' It was still called Dhibban at the beginning of that year.

By July, when Marion Welch, now Mrs Lampard, paid her last visit, the hospital had become Habbaniya. The *Iraq Times* tells the story: 'We much regret to announce the death of Mrs Lampard, the wife of the Secretary of the Young Men's Christian Association in Baghdad. Mrs Lampard had been indisposed for only a few days. On Tuesday she went to Habbaniya where (as a former Matron of the Royal Air Force) she was admitted to the hospital. She died yesterday from the effects (we believe) of septi-caemia . . .' She was fifty years old and had been married for seven brief years.

Gwen Butler's sojourn in Iraq had a dramatic ending, too. While holidaying at Ser Amadia in August 1939, she and other RAF personnel took lunch with the Regent of Iraq and his ministers – a rather glamorous occasion. On their return to the rest camp, they found it rife with 'desert rumours' of war and news of an immediate recall, though no one knew anything for sure. They had all been aware of growing political tension in recent years: a reserve force for the PMRAFNS had been started in 1937; the Munich crisis had occurred just twelve months before; back in the spring Germany had annexed Czechoslovakia, then Italy invaded Albania . . . Had the crisis escalated beyond all hope?

They set out at 4 a.m. to ride down the mountain, their mules picking a way down sheer hillsides amid scenery made breathtaking by the rising sun. And when eventually they reached the nearest RAF airfield, they discovered that war had not, after all, been declared. 'We learned with relief that Mr Neville Chamberlain was on a fishing trip,' Gwen Butler recalled.

Their relief proved premature. A week later, Britain was again at war.

PART III

The Sternest Days

'Do not let us speak of darker days; let us rather
speak of sterner days. These are not dark days,
these are great days – the greatest days our country
has ever lived.'

Winston S. Churchill, speaking at Harrow School,
29 October 1941

ONE

Preparing for war

In 1937, responding to the growing threat from Nazi Germany, the Air Ministry began to recruit a war reserve for all branches of the air force, including the PMRAFNS. Fully trained state registered nurses (SRNs) aged between twenty-four and forty-five were invited to sign on and stand ready to be called up for service should a national emergency arise. That first appeal brought in 200 immediate enquiries.

The following year, on 25 October, four PM sisters were part of the thousand-strong force of RAF personnel which gathered aboard the troopship *Nevasa*. This is believed to have been the largest RAF contingent ever sent overseas in one ship, with personnel destined for such postings as Malta, Aden, the Sudan, Iraq and India.

Meanwhile, at home, two new RAF general hospitals were under construction, one sited at Wroughton, near Swindon in Wiltshire, the other at Ely, near Cambridge. These large, brick-built hospitals would provide full medical and surgical facilities for patients, plus refresher courses for medical officers and training for medical airmen and airwomen. While Ely hospital was being built, beds for RAF personnel in East Anglia were provided at a former convalescent home of the Transport and General Workers' Union, at Littleport. This unit later continued as an annexe for Ely hospital, which boasted the most up-to-date equipment and facilities. Its operating theatre, built to be blast-proof, was the first in the RAF to have twin air-conditioning.

Across the country, aspiring new members of both the RAF and the reborn and renamed Women's Auxiliary Air Force (WAAF) arrived in droves at hastily erected recruiting stations. Large hutted station sick quarters (SSQs) – mini-hospitals, equipped for swift expansion as needed – looked after the health of thousands of young trainees. All of these SSQs had nursing sisters of the PMRAFNS on their staffs.

Other PMs found themselves posted to sick quarters at initial training wings and schools of technical training which were housed wherever a suitable building might be made available. Some sisters were assigned quarters in seaside boarding houses in resorts such as Blackpool, Bournemouth, Newquay, Scarborough and Yarmouth. Wherever they might be located, they worked in tandem with men and women of the medical branch and dental and psychiatric trades, of all ranks from medical officer to what was fondly known as 'AC plonk' (aircraftman second class).

As yet, the PMs themselves held no service rank, but, as one merry recruit remembers, 'we were saluted by all and sundry and we gave back a gracious smile (or grin)'.

Bog rats and battleaxes

The influx of hundreds of modern young women with new ideas came as a shock to some of the long-established sisters, who heartily disapproved of the 'giddy young things' now joining up.

When 'Jenny' Jenkins first joined the service, 'new members were unofficially referred to as "bog rats" and we thought the senior sisters very old. They were about forty, possibly younger.' Iris Jarred (Mrs Bartram) had the impression that new recruits were 'very much looked down upon – "little whipper-snapper" sort of attitude. [We kept] coming up with new ideas, where "they" were still nursing in their day.'

The Halton matron frowned upon too much lipstick and short skirts. She required new members to bend over and demonstrate that their popliteal spaces (the backs of their knees) were not showing. And new member Rona Black (Mrs McAlpine) felt sorry for Principal Matron Gladys Taylor:

Poor Miss Taylor . . . dealing with all these non-conforming volunteers. You would have seen one little curl peeping out from under the beautifully laundered caps, then a gradually increasing quantity of curls ... I wouldn't say we were received with open arms – at best we were tolerated. I suppose my worst offence was to be seen in the Sergeants' Mess, where was the only piano, practising my songs for a concert.

It was, of course, not done for a nursing sister to be caught fraternizing with NCOs.

With five or six other applicants, Kathleen 'Kay' Cranston (Mrs Slim) appeared before the Appointments Board at Adastral House in October 1938. After registering, she remembers being led 'right to the top of the building, over the roof, all among the chimneys . . .' and down into what might have been the same or another building, for a medical examination. 'They treated us as if we were pilots and they spun us round, jumped us up and down, made us breathe into all sorts of things . . . evidently they had never examined Sisters before.'

New recruits also brought their own ideas about fashion. Sister Cranston had acquired her indoor dress, but still needed her outdoor uniform. As instructed, she reported to 'the special tailor's shop which had what they called the "sealed pattern" of the outdoor costume.'

I was horrified. It had not been changed since the 1920s . . . a type of Norfolk jacket with a waistline way down round your bottom . . . awful. So, being a tailor's daughter and knowing what was right, I said, 'I'm not wearing that.' With this nice tailor we devised a very smart (for those days) fitted jacket and skirt. Well, there was mayhem when I wore that back at Halton. The Matron-in-Chief was sent for. I paraded in front of them all like a mannequin, but they all liked it and said, 'Oh, we'll change it.' So everybody had the new uniform.

In those early days each new member received a copy of the 'sealed pattern' and took it to her own tailor to be made up. Close examination of photographs reveals that Kay Cranston was not alone in making adjustments. Particularly variable features were the position of the belt and the length of lapels.

Finding itself with two vacancies for regular (permanent, as opposed to temporary reserve) members, in June 1939 the PMRAFNS interviewed twenty hopeful applicants. Most of them were well-qualified sisters, trained at big London hospitals, and Welsh-born Iris 'Fluffy' Jones (Mrs Ogilvie, now Mrs Bower), from St Mary's, Paddington, felt rather awed to be in this company. She was twenty-four years old but looked much younger, being only five feet two and slightly built, with a halo of fluffy golden curls which had earned her her nickname. Confronted by a board which included Matron-in-Chief (MIC) Emily Blair and the Director-General of Medical Services (DGMS), Air Marshal Sir Victor Richardson, she did not feel she was doing particularly well.

When the board asked if she spoke any languages, Fluffy hesitated to mention her schoolgirl French but declared instead that she spoke Welsh. She fancied that the Air Marshal gave her a very odd look. Convinced that she had blown her chances, she went to sit outside and await the verdict. To her astonishment and delight, she was chosen. Her Welsh connection had done the trick – the DGMS's mother was Welsh, too.

But for her accident of birthplace, she says, 'my whole life would have been different'. The story of the PMRAFNS would have been different, too. Today, Mrs Iris Bower, well over eighty but still known as Fluffy, remains one of the service's best-loved and most distinguished heroines.

Tension grows

The reality of war came nearer when station orders called for exercises of air-raid and blackout precautions. During air-raid practice at Halton, all personnel – except nursing sisters – wore gas masks. As one Flight Sergeant Peach dryly explained to young Sister Cranston, 'Lethal gas goes round Matrons, Group Captains and Wing Commanders, but *not* Sisters!'

After a few days' leave, Kay Cranston came off the train to find the village of Wendover in total darkness. Bewildered, she walked the lanes to the darkened hospital, groped her way to her room and lit a candle to see her to bed. Next day the CO sent for her to ask why she had been showing a light – and such a bright one, too. When she explained that she had not realized there was a blackout practice, and that all she had used was one small candle, he said,

'That's amazing. That little light could be seen for miles!' A good demonstration of the need for total blackout.

Despite growing tension in Europe, the minutiae of nursing life went on . . . Minutes of a matrons' meeting at the Air Ministry in March 1939 record Matron-in-Chief's reminder that two days off per month should be taken to mean per calendar month and not one day per fortnight. A nice distinction. But in those days 'off-duty time' was a precious privilege; with only two free days every calendar month, each minute counted. That was the norm. No nurse complained. And the patients seemed happy.

Wilfred Gooch has nothing but praise for the care he received in Halton when, as a young airman at Upper Heyford, he was badly burned when an old field-kitchen boiler exploded. He remarks on the number of boy apprentices who would come into the hospital 'trying it on' to get away from parades over at the training school. But the sisters' remedy 'a dose of cod liver oil and a charcoal biscuit' soon sent the truants back to work.

As Germany continued its provocative march towards confrontation, the recruiting drive for nurses grew urgent. The nursing press reported how the administration class of the British College of Nurses had paid a visit to RAF Halton, where the hospital stood in beautiful grounds among the Chiltern Hills. In the sisters' mess, a sitting room with a sunny bay window overlooked 'what is to be a glorious garden . . . when the demolition of the remaining huts of the original camp is completed'. The windows of the second floor boasted 'a view of Halton Camp Airport, extending for miles . . . Workshops, where thousands of boys are in training for the Force, the Schools, the Barracks, married men's houses, and finally, situated on a rising eminence . . . Halton House, once the home of a member of the Rothschild family and now the Officers' Mess.' Articles such as this one tempted more young women to sign up.

Early in 1939 Jessie Higgins was happily nursing on the private wards of Queen Charlotte's Hospital in London. Disturbed by events in Germany, she decided to apply to join the PMs. Her aunt had nursed in the First World War, in the reserve of QAIMNS, but had advised, 'Whatever you do, don't go in as a reserve – join the service!' Jessie Higgins took that advice, launching herself into a career that was to last for thirty years and see her rise to be a well-loved and respected senior matron. However, that career had a somewhat anticlimactic beginning: recruits signing on in April 1939 were told to go home and wait to be called. This was mostly because of insufficient accommodation.

To counter this problem, as we have seen, a huge building programme had begun.

Station Hospitals

The first RAF station hospitals (RAFSHs) grew up at three recruit reception and training centres which opened in western Britain. At Cosford, in Shropshire, a large SSQ with a capacity of ninety beds had a senior sister in charge and five sisters among the staff. It opened in September 1938, dealing with both RAF and WAAF recruits. A year later it became a station hospital, with extra sections opening as builders finished erecting more huts, and by June 1940 it was large enough to be designated Royal Air Force General Hospital Cosford. It developed into one of the largest and busiest of RAFGHs, including a rehabilitation centre for technicians and an important burns unit, staffed by ten doctors, twenty-seven nursing sisters, twelve VADs and eighty-three airmen and airwomen.

Another wooden-hutted hospital, at the recruit unit at Padgate, near Warrington in Cheshire, opened in May 1939. On arrival, many recruits proved unfit for service despite their initial medical clearance; they had to be treated, in or out of hospital, before taking up their duties. The hospital also ensured the fitness of personnel drafted overseas when RAF Padgate became one of the main personnel despatch centres. Later, when it served as a quarantine centre for suspected smallpox contacts disembarking from troopships at Liverpool, its latrines proved inadequate and buckets were provided, to be emptied into the local sewer.

At the new hutted recruit-training camp of RAF St Athan, Glamorgan, the SSQ was still under construction when, in January 1939, measles broke out. At first the nearby civilian hospital provided beds, but it couldn't cope when six more cases occurred among men on a flight riggers' course. Two sympathetic PM sisters hurried to get ready what beds they could, with the result that the patients, much to the ribald appreciation of their mates, found themselves in what would become the maternity ward. Alfred Thorne, one of the six men involved, says that he was admitted again later, with toxaemia, which a medical book informed him was a condition of pregnancy. At which point 'I began to wonder if I was having a sex change!'

St Athan SSQ was upgraded to a station hospital in 1940 as the opening of more RAF stations nearby called for extended medical facilities. The increased complement of staff included fifty-six PMs, led by a matron and four senior sisters. As with many wartime units, the St Athan hospital was a sprawl of wooden huts linked together by walkways, some covered and some open to the elements. The old SSQ turned into an infectious diseases centre and annexe for the busy new hospital whose patients came from RAF stations throughout Wales and across the Midlands.

I have to tell you now . . .

On 3 September 1939, Prime Minister Neville Chamberlain's sombre broadcast announced the end of all hope for a peaceful solution to the problem of Nazi Germany. Within minutes air-raid sirens sounded across the south-east of England and people headed for newly built public shelters beneath a sky devoid of German aircraft – that first air-raid warning, and many that followed, turned out to be a false alarm.

The PMRAFNS had, at this time, 400 women on its strength: 184 regular members plus reserves and a pool of VAD nurses. Many of the VADs had been trained at RAF hospitals at Halton or Cranwell, forming a valuable addition to the reserve. On the declaration of war, 6,000 volunteers applied for 460 vacancies. 'The Royal Air Force, youngest of the services, is, with the Navy, most active at the present stage of the war, and the life of the Sisters in PMRAFNS has become hazardous and full,' observed the *Nursing Times* that October.

The wartime PMRAFNS

After the Second World War began, no new members were appointed to the regular service: each new recruit entered as a member of the reserve. She remained in her civilian post until called to duty, at home or overseas. On call-up, she began a six-month probationary term at one of the three main RAF hospitals, where she learned about service routine and practice, ward administration, and what one new recruit called 'those wretched forms'. This initiatory period could include specialist training in areas such as infectious diseases, burns treatment, rehabilitation, electrotherapy and thoracic surgery – the RAF offered its nurses a wide range of experience.

From her training hospital the new PM moved on to wherever need arose. It might be a station hospital or a sick quarters, in rural Wales or on the south coast, or up in the windy wilds of north Scotland; it might even be, and increasingly was, some overseas spot that she had never heard of and possibly couldn't spell, let alone pronounce.

At home, PMs based in SSQs looked after the day-to-day health of serving men and women, while at the big RAF hospitals they prepared to accept casualties brought from the front by flying hospital units staffed by men of the Medical Service (RAFMS). These units were equipped with blood-transfusion equipment which could be taken right to the front line and even used in transit, as necessary. The nursing sisters, their equipment, their hospital beds, all waited . . . and waited . . .

By day silver barrage balloons decorated the skies; by night silver searchlights stabbed up at the clouds. Evacuees left London in their hundreds. People carried gas masks and responded to the wail of air-raid sirens, expecting hourly the first assault from German bombs. But the bombers failed to arrive. The country had entered a deceptively quiet period, often called the phoney war.

The phoney war

During eight long months when the enemy's attention focused on eastern Europe and Scandinavia, British involvement in the war remained peripheral. A handful of bombs dropped in the far north of Scotland, but the most violent encounters occurred at sea, including the sinking of the *Royal Oak* in the harbour of Scapa Flow, Orkney, and the scuttling of the trapped *Graf Spee* in far-off south America. In response the convoy system began, to guard supplies across the Atlantic from prowling U-boats. Certain provisions grew scarce and the government issued ration books, but the war itself seemed unreal. Evacuees returned to the cities; gas masks

PMRAFNS sisters queue for soup at an improvised kitchen of an MFH in France, 1944 (© British Crown Copyright/MOD)

What the well-dressed sister was wearing, MFH India 1944/5: mosquito boot (*left*); trousers (*below*); and dress (*bottom*) – as demonstrated by Sister Rona Black, India 1945

Heading into Burma, 1944

Sister Rona Black, India, 1945

Sister Tessa Lawless in Hiroshima, May 1953

Sister Susan Armistead with staff and patients, RAFH Tel Litwinsky, Palestine, 1946 (© British Crown Copyright/MOD)

began to seem an unnecessary encumbrance; with every quiet night that passed, feet trailed more reluctantly to air-raid shelters. In France the British Expeditionary Force played cards along the Maginot Line, and the RAF, prevented by the rules of fair play from attacking any but military targets, had to content itself with dropping not bombs but millions of propaganda leaflets over Europe.

At RAF hospitals, too, staff watched and waited. Geared up to expect hundreds of war casualties, they found themselves dealing instead with the usual run of health problems.

The wartime nurse worked long hours without complaint, despite hardship and sometimes personal danger. In the blackest days she tended the wounded, learned how to heal burns and shattered jaws, taught crippled men to walk again or to function without hands, and comforted those whose psychological wounds lay too deep for the surgeon's knife. But mostly, and especially during those quiet early months of the war, she confronted old familiar foes – infections of eyes, ears, nose and throat; stomach upsets of all kinds; hernias, cuts and grazes, varicose veins, blisters and, of course, the common cold. In fact, as records reveal, over the whole six years of conflict disease caused far more casualties than bombs and bullets.

When modern central heating began to be installed in RAF premises, hospitals took priority. Personnel lodged in hutted billets took comfort against winter weather by huddling round a coal or coke stove. As a result, colds and other respiratory infections spread happily. At RAF Hednesford, in the bitter winter of 1940/1, scarlet fever, flu, mumps, measles and meningitis rampaged through huts each heated by a single 'tortoise' stove, with fuel severely rationed. Two-thirds of the camp's 6,000 men fell sick and a nursing team was seconded to Hednesford to tend them. John Limmer, one of the medical orderlies on the team, writes of 'all the water pipes frozen, ambulances immobile [because of] two feet of snow . . . we had to carry the worst cases into sick bay by stretcher. Most huts had the skull and crossbones chalked on the door, putting them in quarantine.'

And when germs took a break there were other hazards – boots, for instance. Long hours of drill on hard parade grounds took their toll on tender feet accustomed to softer civilian footwear, and many a keen drill-instructor failed to understand the damage that could be inflicted by foot-stamping and heel-clicking (both were officially banned). At WAAF depots, too, recruits complained of blisters and sore feet caused by heavy shoes.

Increasing numbers of airwomen on all stations created problems for the relatively inexperienced WAAF sick quarters' attendants (later called nursing orderlies). Early in the war, PMs were sent in to improve the quality of care for airwomen and ease demand for female medical officers. On stations where large numbers of WAAF required an SSQ of more than fifty beds, two sisters were assigned; home stations employing more than 350 WAAF had one sister added to their strength. These experienced nursing sisters helped in the training of both male and female sick quarters' attendants; they were able to visit WAAF who lay sick in billets; they gave lectures in hygiene and conducted the infamous FFI (free from infection) inspections – which did wonders for the incidence of head lice and for standards of personal hygiene. In general, they acted as friends and advisers to young airwomen who were often far from home and in need of wise counsel.

Nursing sisters also discovered the inevitable cases of venereal disease, along with the allied problem, endemic among naive young women suddenly plucked from home and facing an uncertain future – the unplanned pregnancy.

Innocents on the loose

The call to arms took thousands of young men and women away from their homes and families and plunged them into strange situations, unusual occupations and, often for the first time in their lives, into one another's company without benefit of chaperones.

Joan Metcalfe, who joined the service after the war and stayed on to become matron-in-chief, well remembered her own days of innocence: 'Our schooling was limited . . . [We had] no television, and there were only two radio programmes. We were not as knowledgeable as they are today . . .'

Not in geography, history, dealing with heat and dust and snakes . . . and certainly not in sexual matters. Some late developers had not been told about menstruation, let alone warned of the dangers of intimacy, as Jessie Higgins discovered after being posted to Cosford:

They put me on to what they called WAAF Welfare, that was looking after 'naughty girls'. We had the main STC – Special Treatment Centre (in other words VD) – unit at Cosford, a separate hospital completely, and the girls that were diagnosed with it were sent to a hospital at Evesham. When they were taken off the treatment, whatever it was – in those days we had no penicillin, of course – they were sent to me.

There were about two thousand WAAF there – not all of them naughty girls! I was posted from the hospital staff to the station staff and I had a nice Warrant Officer's married quarter as a little sick quarters. I was also responsible for seeing the WAAF had their FFI inspections. It was just nits – and spotting pregnancies, of course. The WAAF Officers couldn't cope, didn't know what they were looking for.

I did this FFI and it took me about a fortnight to get through them all. I reckoned there were twenty-two girls pregnant amongst all this lot – all stages, from six or seven weeks to a good, what I call nine and a half months. Half these kids didn't know what was happening. So of course I had to tell the WAAF officer, and of course she went running to the CO ... I was hauled up there – phone call – CO's Adjutant – 'You will be here within fifteen minutes, sistah!' – so I hops on my bike ... went in, WAAF Officer, CO ... he says, 'What's this I hear? Twenty-two girls pregnant on my station? You've got a dirty mind, sister!'

So I said, 'Well, time will tell, won't it?' ... Anyway, they all had babies.

The RAF hospital which opened in 1940 at Evesham, Worcestershire, developed special wards where discreet women doctors dealt with cases of venereal disease and pregnancy among members of the WAAF. With women by the thousand stationed nearby – at Bridgnorth, Innsworth, Gloucester, and the WAAF Officers' School, Loughborough – during its six years' existence Evesham treated women of all types. Gossip renamed the place 'Eve's Shame' and made it a source of grievance among the local community. Any WAAF found to be pregnant would, of course, be discharged 'on compassionate grounds'.

Evesham also had the usual medical and surgical wards. Pilot

Officer William 'Dutchy' Holland, injured when his Whitley crashed near Stow-on-the-Wold, was rushed to Evesham Hospital, where he met his future wife, Sister Ethel Littler. He remembers a Sister Fanny Baldwin, a pre-war regular who, he says, epitomized the 'Sarah Gamp' type of nurse. She would 'enter the mess, line herself up with one of the red leather armchairs and flop with a whoosh into it, legs akimbo, displaying blue issue bloomers! But she had a heart of gold. She specialised in working on 'VD' wards for WAAFs, to whom she gave unstintingly not only of her compassion and care but also much of her meagre pay to buy clothes and necessities for their babies.'

The end of the 'Sitzkreig'

During that first winter, 1939/40, the war centred on Scandinavia. Finland fell to the enemy; then Denmark and Norway. Suddenly, shockingly, war came home to England when the first bombs dropped on Canterbury. The next day, panzer divisions invaded Holland, Belgium and Luxembourg, sweeping through the Ardennes to bypass the Maginot Line where British and French forces waited. Caught out, British troops were obliged to withdraw in haste to the French coast.

Only the bravery of the Royal Navy and the crews of a fleet of individual little boats saved the British Expeditionary Force from decimation at Dunkirk. Some of the men brought back nothing but the clothes they wore. Some were so exhausted they came home and slept for two solid days, cared for by willing nurses. But such had been their haste that they left most of their equipment – tanks and guns and lorries – behind them. Much of it they had destroyed themselves to prevent the enemy from using it.

Holland fell. Belgium surrendered. The *Luftwaffe* raided Middlesbrough and Italy allied herself with Germany. Within days, France had fallen; then German troops took the Channel Islands. Since America remained aloof, refusing to be drawn into the conflict, and Russia maintained a treaty with Germany, Britain stood alone. Ever the rhetorician, Churchill declared it the 'finest hour'. But in truth it was probably the most desperate, desolate period of the war, for the prime minister as well as the British nation.

Hitler again offered peace – on terms that Churchill found unacceptable – so the German chancellor decided he would batter this arrogant little offshore island into submission. He planned to start by destroying her airfields.

First bombs at Cranwell

That spring of 1940 the RAF College Service Flying Training School at Cranwell was filled to capacity with new recruits and trainees all eager to join the aerial defence of Britain. But after the long lull of the phoney war they had relaxed their guard.

According to Kay Cranston (Mrs Slim), Cranwell at that time did not observe any blackout.

> Lights were on all the time, there were no curtains and the flare paths were lit up because they discovered they had accidents with the boys who were learning to fly, and the blackout meant more accidents. So they gave them every light they could and occasionally a German plane would come in at the tail end of their exercises.

The 'boys' had begun to regard the war as a bit of a bore, and to long for something exciting to happen. Their wish was granted on a night in June.

> We had our first air raid there and the bombs fell right down the runway – which was lucky, for had they gone a little more to one side they would have hit the Officers' Mess, the Sisters' Mess and the Hospital. As it was, it didn't cause much damage. All they did was fill in the holes and all was right again. Three bombs did not explode and the naughty Officers put them in front of their Mess in the garden and were having bets on which one would go off first.
>
> All the bits of bomb, shrapnel, etc. which were lying around were gathered up by everyone as keepsakes. Little did we know that everyone could get a bit of bomb eventually, but at that time it was all new and everyone wanted a souvenir. When the bomb disposal people came down they were furious because there were no bits of bomb left for them. They were

angry with the Officers for treating the unexploded bombs so casually . . .

I remember after the raid asking one of the Officers if anyone had been hurt and he said, no, only one casualty, and that was the Padre – his knees were sore because he had been down on them praying all the time . . .

This attack, the first of many in the area, took place at 10.30 on the evening of 6 June 1940. One German aircraft flew across the aerodrome and dropped thirty bombs, of which only fourteen exploded. Of those, nine dropped ineffectually in fields; only five hit the runway.

The authorities had already decided to move the RAF hospital – Cranwell offered too tempting a target for the enemy and, besides, once the war began in earnest the concentration of Bomber and Fighter Command bases in Lincolnshire would call for larger medical facilities than the training station could offer. Even as those first bombs fell, plans were in hand for transfer to a less vulnerable site a few miles away, at what had been the Rauceby Mental Hospital.

The building at Rauceby was already in use as an annexe for Cranwell. Kay Cranston had helped with the cleaning: 'The place smelt horrible, stale urine, horrible pictures drawn on lavatory walls . . . We soon had it cleaned up. But it was great fun at first because as we got the wards ready, making up beds etc. the self-locking doors would lock us in the wards and we couldn't get out. Fortunately there was a telephone!'

When the building was ready – and all the locks changed – an ambulance convoy transferred patients and stores the few miles from Cranwell.

But we kept losing some of the patients. We discovered they were having a whale of a time locking each other in the padded cell and not telling anyone! The inmates of the mental asylum, who worked in the hospital laundry and on the farm, still remained. Our CO gave us a talk and said we were to be polite and considerate to these men and women. He concluded . . . 'These people have certificates to say they're sane, which is more than any of you lot have!'

Iris Jarred (Mrs Bartram), who worked on the burns and orthopaedic wards at Rauceby, remembers that 'they kept a few inmates and the more normal ones ran the laundry. There used to be a little man pushing a trolley and whenever he saw you – "Ooh, little blue eyes! Dear little blue eyes!" He used to totter around the grounds . . .' She describes the hospital as a huge place with several detached buildings, holding four hundred beds.

> The private wards we had for officers and burns were across the garden. The rest was very dour, long corridors with padded cells at the bottom of all of them, it really was awful. Yes, grim . . . they'd got what I thought were rhododendron, but they were laurels – the place was smothered in laurel . . . The only redeeming feature was a golf course across the road, but then it was a question of just knocking a ball around on your own, more or less, the only time we could get into mufti . . .

While stationed at Rauceby she learned of the death of her brother, a test pilot for Vickers-Armstrong.

Some aircrew patients, having recovered from their wounds, needed psychiatric care. Kay Cranston adds with sympathy, 'They were just tired and wanted a rest and understanding and a chance to recover. We used to send a lot of them down to Devon, to Torquay.'

Shelter for the shell-shocked

The RAF Officers' Hospital had moved from Uxbridge to Torquay, on the balmy south coast of Devon, a location considered to be relatively safe from the threat of German bombs. Along with convalescent and rehabilitation facilities, it provided neuropsychiatric wards for those suffering nervous disorders. And in central England a similar haven, this one for non-commissioned aircrew, nestled among the beautiful Derbyshire hills at the spa resort of Matlock. The luxurious Rockside Health Hydro, with its ballroom, tennis courts, croquet lawns and bowling green, had once again, as during the First World War, been requisitioned by the RAF.

Patients with notes marked NYDN (not yet diagnosed, query

neuropsychiatric) came to such centres to rest and be assessed. John Limmer served as an orderly at Matlock, working with nursing sisters and doctors in a small unit of about forty personnel whose CO, Sir John McIntyre, had been physician to King George V. He remembers the place as 'very impressive [and] very luxurious . . . taken over complete with staff i.e. lady cleaners, waiters, gardeners, boilerman, receptionist . . . three chefs and a masseuse . . . Patients were encouraged to record their dreams and hypnosis was also used a lot.' Sisters' quarters lay in another small hydro at the bottom of the driveway with the main building on the hill above, built of stone in five storeys. Its facilities offered mostly single rooms, not ideal for nursing but appreciated by some patients who, under severe stress after terrible ordeals, enjoyed their privacy.

More and more such patients began to need treatment.

New treatment for burns

Prior to 1939, records show only thirteen non-fatal burns cases among RAF personnel. From 1940 they became all too common.

That summer, the blue skies over England staged a terrible aerial ballet full of the rattle of gunfire, the drift of smoke and the death-dives of burning aircraft. The young pilots of the RAF defended their aerodromes with skill and courage, but at terrible cost. Burning planes fell out of the skies, flaming with an intense heat that virtually melted human tissue. Those who survived suffered dreadful disfigurement. Doctors tried all manner of ointments and unguents but, whatever method they used, still the unavoidable changing of dressings caused patients the most terrible pain and left them badly scarred.

At PMRAFH Halton, a VAD nurse walked into a side room one day and discovered two men engaged in a strange ritual: one of them, wearing what appeared to be a pair of cellophane trousers, lay in a pool of water on the floor while his colleague knelt over him. The men turned out to be two young RAF doctors, Bunyan and Stannard. They were experimenting with coverings designed to contain an antiseptic mixture of Milton fluid and saline solution which would keep burned flesh constantly irrigated and prevent dressings from sticking to the wounds. As more aircraft went down in flames, and ships and tanks caught fire, the Bunyan-Stannard irrigation envelope, as it came to be called, was soon being used on hospital wards all over Britain.

Not all the burns victims were aircrew, or even servicemen. At Halton's burns centre, a woman was brought in with 75 per cent burns on her body. A barrage balloon had been shot down in flames and engulfed her. Joan White (Mrs Cool) was on duty. 'I can't describe how she looked. It was awful, tragic.'

That patient did not survive, but many did. The RAF's chief consultant in plastic surgery, Mr A.H. (later Sir Archibald) McIndoe, won acclaim during the Second World War for his treatment of badly burned aircrew, for whom he formed the Guinea Pig Club. Working out of the Queen Victoria Hospital at East Grinstead, Sussex, he pioneered the use of saline baths to replace treatment by tannic coagulation. The new method – constant-temperature immersion in brine combined with the new relatively pain-free dressings – aided healing and greatly reduced the severity of scarring.

As an accessory to their general training, PMs attended brief training courses at East Grinstead to observe these new techniques. Those who were to specialize in 'plastics' went on to complete their training, in resuscitation and the principles of early skin coverage and healing by skin grafts, at the new burns centres which opened at Halton, Rauceby, Cosford and the brand-new RAFH at Ely.

Sergeant John Hannah

Films and TV programmes depicting the war often fail to portray the fact that a great many of our gallant aircrew were non-commissioned officers, sergeants and flight sergeants. The story of one of them will exemplify them all.

Sergeant John Hannah, an eighteen-year-old wireless operator and air gunner, was admitted to RAFH Rauceby with burns to his face and hands. He had used his bare hands to battle the flames in a stricken Hampden bomber, which he and his Canadian skipper were nursing home to RAF Scampton. Later, promoted to Flight Sergeant, John Hannah wrote to the *MTE Journal*, a magazine published by the RAF Medical Training Establishment, saying that he used to have a dread of hospitals and everything connected with them. Now, however:

I have come to regard with admiration and profound thank-
fulness the wonderful work of the surgeons, and the devoted
attention of the Sisters and nursing orderlies . . . I was fortunately afforded the opportunity of earning the Victoria Cross
on one of my return trips from Germany – this time over
Antwerp in September 1940 – by extinguishing a number of
fires which broke out in the bomb compartment and rear cock-
pits, and thereby, I understand, I 'saved the aircraft'. I was
severely burned as a result and spent two months in RAF
Hospital 'R' . . . The painstaking care with which I was
attended on that occasion has been equalled only by similar
instances on a subsequent occasion . . . in RAF Hospital 'Y' . . .

I should like to be allowed the privilege of here expressing
my heartfelt thanks . . . in particular to Wing Commander
Handley and Sister Marshall . . .

The hospitals whose identities he shields, because of wartime security, were Rauceby and Yatesbury.

In October 1940 the press published pictures of Sergeant
Hannah as a patient at Rauceby, standing beside Sister Marshall and
holding the telegram which told of his award. He was the youngest
man ever to win the VC, being still a few weeks short of his nine-
teenth birthday when he went to Buckingham Palace to receive the
medal from the King. Because of his injuries he was never able to
fly again. He became an instructor but was discharged as medically
unfit in December 1941. His lungs had been affected by the smoke
and heat and he developed tuberculosis, from which he died in June
1947, aged twenty-five.

By August 1940 the Battle of Britain had been won. But the Blitz
was only beginning. Before the end of the year, London itself would
be in flames.

TWO

Air Raids

As the months went by, every centre of industry, every port and every railway came under attack. No one in Britain could sleep easily – not even while lying in a hospital bed.

RAF Hospital St Athan, in South Wales, found itself too close to the docks of Cardiff and Swansea. Four bombs struck in July 1940, causing one fatality and some damage to the infectious diseases annexe. In August two more raids occurred. The first hit outside the station perimeter. The second . . .

Iris 'Fluffy' Jones (Mrs Ogilvie, now Mrs Bower) was a junior sister at the time:

> But it so happened that on this particular night I had been detailed to be in charge . . . Suddenly we heard bombs dropping . . . the siren started wailing in the darkness. I heard Nurse Traherne shouting, 'Don't run!' In a few seconds I had reached a ward full of patients and found the entrance vanished. It was pitch black; shouting, moaning and rushing water could be heard. Suddenly I seemed to be falling into a deep hole – a bomb crater. I climbed out pretty fast, and the first patient I came to was still sitting on a lavatory seat. All the walls had disappeared. I could see by the light of my torch that blood was streaming down his face. He was shocked, but by some miracle was not badly hurt. In no time at all, we could see the funny side to the situation, that he was still sitting on the 'loo' . . .

Groping her way in the darkness, wading through water from fractured pipes, Fluffy Jones found other patients, 'injured and in obvious pain. Fortunately most had minor injuries, only due to the fact that the wards were wooden huts and there was no heavy masonry. The most menacing sound in the darkness was that of rushing water . . . Ghostly figures running about and the ambulances coming and going made it a hectic night . . . We were all glad to see the dawn.'

The 'Nurse Traherne' she mentioned was, in fact, Lady Rowena Traherne, a Red Cross member of the VAD. Her impression, quoted in the history of St Athan, *Twenty-One Caring Years* by Dillwyn Rees, was that 'on a quiet evening in August a lone German plane came over Glamorgan and stupidly dropped all its little 250 lb bombs on our Hospital. We were all furious . . .'

Although, miraculously, human casualties were few, so much structural damage occurred that the entire place had to be evacuated, patients being transported to civilian hospitals at Whitchurch, Llandough and Cardiff. But as soon as essential repair work had been completed, RAFH St Athan reopened for business.

Over on the south coast of England, the resort town of St Leonards-on-Sea, near Hastings, lay in a far more vulnerable area: it faced the Channel, with only a few miles separating it from the coast of Nazi-occupied France. The town itself had become a prohibited zone, its residents dispersed to other counties and forbidden to return except by official permit. Only a few essential services, including those at the Buchanan Hospital, kept the place ticking over.

A huge block of luxury flats dominated the promenade. Shaped to resemble the liner *Queen Mary*, painted white and nicknamed 'the skyscraper', Marine Court had been commandeered in 1939 by the Air Ministry for use as an initial training wing (ITW). As the name implies, it housed fresh recruits, turning them from raw civilians into 'erks' fit for more specialized training elsewhere.

The windows of No.14 ITW commanded wonderful views across the Channel, sea and sky ever changing with season and weather. Conversely, viewed from the sea, and from those skies, the tall white mass beckoned the eye like a beacon. It made a tempting target for 'tip and run' raids by enemy aircraft.

At the sick quarters up on the sixth floor, Mary Moultrie (Mrs Nicholson) experienced her 'most exciting posting'. While making her morning rounds of the wards, she 'heard the unmistakable sound of an aircraft very close by. I was at a window by one of the beds and, looking out, I saw, almost directly above, a German aircraft, probably a Heinkel, the Swastika large and menacing . . . the pilot literally staring into my face . . .'

A deafening explosion rocked the building and she rushed out to see smoke and flames belching along the hallway. Several of the maintenance staff were 'seriously injured, I believe two died, and the airmen doing physical training were also machine gunned . . . The male orderlies were a source of strength.' Those orderlies evacuated the sick quarter wards, transferring patients from the sixth floor down to the basement. 'The lift only took three people at a time so it wasn't too efficient . . . The Buchanan Hospital was able to admit some of the many injured. Sqn Ldr Mitchell and myself worked all day . . . stitching wounds went on well into the night, and extra emergency beds were lined up along the floor.' After this, No.14 ITW moved to less exposed quarters at Harrogate in Yorkshire.

Some nursing sisters came under fire even before they joined the service. In autumn 1940 civilian matron Noelle Horrocks completed a contract in Cyprus and travelled back to England aboard the troopship *Empress of Britain*, intent on joining the PMRAFNS. The western Mediterranean being closed to Allied ships, the liner had to go round the long way, via Suez, down the Red Sea and all round Africa. Finally, on 26 October 1940, she was sailing off Donegal, only hours away from home, when a German plane attacked. Incendiary bombs set the *Empress* hopelessly afire.

When the call went out to abandon ship, Noelle Horrocks was having breakfast in the dining room, five decks below sea level: 'As a staircase had collapsed and all the lights had gone, we only got out . . . by a miracle. General Legentilhomme (the Fighting French leader), who was also a passenger, happened to come along with a torch when we were being stifled by the smoke and had almost given up hope . . .'

On deck, fire and smoke cut them off from the lifeboat stations. 'There was nothing for it but to slide down a rope to the sea below . . . There had been no time, of course, to return to the cabins . . . so of course we lost everything we possessed.' Having made it to a lifeboat, they were eventually picked up by a destroyer. 'We felt very chilly and inadequately clad standing on Greenock quay at the end of October . . . However, we had much to be thankful for.'

One small step for woman . . .

Nursing sisters enjoyed high respect and privilege simply because of their calling. What better title could they have than the time-honoured 'Sister', or 'Matron'? 'In the early days,' says Marianne Galletly (Mrs Hollowell), 'we were just proud of being "Nursing Sisters" and not expected to salute. We wore our smart "DICKS" when in restaurants, etc.'

Even so, their status had become more and more anomalous. Their curious blue and maroon rank markings, allied with their unusual quatrecorn hats, caused speculation in the streets. Because they were not officially commissioned officers, they did not return a salute but acknowledged it with a spoken greeting – 'Good morning,' or whatever might be appropriate to the time of day. This 'really confused the Americans', says Joan White (Mrs Cool). She heard people wondering whether she and her friends were in the Fleet Air Arm or something even more exotic. One particular waitress took her for an 'Aircommodoress'!

This confusion was about to end.

Under Defence (Women's Forces) Regulations published on 25 April, 1941, all members of the WAAF and the PMRAFNS – the VADs who worked with them – became legally part of the armed forces, subject to King's Regulations. At the same time, officers of the WAAF won the right to hold the King's commission. Although the Director-General of Medical Services requested that members of the PMRAFNS should receive the same privilege, not until March 1943 did the authorities agree to grant emergency (wartime) commissions to nursing sisters.

However, one concession was made in July 1941: since too many excellent young women were being forced to leave simply because they fell in love and got married, the ban on married members was lifted. The change took some time to be effective – in those days it was still 'not done' for a married woman to go out to work – but eventually more nurses did choose to stay on in the Service after they became 'Mrs'.

Overseas, 1941-2

When the RAF hospital in Palestine closed, in 1940, only Habbaniya and Aden remained as overseas postings for PMs. But they too saw their share of troubles in the early years of the war. Reaching these outposts could be quite an adventure. Lurking U-boats and vigilant German planes made voyages out from Britain slow and hazardous, and after Italy's entry into the war the Mediterranean became highly dangerous. Wherever possible, merchantmen and troopships avoided what Mussolini liked to call the 'Italian lake' and, travelling in convoy, went round the long way, via the Cape of Good Hope. A voyage to Cairo, for instance, instead of taking a week or two could go on for months. Joan Botting (Mrs Peake), posted to RAFH Aden in autumn 1941, was at sea for nearly eight weeks.

Together with Senior Sister Alice Lowrey and seven other nursing sisters, Joan Botting had been sent to RAFH Wilmslow to await embarkation. Annual pay in those days was, she recollects, 'a hundred and seventeen pounds a year. We were given twenty pounds . . . to supplement our indoor uniform by six. White shoes – extra shoes because the tropics rotted them – a white felt hat . . . plus a white topee and two poplin dress uniforms . . . We also had to provide ourselves with two suitcases and a tin trunk.'

On a Friday morning they rose at 4.30 to catch a train for Liverpool, where they had breakfast aboard the ocean liner-turned-troopship *Empress of Australia*. Personnel of officer rank had cabins, but below decks the ship carried 2,500 troops. They were part of one of the largest convoys yet to sail, three miles long and guarded by forty naval vessels.

This huge convoy split as it plied south, some of the ships heading off westward towards America, looking, as Joan Botting puts it, 'like elephants on the horizon', while the others continued south, into warmer weather. Within a week the PMs 'went into whites for dinner'. Social life was good, with officers of all three services mingling over quoits and cards and cheap drinks, with plentiful food served by the liner's stewards. A leading aircraftman had volunteered to 'look after our buttons, which were brass, all our uniforms, plus cleaning our shoes . . . it got him out from below decks!'

They paused for a few days in West Africa, anchoring in the river at Freetown, Sierra Leone. The passengers did not go ashore, but extracts from Joan Botting's diary give a flavour of what ship-board life was like.

Monday. Up 6.20 a.m. . . . clouds enveloping mountain tops,
with sunlight sparkling on water, flying boats round and
taking off, it's good to be alive. Sat on deck and wrote. On
deck all morning and slept all afternoon. Chatted with
Hancock and the Navy after dinner. Drinks with Young later
. . . Wonderful sunset. Molten gold stretching over the sky,
turning to flames. Large and little ships as objects against the
horizon. Battleships, foodships all as a silhouette . . .

Thursday – leaving Freetown . . . Going out into the bay
one passes charge ships, passenger, warships and hospital
ships, all waiting their turn to venture forth . . . little penin-
sulas with odd temple-like buildings and palm trees against a
vivid background, till outside the boom nothing remains but a
memory of mountains . . . with European houses at their feet
– heat of about 90 with 80% humidity . . .'

After another week or so they rounded the Cape and turned north,
pausing again at Durban where they were able to go ashore and do
some shopping. Since some of the ships were heading off east, the
PMs, bound for Aden and Iraq, transferred to the smaller mail ship,
SS *Llandaff Castle*, which took them up round the horn of Africa,
into the Gulf of Aden.

At this time Aden provided a base for troops and aircraft opposing the Italians in Ethiopia and British Somaliland. Minutes of the
Advisory Board in 1941 record that 'RAF sisters are employed in
the hospitals at Steamer Point and Sheik Othman (500 beds)'. These
hospitals served personnel from the colony, from RAF Khormaksar,
and from Sheik Othman (Shaykh Uthman), where more RAF
squadrons were based; they also took in patients among South
African and Polish troops passing through Aden on their way to the
western deserts of North Africa.

At Steamer Point, says Joan Botting, the complement of staff
'was supposed to be nineteen, but if we were fourteen we were very
fortunate and usually one or two of those were off sick . . .' The
sisters' mess was very comfortable, two sisters to a room with a
bearer to look after them, but 'no sanitary drainage . . . The bathrooms were large and in each bathroom there were two commodes.
You had your own commode . . .' Hot water came via buckets
carried by the bearer. Ants were a problem, so furniture legs stood

in tins of kerosene. But the food was good, fresh vegetables and salad crops brought by camel train every day from Lehej, about thirty miles away. And with so few women among so many men, social life could not have been better!

Ships came through carrying troops towards Suez to join the fighting in Egypt and Libya, and RAF pilots stopped off to learn how to fly Hurricanes before they too went north to the desert. Joan Botting remembers many funerals.

> They either acted the goat and they got killed, or crashed the plane and got killed, or they got some complaint and died. There was no sanitation, either at the hospital or at the camps ... At one stage I had about four typhoids in a ward. Well, in that climate, at that stage, they just died ... Also you got the ships going up to Suez and anybody sick on board, they loaded them off onto the Air Force hospital. All burials were at six o'clock in the morning because it was hot ...

The RAF hospital at Habbaniya, in Iraq, came under siege in 1941 when pro-Hitler rebels led by Raschid Ali surrounded the vast desert base. Heavy shells bombarded the camp for several days and some of the flying school's aircraft were hit, student pilots being among the casualties rushed to the hospital. Chief surgeon at RAFGH Habbaniya at the time was Lewis Mackenzie Crooks, the 'father of orthopaedics in the RAF'. Despite the fact that the light British planes – Airspeed Oxford trainers and Fairey Gordon bi-planes – were vastly inferior to Iraqi Air Force fighters, the RAF eventually drove off the attack.

Dope

Back at home, while the *Luftwaffe* rained daily destruction, less expected hazards lurked for those engaged behind the scenes of Britain's defence. Barrage balloons, for instance, not only erupted in flames on occasion but in high winds their steel guy ropes could whip through the air like swords, or foul high-tension grid wires and become electrically charged. Even when brought to earth and under repair, the huge balloons caused problems.

At RAF Chigwell, in Essex, young WAAFs and airmen worked in

vast hangars rigging and doping barrage balloons. The rubber solution used for cementing patches was made up in benzol, whose fumes could cause fainting and dizziness, or even death, especially when working in a confined space. The dopers sometimes had to clamber right inside the balloon to effect repairs. It was hard, physical work. For the nurses who worked at Chigwell SSQ, preserving the good health of these essential personnel was a priority.

Florrie Buck, a WAAF corporal nursing orderly, recalls, 'The girls had to be especially cared for . . . The paint for doping the fabric had a lead content and the girls had to be given extra milk ration and have a chest examination once a month. I would accompany the MO out to Balloon sites to mete out inoculations etc.' The camp was somewhat isolated, with buildings set far apart to allow balloons room to manoeuvre. Personnel had to walk long distances from the hangars to their billets and messes. 'Some of them were very young, rather scared. Some of them acquired dogs to make them feel safer.'

Around the hospitals

By 1942 twenty-six full-size RAF hospitals had opened in Britain, with nine more established overseas. Princess Mary continued to do her bit to raise morale and foster *esprit de corps* among 'her' nurses by visiting as many of them as she possibly could. In one period of four months she managed to visit seven separate RAF station hospitals. Nor was she alone. Many other members of the Royal Family went along hoping to brighten the spirits of both patients and hospital staff.

A visit by the Duchess of Gloucester to RAFH Henlow, however, caused one patient to feel less than happy. WAAF Sergeant Edith Francis, fresh out of theatre after an appendicectomy, proudly displayed by her bed a vase of fresh flowers, a wartime rarity brought some distance, by bus, by her young husband. Since they were the only flowers around, a nurse appropriated them to decorate the hospital foyer for the royal visitor.

Mrs Francis was, 'feeling very low after the op . . . and when HRH stopped at my bedside to enquire how I was, I dissolved into floods of tears and sobbed, "The nurses have taken my flowers." The lovely RAF Nursing Sister, in her blue-grey cape and white head-dress, came to console me after this embarrassing episode, and from then on she was always so kind, and sat beside me during the night. But I didn't get my flowers back!' Nevertheless, Mrs Francis retains fond memories of the 'super ladies who were in that branch of the Service'.

The Duchess of Gloucester may have thought she was jinxed when, as she left after paying a visit to another RAFH, at Ely, loud and clear from the tannoy came the call, 'Three cheers for the Duchess of Kent!'

Answering the call to 'dig for victory', PMs at Cosford decided that the land around their mess huts should be ploughed up and sown with potatoes. Minutes of their mess meeting, dated 6 May, 1941, note that this will cost £4.15s [£4.75] – £2 for ploughing, the rest for seed potatoes. Called to economize in the use of electricity and water, the sisters decided to restrict themselves to having break-fast toast only once per week; and bath water would be four inches deep, as advised by the government, level to be marked on the baths.

Amid economies, hard work and grim routine, many lighter moments occurred. Valerie Blackwell (Mrs Cornford) attended a dance at Ely hospital, at which the hats of three group captains went astray, to be found next morning in the lavatories at the sisters' mess. On another occasion, she accompanied the CO on his rounds of the hospital at Locking. While inspecting the toilet facil-ities he observed, 'No toilet paper in this one.' From the next cubi-cle came the answer, 'Coming over!' and a flying toilet roll just missed the CO's hat.

From the sick bay at RAF Weston-Super-Mare, Aircraftman P.R. Richards, recuperating from double pneumonia, was trans-ferred to RAF Hospital Locking where the sisters were 'charm-ing, very efficient "no nonsense" young women'. He and the other 'up-patients' helped out with bumpering ward floors, distributing food, even turning patients to alleviate bedsores. Up-patients had to wear a uniform of 'hospital blues' with white shirts. They also wore pink-red ties whose shape suggested they might look well done in a bow. One day, playing a joke on their popular day sister, the patients all tied their ties as bows, but 'before the Day Sister had time to see us, Matron called a snap inspection of the ward'.

As she swept in with her entourage of Senior Staff, Up-Patients stood to attention at the foot of their beds, whilst the Bed-Patients tried as well as they could to lie to attention. The Matron inspected us all, gazing with horror at our Bow Ties, said not a word to any of us and swept out. We could hear her haranguing the Sister in her office for over 10 minutes. Later our Sister returned very upset and holding back tears . . . The Matron had threatened to demote her and post her to another hospital . . .

The patients wrote to Matron to explain – every man on the ward signed the letter. Nothing was ever said, but the day sister stayed on. However, the chaps did notice that for three weeks the tannoy failed to play the usual popular records, and the orderly who took blood samples (they referred to him as 'Dracula') came four times in a fortnight instead of once a week!

At another initial training wing full of new recruits, RAF Bridgnorth in Shropshire, the station hospital became a posting for Barbara Rampton (Mrs White), who often worked on night duty.

The Isolation ward was well and truly isolated across a field and had to be visited at least twice a night, which could be a little scary, particularly if the mist was rising from the River Severn and the owls were hooting. The staff there had surreptitiously adopted a cat and used to add him to the Ward report, on a separate form, under the name of A/C Tibbles . . . Once, when taking the Day Report from matron, prior to going on duty, I was shocked to read a report on A/C Tibbles, but said nothing. On going on my first round of Isolation I was relieved to find that there actually was a patient by the name of A/C Tibbles.

Staff at Bridgnorth loved to play practical jokes on the duty medical officer, whose bed was in a room next to Matron's office. One night he climbed into bed only to shoot out again on coming into contact with a wet frog. While the duty room was being redecorated, the duty MO used a twin-bedded *en suite* side ward, except on one occasion when no spare beds could be found in the officers' mess for two visiting senior officers. The side ward was allocated to them, the MO being told to sleep in his own room in the mess.

Barbara Rampton came on night duty and discovered that 'the day staff had already prepared an "apple pie bed" with Prickly Spinach seeds under the bottom sheets'. The guests arrived before she could change the beds, but she did manage to warn the more junior visitor that he had better use the 'apple pie bed' himself and perhaps remove the offending seeds while his superior used the bathroom.

> Imagine my horror the following morning, when I took them a cup of tea, to find the more Senior officer in the 'apple pie bed'. The pair of them roared with laughter . . . and said that they'd never had such a trick played on them so innocently before. In spite of all my efforts the Junior hadn't done as I had suggested, but left his Senior to get into the bed . . . and had thoroughly enjoyed seeing what happened – those seeds have really sharp spines.

Those days of sixty years ago seem imbued with charming innocence, despite the horrors being perpetrated all around.

At Church Village, in South Wales, the hospital had been taken over by the RAF from Glamorgan County Council while still under construction. The brand new building, two storeys high and made of bricks rather than wood, was an airy place with big windows overlooking lovely countryside. One of the sisters stationed there was herself a patient, in a side ward on her own, when her friend John Rees paid a visit. 'Within a very short time,' Mr Rees recalls, 'the ward sister stormed in and reprimanded me for visiting a female patient unchaperoned. She reported me to the CO.'

And poor Cliff Hardy, an aircrew trainee with tonsillitis, was whisked into RAFH Bridgnorth delirious with fever. Having led a very sheltered life, he was horrified to find himself 'waking up in the middle of the night absolutely soaking wet and trying to fight off a young woman who was trying to take off my pyjamas'. Worse awaited him next morning when two young nurses descended on him to give him a blanket bath: 'the most embarrassing moment ever, for me'. Yet he and many other young lads were being trained to fly into enemy flak.

Sergeant Pilot Sharp, aged twenty-one, walked into the blade of an idling propeller on his Whitley bomber and suffered a terrible injury to his head. Colleagues helped him to the nearby dispersal hut, from where he was taken to RAFH Rauceby. Fellow patient Hugh Aitken recalls how, at night, Sergeant Pilot Sharp was put into a small isolation ward where he would 'sing and whistle, to help him through his great pain and suffering'. Though swathed in bandages with holes for his nose, mouth and one eye, he still managed to plague the nursing sisters, especially one young Irish girl. When she told him to lie straight instead of with his knees up, he replied, 'Sister, it's not my knees!', which set the other men roaring with laughter while the sister walked out pink-faced.

Was Sergeant Pilot Sharp tended by surgeon Squadron Leader Fenton Braithwaite? PM Maureen Lumley, then nursing at Rauceby, remembers a patient who had walked into a propeller and received a terrible brain injury. She says that Squadron Leader Braithwaite, 'a marvellous surgeon', patched up the damage 'with a bit of placenta from the maternity ward'.

Air ambulances

Civilian hospitals readily accepted RAF aircrew casualties forced down in their local area, but the injured men were usually transferred as soon as possible to RAF hospitals. Since the most speedy method of achieving this transfer was by air, the RAF established an air ambulance service early in the war.

In 1940, Princess Mary, the Princess Royal, presided at a ceremony to receive the first two specially designed Airspeed Oxford air ambulances, a gift presented by the Girl Guides of the Empire. Two years later a squadron of seven air ambulances, of various types, covered the whole of the United Kingdom from their bases at Hendon (north London), Abbotsinch (Northern Ireland) and Wick (Scotland). The aircraft all bore the identifying mark of the Red Cross but, being small, could carry only a few stretchers at a time. To cope with greater numbers, it became the practice to modify normal troop-carrying aircraft so that most of them could convert to air ambulances within ten minutes.

Selected orderlies of the RAF Medical Service undertook a course which taught them how to load and unload aircraft with stretchers and medical necessities, and how to prepare patients for air transportation. It also gave them a chance to familiarize themselves with the effects of air travel.

Pioneering work

As yet, no members of the PMRAFNS flew on casevac missions, but in many other areas their expertise expanded hourly. Health problems created by the war forced the evolution of new techniques to deal with them and departments dedicated to the treatment of burns, shattered limbs and specific diseases developed at most of the RAF hospitals.

Larger hospitals became centres for many areas of specialization. Halton, for instance, specialized not only in burns and plastic surgery but in cancer therapy and renal medicine. It pioneered the use of radiation as a means of locating foreign bodies in the eye. As more personnel went overseas and contracted exotic diseases, their treatment greatly widened the knowledge of Halton's Institute of Pathology and Tropical Medicine (IPTM). When it became evident that the health of troops in foreign climes depended greatly on the efforts of individual medical officers in the field, the Halton IPTM inaugurated courses in tropical medicine and field hygiene for recently-qualified doctors. In turn the doctors passed on their new skills to nursing sisters who later worked with them in the desert or the jungle.

The war produced so many jaw injuries that specialization in that field too became imperative. At Ely the RAF's first maxillo-facial centre opened in summer 1942, employing the first dental officer to be specifically trained for such work.

Nervous disorders – another problem – affected two-thirds of WAAF members who were invalided out of the service; but men suffered almost as badly from these illnesses. In the eastern area alone, six neuropsychiatric centres treated operational personnel, while another eight or nine units opened in other hospitals. Before being posted to these units nursing sisters were, of course, required to hold qualifications in psychiatric work.

Similarly, rehabilitation centres in Halton, Ely, Cosford, St Athan, Wroughton, Weeton, Yatesbury and Torquay employed sisters with orthopaedic qualifications. These essential units might be described as the most up-to-date human repair shops in the world, every amenity designed to restore patients to their operational posts with all speed.

On Halton's orthopaedic wards, WAAF nursing orderly Joyce Hooper came to know the long-term patients very well. She hurt her back while lifting a patient and was put on light duties in the occupational therapy department. She loved it; 'teaching men with hands like shovels to do embroidery . . . make belts from macramé twine, and soft toys . . . One patient even knitted a beautiful layette for the baby his wife was expecting, and some of the long-term patients made beautiful regimental badges with silks . . .'

In the welfare field, a total of sixty-three sisters were appointed, some to large WAAF SSQs and some with a peripatetic role covering smaller outlying units in remote areas. They helped to supervise nursing orderlies and acted as health confidantes to WAAFs. As doctors all agreed, the right type of nursing sister could prove invaluable: the wrong type could do more harm than good! However, after D-Day the welfare scheme was to be abandoned; those experienced sisters were needed for more urgent duties.

First use of penicillin

WAAF clerk Biddy Spencer (Mrs Wilson), working as secretary to the ophthalmic surgeons at Halton, enjoyed some varied duties, including conducting colour-vision tests for 300 Polish boys who had endured 'a very arduous trek from the Russian-occupied part of Poland'. She also helped to choose the colour of artificial eyes. But perhaps her most unusual task was 'collecting empty face-cream jars for despatch to Professor Florey (Sir Alexander Fleming's assistant) in Oxford, who returned them filled with precious penicillin, still in its trial stage, for use in the Ophthalmic Ward. Progress reports would be typed weekly and returned to Oxford with the next batch of jars.'

Although Sir Alexander Fleming had discovered penicillin in 1928, its full value only became clear eleven years later, when Australian Sir Howard W. Florey and German Dr Ernst B. Chain, working at Oxford, isolated and purified the active ingredient of the mould. The first precious drops, made available by the Medical Research Council, went to RAF doctors who, hours later, used it to save the life of a soldier with septicaemia.

Joan White (Mrs Cool) first used penicillin 'in the form of a drip, intramuscularly at three drops a minute. This was a nightmare as the apparatus was very hard to regulate . . .'

Halton also conducted experiments using penicillin in burns creams, under the supervision of consultant surgeon Archibald McIndoe. Fran Keech (Mrs Judson) worked with this 'great character who would always sit on the bed to talk to his patients. Matron's strict rule did not really allow such frivolity, but he was a law unto himself.' McIndoe's ward at Halton was intensely busy, 'treating aircrew who had suffered horrific injuries. Faces were rebuilt, as were ears and eyes, etc., by the formation of pedicle grafts which needed daily injections of penicillin. Penicillin had only just been discovered and was as precious as gold dust. Two staff were needed to measure out the appropriate drops and double check – not as today, where popping the pill is commonplace.'

Their work with penicillin earned Fleming, Florey and Chain the Nobel Prize for Medicine in 1945.

Sunday horror at Torquay

The Officers' Convalescent Hospital now flourished near Torquay, in the former Palace Hotel at Babbacombe. By the end of 1939 it had achieved its full capacity of 249 equipped beds and, after minor alterations, four bedrooms on the second floor had become an operating theatre. Patients recuperating in cosy rooms holding two or three beds, rather than in crowded wards, found the hospital a pleasant spot. This being good for morale, nursing staff put up with the slight inconvenience which the warren of small rooms and long hallways brought for them.

Matron W.M. Coulthurst led a nursing team of twenty-one members of the PMRAFNS – four senior sisters, ten junior sisters and some VAD nurses – plus a number of nursing orderlies. Other staff included RAF doctors and dentists, administration and supporting personnel, and about eighty civilian ancillary workers, most of whom were former hotel employees. Altogether, Torquay gave employment to around 200 people.

The hospital became known for its lively and optimistic atmosphere. BBC correspondent Macdonald Hastings, writing in *London Calling*, the overseas journal of the BBC, in October 1941, describes it as being like a country club, but with incomparable amenities: 'wooded grounds with velvet lawns, tropical trees, luxurious flower beds ... golf course, tennis courts, squash courts, swimming pool, archery butts, and gymnasium.' In the mornings the gymnasium and its milk bar, run by officers' wives, provided a popular rendezvous. Other facilities included a cinema where the latest films were shown, a concert hall where patients and staff put on shows, a dance floor, sun lounges, writing rooms, libraries, and a fully licensed bar: 'the essence of these RAF establishments is [to] presume that a man who is old enough to fight for the rest of us is old enough to decide how he will comport himself when he himself is in trouble ... a man who has been accustomed to shooting down Messerschmitts before breakfast won't take kindly to being tucked up in bed with a jig-saw.'

As director of games, RAFH Torquay had the famous tennis player (later to be the well-known tennis commentator) Dan Maskell. His athletic presence must have inspired the men to get fit again, and his wife did her bit by acting in shows. Mrs Edith Payne, who met and married theatre assistant Fred 'Blondie' Payne while he was working at the hospital, recalls that Mrs Maskell 'nearly brought the house down with her dress, or should I say lack of it?' while 'taking off' the exotic South American film star Carmen Miranda.

Among the nursing sisters was newly-wed Iris 'Fluffy' Ogilvie, née Jones. In April 1942 she had married one of her patients, a squadron leader flyer of heavy bombers. Thanks to the new regulations permitting married women to remain as PMs, she stayed at her post while her husband, recovered from his wounds, returned to his squadron.

Patients were encouraged to take as much exercise as was good for them, to enter tournaments and races, to entertain wives and girlfriends if they wished, to go off for a walk if solitude seemed beneficial, or to join an outing to some local beauty spot or theatre. Fluffy Ogilvie and her colleagues would take the convalescents on country rambles and occasionally accompany them 'in a coach lovingly known as "the drunks' bus", which had been donated by the Dewar Whisky family.'

The bus would take us down to the Imperial Hotel. I still remember how some of the guests would, understandably, look away when they saw the badly burnt faces.

I remember, too, the good-looking young pilot whose legs had been badly injured . . . saying to me, 'When we get to the bar, Fluff, sit me up on a stool . . . I want to chat up the girls, but watch their faces when I get off the stool!' These young men had such wonderful spirit and courage . . .

The Torquay area seemed an ideal location for such men to recuperate. It was easily accessible; it had swaying palm trees, lovely views of the sea and a balmy climate; and it was relatively well away from the 'bomb alley' that invisibly linked London with occupied Europe. At least, that was the theory. In reality, as Mrs Payne remembers 'we used to get the German planes coming over . . . flying low over the front, gunning along the coast. Other times . . . if they had not dropped all their bombs on Plymouth they would discharge them over Torquay . . .'

Disaster struck on the bitterly cold, wet morning of 25 October 1942. A Sunday morning, around 1100hrs.

Most of the patients were in their rooms, shaving, dressing or reading the Sunday papers. Domestic staff tidied up, kitchen hands prepared Sunday lunch, and nurses readied themselves for doctors' rounds. Fred Payne, gowned and masked, was assisting in the operating theatre. Fluffy Ogilvie was on the first floor, with her friend 'Tinkle' Bell, 'a very young, delightful, pretty Australian VAD . . . A Medical Officer asked me to accompany him to see four patients in a nearby room. I told the VAD that I would join her as soon as I could.' As Fluffy and the MO went into the patients' room, 'we both saw, through the large windows, German planes, with their Swastikas clearly visible. There was no time to be brave or heroic, we dived under the bed . . .'

After preliminary machine-gun strafing, the enemy dropped high-explosive 500 kilo bombs. The first scored a direct hit on the east wing. The second landed in the road, its blast shattering windows, doors and partitions in the west wing and severely damaging the operating theatre. Lamps over the operating table fell on to the unconscious patient and a door flew across the room and knocked out Fred Payne.

The room where Fluffy Ogilvie had taken cover lost its door and windows. Rain and cold air rushed in, but all four patients, plus doctor and nurse, had survived. The latter pair dashed out into the hall to find 'dust and rubble everywhere and, where there had been a further room, just one big gaping hole . . . The first body we came to was that of 'Tinkle' Bell. I saw her hand and arm sticking out beneath the heavy masonry. I also saw . . . two bodies which seemed to be hanging from the girder. The bomb had gone through all the floors down to the basement . . .'

Two platoons of the local home guard had been carrying out exercises close by. Two of their number died in the attack but the rest came to help, along with local air raid precaution volunteers.

Since the most obvious gathering place – the ballroom – had been badly damaged, the CO ordered that casualties should be taken to the sisters' mess. Through the rubble and dust, shivering against the cold winds that swept through shattered windows and gaping holes in brickwork, men carried laden stretchers to where doctors and nurses made rapid diagnoses, applied dressings and splints, and administered what drugs they could; amid such chaos and destruction they could offer little more than first aid. Fortunately they found ample blankets and hot-water bottles to combat shock, and the kitchens still functioned sufficiently to provide hot drinks, so vital on that bitter day.

Nineteen people died, one was missing, another forty-five suffered injury. Had it not been a Sunday, casualties would have been even worse because many patients would have been in the basement gymnasium and its milk bar, which had been flattened. The Torbay hospital took the more serious cases; others went to RAFHs Wroughton or Melksham, and uninjured patients were sent home wherever possible. Within four days the Officers' Convalescent Hospital was empty.

Fluffy Ogilvie, like many of the nursing staff, spent the night after the bombing with a kindly Torquay family. Next day she accompanied a group of patients on their journey to Wroughton. 'I had the unnerving experience of feeling the closeness of the little VAD 'Tinkle' Bell. Her presence was with me everywhere I went for about three days, then it seemed to leave me suddenly. I have never in my life experienced such a feeling . . .

'What a sadness it was to all of us involved. The Palace Hotel had been such a happy place . . .'

The battered hospital remained in the care of maintenance staff until another raid, three months later in January 1943, destroyed part of the central block. The building was considered beyond repair. The work of the RAF Officers' Convalescent Hospital moved to Cleveleys Hydro, in Blackpool, Lancashire.

And the war ground on, spreading its evil tendrils across Europe, and beyond.

THREE

Faraway places

The Blitz went on. Over occupied Europe, RAF planes flew deadly sorties. Everyone's geography improved as they studied newspaper charts of events taking place in the Balkans, Greece and the deserts of North Africa. Most of the news was bleak. But subtle changes began when Russia changed sides in the summer of 1941 and, in December, Japan made the mistake of attacking Pearl Harbor. As the first American GIs arrived in England, the conflict began to spread, drawing in Malaya, Burma, Borneo . . .

By the autumn of 1942 total war, by air, sea and land, engaged much of the world. Newsreel commentaries tried to bolster morale, remaining relentlessly optimistic despite terrible loss of life, appalling barbarity, and the continuing toll taken by disease.

Some PMs were posted overseas within days of being called up from the reserve. For days, and sometimes weeks, they waited at personnel holding units such as Blackpool, before embarking at Liverpool or going up to Glasgow by train to sail from Greenock. Most had never been outside England before; some had hardly stirred from their home towns; few knew exactly where they were heading. Their emotions can be imagined – apprehension, excitement, curiosity . . . Amazingly, most of them remember it as being, overall, 'great fun', a chance to travel and share an adventure which many could never have experienced in normal life.

Iris Jarred (Mrs Bartram), still nursing at RAFH Rauceby, was sent for and asked if she was prepared to go abroad – 'India, they were talking about. I said I didn't think it was fair, with elderly parents, in Norfolk, to go all that way. So, for my sins, I went to Wick!'

Windswept Wick

Units of all three armed services, dotted about the north of Scotland and across the Western Isles, enjoyed a relatively mild climate, thanks to the benevolent lapping of the Gulf Stream. But, however mild it might be, the weather was habitually wet and windy. Sister Jarred found it trying: 'You've never known such wind. You couldn't walk without something in front of your face. It never stopped! In fact, you walked backwards to get your breath.'

The sick quarters at RAF Wick, only a few miles south of John o'Groats, expanded when an operating theatre with X-ray opened in 1943; then in January 1944 a nearby cottage hospital became Wick Station Hospital. It lay about half a mile outside the camp, obliging staff to walk to and fro, often soaked to the skin despite being swathed in oilskins and rubber boots. To add to their troubles, they had no proper drying facilities!

Nursing sisters based at Wick would visit outlying stations and offer treatment and advice, but during Iris Jarred's posting the hospital was never really busy.

Somebody would come down from Shetland, or Orkney . . . They'd say, 'No, both my men are quite well.' We had to take civilian people in. One drunkard walked off the end of the jetty . . . It was supposed to be a 'dry' town, too.

And one of the WAAFs suddenly produced this tummy-ache in the middle of the night, and next morning there was the baby. That rather put the cat amongst the pigeons because the two medics we had hadn't dealt with a baby since training days . . . I [had done] orthopaedics – 'midder' [midwifery] never appealed to me. We didn't know where to put it. I think we found a linen basket.

The RAF squadrons based at Wick occupied themselves 'chasing the battleships in the Norwegian fjords. We had two or three squadrons, and Catalinas coming in from Reykjavik. Of course,' she adds, 'that was a home posting – no, not Wick – Reykjavik!'

On the edge of the Arctic

In Iceland, even the summer is cold and damp. In winter, for months at a time, a thick coat of snow and ice covers a landscape of low, scrub-covered hills, hot springs and mud ponds.

The bleak, windswept bay outside Reykjavik provided anchorage for merchant ships of many Allied and friendly nations. Every ten days convoys set sail, laden with raw materials such as jute, tin and rubber for Russia's manufacturing plants. Others plied the Atlantic, bearing cargoes of refugees and raw materials and bringing home crated aircraft and munitions, and food. Royal Navy ships rode escort, on watch for German U-boats.

In order to offer better aerial cover for the convoys, RAF presence in Iceland grew until it stood at 3,000 personnel. The original army hospital, adapted from part of the university buildings, was taken over by the RAF early in 1942. It had a hundred beds but could double its capacity if needed. Staff included several doctors, twelve members of the PMRAFNS, and around twenty male nursing orderlies – their numbers went up as the months passed and workload increased. Patients came not only from the Royal Air Force and the Royal Navy, but from Dominion and Allied services, including a Norwegian float-plane squadron.

If prowling U-boats were a menace, Arctic storms provided another. A particularly violent hurricane, reaching 133 m.p.h., swept over Reykjavik in 1942. It sank five American flying boats, smashed many smaller craft, destroyed the RAF station workshops and damaged other buildings. Nursing orderly John Limmer witnessed this storm: 'The Aerodrome Log Book records a Nissen hut proceeding in a northerly direction, height approx 60 ft, in spite of being fastened down with a steel cable and earthed up halfway.'

For insulation, the huts were buttressed with earth and their entrances draped with tenting or given makeshift porches to keep out the cold. Long and gloomy nights created huge demand on small electric generators and, with both fittings and light bulbs scarce, paraffin lamps came back into their own: their light reflected from walls lightened with lime wash to alleviate the gloaming. John Limmer writes, 'In spite of a tortoise stove going night and day our boots were frozen to the floor each morning ... This was where I had to identify my hut-mate, killed with 8 others in a Liberator crash ...'

But PM Noelle Horrocks remembers it rather fondly. 'Nissen huts can be made quite comfortable . . . [but] once the stoves went out, the huts got cold very quickly, so that when we got up in the morning our sponges and face flannels were frozen and all water in the jugs or tumblers turned to ice.' However, despite years spent near the Equator, she 'did not feel the cold very much . . . Some days the air was like a tonic. One would go for a walk on crisp snow that crunched under one's feet [and] come in with glowing cheeks. Of course, we got blizzards and sometimes . . . one would lie in bed at night and feel that the roof of the hut would blow away any minute [or] one would be greeted by a hut thick with smoke and black smuts . . . But, on the whole, I loved my year in Iceland.'

To combat freezing winds and driving snows, issues of special clothing saw PMs clad in hooded duffle coats or waterproof great-coats, clumping about in rubber knee boots, their hands kept warm by lambswool gloves covered in waterproof material. But, off duty, they had cinema shows, mountain climbing, whist drives, concerts, bus trips, sports, hobby workshops and a library. Hot springs provided a venue for bathing parties all year round; winter added the delights of skating and skiing.

A party of twelve PMs set out for Reykjavik in March 1943. They included Mary Allen and her friend Barbara Burgess, both Red Cross nurses of the VAD, attached to the PMRAFNS. Since only four VADs had been selected, Mary and her friend 'thought it marvellous to be two of the four . . . We could not believe our luck as we travelled by sleeper from Euston to Greenock . . . Four new PM Sisters accompanied us, plus a few hundred RAF personnel. The voyage to Iceland took about three days. Corvettes accompanied the ship for the first part of the journey . . . [It] was rough, with mountainous seas and stiff winds. We approached our destination thankfully . . .'

Nursing sisters' accommodation – eight Nissen huts – connected with the hospital via a corridor whose walls 'were forever papered by a thin sheet of ice.'

Our sleeping huts (we four VAD nurses shared one) were heated by Tortoise stoves, the living rooms by large fires, and a team of Leading Aircraftmen came in handy for domestic duties . . . The huts contained a very comfortable bed each, a chair, rug and wooden box, contraptions for bedside locker and hanging space, and of course a mirror. With the purchase of some printed cretonne, we added curtains to our packing-case furniture . . .

Apart from sleeping quarters, the eight Nissen huts each had a sitting room and dining room, but no plumbed-in ablution facilities. The twelve PMs had to share a single lavatory, wash-place and bathroom.

We did have an alcove for washing effects, but as most items in our quarters became frozen, we generally used the bathroom at the entry to the hospital, which had been designated for our use. Oh, lovely hot water to wash, to bathe, to launder – it was precious to the extreme. It was quite usual when I was taking a bath to hear a gentle tap on the door and a, 'Let me in, Allen, please, I've got a little washing to do.'

When two of the VAD nurses were replaced by PM sisters, Mary Allen and Barbara Burgess became the only VADs at Reykjavik.

The patients were principally RAF personnel and sick and injured from passing ships. At one time, apart from British Navy personnel, we had a Norwegian, a Russian woman, a Lascar seaman, and even a Chinese. Once we received three Icelandic fishermen – having wrecked themselves on one of the small islands in the harbour, they were suffering from severe frostbite . . .

Long days of light and long days of dark were all new and strange to us. I shall never forget the joy of being on duty to see the sun rise, perhaps about 10.30 a.m., in a blaze of glorious colour, with Sunderland flying boats taking off on patrol, soaring overhead like giant white birds.

Duties were inflexible – we were off-duty for half a day every third day, with a whole day off once a month. But the most important day of the month was 'Boat Day' . . . New personnel arrived and equal numbers left for home and leave, and of course the sick went home. Then, apart from the necessities of life, the mail too arrived. The day was a continual buzz of excitement before, once again, we were left in isolation and our own little world . . .

As the Sisters' Mess was the one female unit in Reykjavik, you can imagine we were at a premium . . . for dances at the Officers' Club, for films, and of course for the more formal parties . . . One really memorable moment was at our Christmas party, I believe on Boxing Day . . . The Admiral of the Island was Matron's guest and we each had our invited guest. It was puzzling to us that they all seemed to be arriving late, but however at last we were all happy and ready to enjoy ourselves. An LAC [leading aircraftman] came into the dining room and asked if a marine might be allowed to enter with a message for the Admiral. Surely nothing could happen to take him away? But with a big smile he rose, saying, 'I think we should all drink a toast to the Royal Navy. The *Scharnhorst* has just been sunk and you are hearing this news three minutes before BBC London.' This explained our guests' late arrival as the air force base was on the alert to go to the aid of the Royal Navy if their manoeuvres had not succeeded. [The *Scharnhorst*, Germany's only remaining battle cruiser, was sunk by HMS *Duke of York* on 26 December 1943.]

RAFH Reykjavik continued to function until 1945, when it was reduced to the status of a sick quarters. Three PMs remained on its strength for the few months before the need for the RAF's presence in Iceland ended.

Warmer climes

While some nursing sisters worked amid ice and snow, others headed for the Equator. During 1942, two more RAF hospitals opened overseas, the first being at Takoradi on the Gold Coast (now Ghana).

Mediterranean supply routes remained hazardous. With the enemy dominating southern Europe and fortunes fluctuating in the western desert, essential supplies bound for the Middle East – including new aircraft, sectioned and crated – went south by sea, to a spot tucked away under the western bulge of Africa. There, at RAF Takoradi, technicians assembled and tested the new planes before ferry pilots flew them east via staging posts across Africa to the Sudan, and then north to join the squadrons engaged in Libya and Egypt. Transport planes took stores and equipment along the same 4,000-mile supply route via Khartoum, while other RAF squadrons, based in the Gambia, Sierra Leone and Nigeria, flew ocean-reconnaissance missions in support of Atlantic convoys. As the number of personnel in British West Africa increased, a full-scale RAF hospital opened at Takoradi early in 1942.

Takoradi has a good artificial harbour backed by fertile heath and bush, but the hot and humid climate can be uncomfortable for Europeans, with a wet season lasting for more than half the year. Frequent squalls and rain-storms lash the coast and low cloud obscures the jungle-clad hills inland – perfect conditions for the mosquitoes and other flies that carry malaria, dysentery and yellow fever. In Takoradi endemic disease was the worst enemy: 80 per cent of personnel went down with malaria, decimating whole sections whose efficiency might mean the difference between operational success and disaster. Preventive measures included the use of the drug mepacrine, which turned one's skin yellow and caused unpleasant side effects such as colic and nausea, but was highly effective.

Tropical sunlight added to difficulties. Godfrey Jones, a civilian-trained member of the VAD, tells how the hospital overlooked the beach – handy for cooling off when off duty, but 'one chap who had just come out from UK went to sleep on the beach and at 6 p.m. at night was on the operating table for treatment of burns'.

The main two-storey part of the hospital had wide mosquito-proof verandahs on both floors. Matron Miss Meikle led a nursing team of fourteen PMs, with appropriate numbers of male orderlies in support. Each nursing sister had her own bedroom and sitting room, a welcome haven from the busy hospital wards. With such a vast area to cover, and with members of all three services as patients, by 1943 the hospital bed-state had increased to over 300. Because of the health risks, nursing sisters stayed for a maximum of eighteen months, and they too had to take mepacrine. Malaria was no respecter of persons.

The Azores

Out in the Atlantic, the steep, fertile Portuguese-owned islands of the Azores provided a staging post for Allied forces from September 1943. The first tented SSQ and a later larger medical centre at

Lagens, on Terceira island, were both badly damaged by hurricanes in December 1943 and October 1944. In between, staff coped with an outbreak of poliomyelitis. Urgent rebuilding saw a more substantial RAF hospital, of 150 beds, functional by November 1944. Seven PMs, under Matron Gwen Butler, the first British women posted to the Azores, arrived aboard an armed merchant ship, part of a convoy, in January 1945.

Sister Dilys Palmer (Mrs Bore) remembers a good social life, with lots of picnics. A serious outbreak of typhoid added to the workload, but mostly nurses dealt with common illnesses. With sport providing a popular pastime, some patients came in with leisure-induced problems, and gossip suggested that many a fearless rugger tackle was prompted by a desire to 'indulge in the comforts of the hospital and receive the sympathetic attentions of our sisters'.

RAFH Lagens was handed over to Portuguese authorities in October 1946.

Cairo

Before the war, the few RAF personnel stationed in Egypt had been treated by army hospitals. As war loomed, tented sick quarters opened at Heliopolis (Cairo) and Alexandria, and from 1939 RAF medical facilities in Egypt expanded, adjusting to serve the needs of the hour as war swept across North Africa. Cairo provided military headquarters for British forces fighting what troops ironically dubbed the 'Benghazi Handicap' – the tug of war in which Wavell and Rommel alternately led advance and retreat in the deserts to the west. The history of those years still resonates with the names Tobruk and El Alamein.

No. 5 RAFGH, variously referred to as 'Cairo', 'Heliopolis' or 'Abbassia', opened in March 1942 in a new maternity hospital and welfare centre, an elegant white building resembling a big hotel. It was still in the final stages of construction when the RAF took it over, but before long new fences went up and grass-seed sprouted, spreading a cool green sward between the hospital and the main Cairo-Heliopolis road. A shortage of living accommodation obliged the matron and thirty-four sisters, most of them straight from the UK, to move into quarters half a mile from the hospital.

Hardly had they caught their breath than the first patients

arrived; the flow of casualties and sickness kept them well occupied. For a time, as the tide of war surged and fell, they lived in constant readiness to evacuate, but by the summer the Allies had begun to drive the enemy back. Step by step, the desert campaign gained ground. In its wake, dotted along the southern shores of the Mediterranean, temporary front-line RAF hospitals opened. No. 5 RAFGH settled down to its primary task of acting as a base hospital for flying personnel from all the Allied forces.

Ranking officers – on paper

After three and a half years of war service, PMs finally received a measure of official recognition. From March 1943, they wore regulation rank insignia and enjoyed what the Air Ministry order called 'the compliments and respect due to an officer of equivalent rank in the WAAF'. Since the title 'Staff Nurse' had been abolished in 1941, equivalents of PMRAFNS to WAAF were: Sister/Flying Officer; Senior Sister/Flight Officer; Matron (RAFSH)/Squadron Officer; Principal Matron (RAFGH)/Wing Officer; Chief Principal Matron (a post established in 1944)/Group Officer; Matron-in-Chief/Air Commandant. However, appropriate braid on sleeve or shoulder was the only outward sign of this change; in all other ways, PMs were still known by their time-honoured professional titles. Rona Black (Mrs McAlpine) writes:

> I was very proud of my stripes. At that time I was Sister Black, Lady of the Air Force – as such I had licence to resign from the service if I wished – but suddenly we became Commissioned Officers subject to King's Regulations ... We soon discovered the reason for the change – a fairly large draft of nursing sisters was required to staff Middle Eastern and African hospitals ...

Defying the U-boats

As the war spread, more and more RAF squadrons flew out of more and more overseas airfields. Each squadron required many supporting staff, both RAF and WAAF, and the only means of transporting them was by sea. As a result, many of the larger ocean liners were called on to act as troopships.

First to come under sole RAF control was the *Queen Elizabeth*.
From May 1943 her crew included two PMs whose work the
Nursing Service Advisory Board commended as outstanding. So
successful was this initial venture that the RAF were given responsibility for two additional ships, the *Mauretania* and the *Nieu
Amsterdam*, with more nursing sisters on their medical teams. Later
the *Pasteur* and the *Andes* also came under RAF control.

As more and more WAAF sailed for duty overseas, separate parts
of the troopships' hospital accommodation were allocated to their
needs, with WAAF nursing assistants to help the PMs. The authorities, somewhat chauvinistically, expected girlish moans and whinges
about cramped conditions and lack of privacy, but the women
proved just as tough, resilient and good-humoured as the men when
faced with adversity and discomfort – not to mention danger, with
U-boats hunting below and German planes circling above.

The Cunard White Star cruise liner *Mauretania*, even when
stripped of her most luxurious furniture and fittings, offered a desirable posting. She plied the Atlantic from Liverpool to New York and
to Halifax, Nova Scotia, carrying thousands of troops to Europe and
bringing British families of American and Canadian servicemen
home to their new countries. The *Mauretania* was staffed half by
RAF and half by US Army officers, with a complement of medical
orderlies of the RAFMS; her two nursing sisters, Beryl Chadney and
Lucy Woodward, covered most eventualities, the one being a children's nurse and theatre sister, the other a midwife – 'Although a
number of the wives were pregnant we managed to get them all on
dry land to have their babies!' Beryl Chadney reports with relief.

Each time they left Liverpool, and on their return, destroyers
escorted them for two days – the Atlantic crossing took six or seven
days each way. The PMs attended occasional dances 'in the beautiful ballroom, when all female personnel were pressed into service
for what could only be called 'excuse me' dances, since we were
totally outnumbered'.

Lucy Woodward had charge of a ward for women and children,
with an RAF medical officer; Beryl Chadney had the men's ward,
with American army doctors. Daily clinics and sick parades
confronted them with the inevitable sea-sickness and infectious
diseases of childhood, and of course there were endless boat drills.
At night the two PMs took turns to be on call and, since a night

seldom passed without some small emergency arising, they were usually desperately tired by the time they reached port.

On arrival in New York, medical staff disembarked a day later than passengers and came aboard again a day in advance; since the ship 'turned around' in about five days, this gave them three days' shore leave, staying at the Governor Clinton Hotel and visiting nightspots such as 'Roger's Corner', opposite Madison Square Gardens in downtown Manhattan. Or they went shopping, armed with long lists of goods unobtainable at home, 'mainly cosmetics and nylons, though I remember having to buy a pair of wellington boots on one occasion'.

The story of the great liners' involvement could not be told until after the war ended. In September 1945 the *Evening Standard* revealed how the security blackout had been even more important for *Mauretania* than for 'the famous "*Queens*". Their greatest protection throughout the war was speed. The *Mauretania* was . . . eight knots slower . . . I have seen a list of her war-time ports of call. Hardly an important name is missing, yet the ship moved like a phantom over the oceans, rumour and report never catching up with her . . .'

Light on the horizon

As the war dragged on into a fourth year, events encouraged the Allies to hope for eventual victory. Russia slowly turned back the German incursions on her frontiers; in the Pacific the USA won victories over Japan; and in North Africa the Desert Rats and their comrades, under Lieutenant-General Bernard Montgomery, had Rommel, the 'Desert Fox' on the run. This was the moment for which the medical branch of the RAF had long been preparing.

As the Allied advance pushed further and further, driving the enemy westward from Cairo, through Libya and eventually out of North Africa altogether, right behind them moved small medical units called mobile receiving stations. These in turn moved on to care for the immediate needs of the wounded, leaving behind a succession of temporary RAF general hospitals. At the first of these, at Benghazi, PM sisters found the old civil hospital badly damaged by bombs and shells, but soon they had it fit to receive the Allied casualties that poured in; the second RAFGH opened at Tripoli, the third on the site of ancient Carthage (in Tunisia). Rumour has it that when the hospital in Tunisia opened a signal came from the Air Ministry asking, 'Carthage? Where's that?'

Sisters sailing out to join the three new hospitals and other units that opened in the Mediterranean area, faced a variety of weather and terrain, from North Africa with its 110°F heat, dust and sandstorms – not to mention plagues of flies – to torrential rains turning battle-scarred land to mud, and deep winter snows in the Italian mountains. In impossible conditions they cared for the sick and wounded of both sides, battling endemic disease such as malaria, typhoid, infective hepatitis, dysentery and, not least, all the varied types of venereal infection. As one of those doughty ladies remarks, 'You didn't worry about that until afterwards. You had a job to do so you rolled up your sleeves and got on with it.'

Hospitals on the move

Mobile receiving stations were conceived at the start of the war, intended to be a primary link in the chain that sped sick and wounded men directly from the fighting front to the safety of base hospitals. Originally only male nurses worked with these units, but in March 1943 they were joined by PMs wearing their new honorary rank insignia. From that date, too – to avoid the ambiguity of the initials MRS – the units became known as mobile field hospitals (MFHs).

As their name implies, these tented medical units were designed to move from place to place at short notice, either by air or by road, their equipment loaded onto a transport plane or a convoy of trucks. Where possible they set up close to a forward airfield; otherwise they chose a site convenient for the evacuation of casualties by sea, rail or river. As wounded men came in, straight from battle, the MFH offered treatment to stabilize their condition ready for the journey back to the nearest base hospital. The units were designed to cater for up to fifty patients at a time, though on occasions – after D-Day, for instance, as we shall see – they coped with very many more. Nor were the patients all Allied troops; many sick and wounded prisoners of war also owed their lives to the front-line field hospitals.

Staff of these mobile hospitals included medical officers and surgeons, dental officers, medical orderlies and assistants, plus non-medical support from numerous drivers, cooks, clerks, carpenters, and electricians. These men were skilled in the swift packing and unpacking of their unit. (At a post-war demonstration at Farnborough, a tented hundred-bed hospital – nine tons of it – was flown in aboard a Beverley aircraft; it became functional, a mile away from the airfield, just twenty-five minutes later.)

In some locations, once the MFH had established itself under canvas, its staff commandeered local buildings to increase bed-spaces and offer more security. Then, with more medical staff posted in, the unit, however makeshift and temporary, might be designated an RAF general hospital. The original MFH might stay, or move on, or split into two separate teams. Even an RAFGH could relocate if necessary. The field hospitals were fluid in both form and function, their work of vital importance both to the men and women actually engaged in the war and to local civilians who needed medical aid.

Twenty-six MFHs formed during the war years, the earliest in August 1939. They served in all theatres of war and lasted variously from a few months to several years. The last of them disbanded in October 1946. Not all of these units had PMs with them; the choice depended on the senior medical officer (SMO) involved. Some SMOs preferred to lead an all-male unit, especially under more adverse conditions in the desert or the jungle; others, appreciating the benefits of a female presence, found nursing sisters invaluable. When requested, at least two sisters would be attached to each MFH. Some went to North Africa and, of these, some followed the troops into Italy, arriving by landing craft, under enemy fire, at places like Salerno. Others sailed for India and Burma. Meanwhile, back in England four PMs stood by as part of two mobile field hospitals whose destination was, as yet, unknown – back in 1943, D-Day was only a gleam in Churchill's eye.

The adventures of No. 30 MFH

The variety of life with an MFH is demonstrated by the story of two particular PMs, Senior Sister Jessie W. Atkinson and Sister Helen Jones. They were with 30 MFH from the day it formed, in March 1943 at RAF West Kirby, Lancashire, until it disbanded in Italy in

June 1945. The unit comprised eighty-one personnel: four medical officers, a medical quartermaster, the two nursing sisters, a warrant officer nursing orderly, twenty-seven medics of NCO and airman rank, the rest made up of supporting staff. They sailed from the Clyde and landed twelve days later, on 23 April, at Algiers, where they had to wait a couple of weeks for their equipment to arrive; in the interim the sisters helped out at RAF Blida sick quarters while the men found duties elsewhere. When their equipment arrived they formed into convoy and drove east to Tunis, arriving as the enemy were withdrawing back through Sicily and into Italy. Thousands of Italians and Germans remained behind as prisoners of war.

No. 30 MFH opened for business on the seashore at Hammamet. A few weeks later medical reinforcements arrived and took over a school and a convent in Carthage. There, PMs Atkinson and Jones were joined by their colleagues Naughton and Ashworth. Clad in khaki shirts without ties, divided skirts made of khaki drill, khaki stockings and black shoes, worn with wide-brimmed white felt hats sporting a 'flash' or ribbon in RAF colours, they helped to establish a busy base hospital, officially No. 1 RAFGH, Carthage.

Contemporary reports from the *MTE Journal* confirm the success of the scheme to evacuate casualties by air via MFHs in the desert.

The huge transport aircraft . . . have been carrying as many as 13 or 14 stretcher cases in addition to sitting cases which, on treatment at base hospitals, have had a surprising recovery rate.

A British pilot flying over Sollum was attacked and severely wounded in the shoulder and thigh, crash-landing his aircraft. Within four hours he was two hundred miles away receiving the blood transfusion which put him on the road to recovery . . . Another pilot . . . was severely burned. In grave danger of dying from shock, he was given intravenous plasma, and in a few hours was speeding by air to base, where a blood transfusion saved his life . . .

A mechanic was blown up by an exploding petrol tank and tore his side severely. Weak from loss of blood, he was brought into the desert SSQ, straight onto the operating table where his pulse was thought to have stopped. The RAF surgeon worked on him and . . . after two hours his radial pulse returned to such a degree that he was considered fit to survive a fifteen-mile journey to hospital.

As the Allies launched their offensive across the hundred miles or so of Mediterranean which separated them from Sicily, 30 MFH gathered its personnel together again. Sisters Atkinson and Jones left the relative safety of the Carthage hospital, staff loaded the equipment and, side by side with the fighting troops, sailed for Sicily in 'landing ships' tanks'. They came ashore at Lacati and drove in convoy to Lentini, south of the volcano Mount Etna, setting up camp not far from the airfield.

Leslie Moore, NCO in charge of 30 MFH's orderly room, writes:

> On the 11th August, it had been a very wet day but the night was as clear as daylight with a full moon. The RAF aircraft were unable to take off in the mud . . . The Germans came over in force and dive-bombed the airfield. They also dived on the hospital, but did not drop any bombs. We felt certain that they saw the Red Cross on the ground in the centre of the camp . . .

German forces pulled out of Sicily the next day and the Allies pursued them into Italy. No. 30 MFH followed. 'The beach was still under fire and we drove about a mile inland and set up the hospital in a field, with our two Sisters supervising.' Italy surrendered but German troops in the country fought on.

Having worked their way across Italy, 30 MFH settled in for the winter in Foggia, just south of the spur on Italy's heel. Here they tended the wounded who came back from the front and airlifted them back to the hospitals in North Africa, or to the new RAFGH which established itself near Naples that December. The next June, as D-Day dawned and the Allied assault on Normandy began, 30 MFH moved on again; behind it No. 4 RAFGH, sited in an old folk's home with more PMs on its staff, took over medical care in that area.

Through the summer of 1944, 30 MFH travelled in stages up central Italy to Sienna, then across to the east coast to spend the winter in a school at Termoli. Extra nursing sisters were sent to help them at various times during the winter. Then, with the Balkans more involved in the war, 'in April 1945 we crossed to Zara in Yugoslavia, where we provided medical cover for the RAF ground crews who maintained the aircraft flown by Tito's pilots . . . We celebrated VE Day in Yugoslavia but were evacuated back to Termoli in a few days.' From there they headed back to Naples where the MFH disbanded and 'we packed all our equipment for despatch to the Far East and Senior Sister Atkinson and Sister Jones left us for a Base Hospital.'

In the twenty-six months which had passed since their arrival in Algeria, they had witnessed the liberation of North Africa, Sicily and Italy; they had travelled, in convoy, 3,571 lurching, rolling, back-breaking miles; and they had lost count of how many times they had packed and unpacked those life-saving tents!

(The war produced twenty-six MFHs, but they were not numbered 1–26. The smaller numbers, 1–11, were used for temporary RAFGHs which set up shop in disused schools, convents etc. Of the others, Nos. 21, 24, 30 and 31 went to North Africa and then into Italy; No. 50 followed the troops into Normandy; No. 52 went to Holland; Nos. 60, 61, 62 and 63 sailed for India; Nos. 65 and 67 went to Burma; No. 80 was in Hong Kong and No. 81 in Singapore. The remaining one, number unknown, was operational in Ceylon.)

Mediterranean memories

Many other PMs were caught up in the unfolding drama, thirty-two at the Benghazi hospital, another forty or so at Carthage, with thirty-five later at Naples and more at Algiers. Forty-six of these had sailed from home aboard the *Orontes*, in a huge ninety-six-ship convoy which departed in August 1943. They left Liverpool, bound first for the Clyde, on Friday the 13th, and when Elizabeth Mansell (Mrs Ogden) discovered that she and another sister had been given a berth in Cabin 13, 'we tried to change it, but nobody would change – it was, however, the Bridal Suite!'

Personnel and stores crammed the convoy to capacity, bound for destinations in the Mediterranean, North, South and West Africa, Iraq, Aden, India and Ceylon. *Orontes* alone carried almost 4,000 troops, plus twenty-two tons of petrol for Algiers and Malta. U-boats menaced the ships; depth-charges boomed from time to time. As so often happened during the war, personnel on board had little idea of where they were heading.

Off Gibraltar, when the convoy split into two, *Orontes* and others sailed into the Mediterranean. They arrived as the Allies were invading Sicily. In the harbour at Algiers, Elizabeth Mansell saw 'two big battleships, the *Howe* and *George V*, waiting to go into the Sicily attack'. Because of the risk of bombers attacking the two battleships, *Orontes* remained outside the harbour all night, to dock next morning to the sound of 'God Save the King'. The PMs took over a boys' boarding school, designated No. 2 RAFGH, 'but it was filthy, filthy. Flies flying into your mouth . . . we had to do away with the flies . . . We got some special stuff from the Americans.'

Elizabeth Smallwood (Mrs Andrews) had earlier served at Halton, where she had danced with legless air ace Douglas Bader to celebrate the arrival of his new improved 'tin pins'. Now she found herself where 'conditions were very bad, flies galore and a shortage of water. We lived on Spam [tinned, processed meat] for one year – breakfast, dinner, tea and supper! We had a canvas bucket half-filled each day by the Water Bowser, in which we washed, and then had to wash our "smalls" in the same water. We were allowed a small flask of drinking water . . . one gulp, but it had to last all day.'

Later, posted to Tunisia, she

> . . . ended up in the ruins of Carthage, in an old and very dirty monastery, which we had to scrub and clean ready for the wounded . . . We sisters were put in a Nissen hut, with temperatures of 100 degrees and it was very difficult to sleep. The sea was near so several of us used to go down behind a large rock and bathe, and also wash our hair. My family sent out some salt-water soap . . .

With few women around, the PMs were in social demand, often dated by Americans. They even attended a party given by General Eisenhower. In January 1943, when 'Ike' and the other chiefs of staff met the British prime minister and the American president in Casablanca, Elizabeth Smallwood encountered General de Gaulle, Air Marshal Sir Arthur Tedder and Field Marshal Montgomery. She actually nursed Winston Churchill, who, 'became ill with pneumo-

nia. [We] treated him with one of the first antibiotics – M&B 693
. . . I was in charge of the hospital on night duty when an Army
Sergeant came to my office and asked for a bedpan. I asked who it
was for and he replied that it was top secret and he could not tell
me . . .' She persisted and, discovering that the needy patient was
Churchill himself, 'I picked out the best of my rather battered
collection.' Next day she learned that the 'great man' had taken one
look at the item and growled, 'Take that damned thing away!'

As the invasion of Italy gathered pace, No. 1 RAFGH, Carthage,
handed over its duties to 31 MFH and packed up to follow the
troops. A full complement of PMs went with it, two days after
Christmas, 1943. Jean Ponsford (Mrs Howell) remembers being
seen off at the airport by Lord Tedder, who had just bidden farewell
to Winston Churchill, off to convalesce in Marrakesh. 'We landed
at Capo de Chino airport in Naples and were then taken to our
mess in the village of Torre-del-Greco. It consisted of two villas, the
main one had been four flats, and the other was situated in its own
grounds, totally different from N. Africa . . .'

The hospital's advance party had taken over a convalescent
home on the lower slopes of a mountain, with three acres of
grounds in which stood several villas now employed both as extra
wards and as accommodation for staff. It was not at all a bad posting, with plenty going on: after the army repaired the bridge above,
the road was busy with convoys going up towards Cassino. But the
PMs did face a few difficulties. To begin with, a typhus epidemic
raged through Naples that winter so the city was put out of bounds
to off-duty personnel. And then there was the volcano . . .

Torre del Greco stands on the lower slopes of Vesuvius; it had
been laid waste when the volcano erupted in 1800. Even as the PMs
arrived, the mountain was rumbling again. It grew ever more active
as the weeks passed. At one o'clock in the morning of 22 March
1944, when the hospital was busy, with over 300 bed-ridden
patients, Vesuvius blew its top. Those whose rooms looked out on
the mountain witnessed a spectacular display of boiling smoke,
sparks, flying red-hot boulders and rivers of molten lava glowing in
the darkness. Fortunately the wind blew most of the cinders and ash
in the opposite direction, but a blanket of hot ash descended on the
roof of the hospital, making evacuation a necessary precaution.
Mary Drew (Mrs Mitchell) was on night duty that night.

The battle for Cassino was on when the volcano erupted, and after a difficult night with windows falling and a minor earthquake, it was decided at 6 a.m. that we should evacuate . . . I instructed my 100 patients to fill one of their pillowcases with their belongings and stay by their beds . . . (They were all taken to Army hospitals, so the War Department owes the RAF 100 pillowcases!) Matron and all sisters [went] to a transit camp in Naples . . . Everything was covered in thick dust, and the village of San Sebastiano was destroyed. The lava flow finished at the wall of a house and the ground was very hot for weeks afterwards . . .

In the windward direction, ash and cinders blocked the roads for twenty-five miles.

While working at Torre del Greco, Sister Elizabeth Mansell received permission to marry her fiancé, Pilot Officer 'Mickey' Ogden, based in North Africa. She flew over to make arrangements for a wedding in the British church at Algiers, then returned to Naples where 'the Catering Officer made a great big wedding cake'.

It was in a big wooden box with 'British Red Cross, Wedding Cake' and I had to take it to the airport – the Americans were in charge at that time. They said they 'couldn't put it down the chute, Mam!' I had to get four of the crew to carry it on to the aeroplane . . . The wedding day was held in the mess . . . 25 bottles of champagne at 2/6d [12.5p] a bottle, which Mickey got direct from the factory! The food was only like you would have at a coffee morning.

Later she returned again to No. 1 RAFGH in Italy and 'Mickey used to fly over in a Beaufighter, circling Vesuvius . . .'
Romance flourished, despite the war.

FOUR

A *new theatre of care*

Just one day after the bombing of Pearl Harbor in December 1941, Japanese troops invaded Malaya. Within weeks they seemed to have a foothold on every island and peninsula in the area. The early months of 1942 saw the fall of Singapore, the Allied defeat in the Java Sea, then the loss of Rangoon and the long bitter trek back via Mandalay as British, Indian and Chinese troops withdrew behind the Chindwin river into India.

The Japanese were in trouble, too, and with supply lines stretched to breaking they halted to regroup. For eighteen months the Chindwin formed an uneasy boundary between British and Japanese forces. General Slim, commander of the Burma Corps, used the time to prepare a base, at Imphal, from which to mount his counter-attack, while the US fleet kept the Japanese occupied in the Pacific.

Successes in North Africa enabled Britain to direct more of her naval and air forces to the Far East. By June 1943 over fifty RAF squadrons were based in India, with modern aircraft replacing old, antiquated machines and more coming in all the time. At last they were in a position to counter the challenge along the border between India and Burma.

This 1,000-mile frontier (which now edges Bangladesh and Assam), runs through impenetrable jungle, among steep mountains traversed by narrow passes, across mosquito-ridden plains and paddy-fields. What roads exist tend to be swept away or turned into thick mud by the monsoon season, which lasts from June to

November every year. This difficult and dangerous country was to be the next theatre of care for the PMs – not that any of them knew it as they waited for the call to embark.

In July 1943, Rona Black (Mrs McAlpine) was at RAFH Innsworth, Gloucestershire, standing by to go overseas. Writing to her mother, she felt able to hint at a possible end to the waiting.

> I may get some leave suddenly . . . as soon as I know I will let you know – but let there be no panic! It's a great life! . . . Have been to the hairdresser and have a glamorous style – bags of curls, frightfully natty! I'm sure you will understand this letter but keep your hopes and fears under your hat. Life is uncertain at the moment. We have been warned.

Later that month, she joined 62 Mobile Field Hospital, under canvas at Chislehurst in Kent.

Boots, mosquito

Jessie Higgins, by now promoted to senior sister, had been told to be ready for overseas duty by June.

> The list of requirements for the posting included tropical kit and, of all things, mosquito boots! No one had heard of these . . . I spent two whole days of my disembarkation leave searching all boot and shoe shops in London. Eventually, at a great cost of £5 I discovered a pair! Made of thick white canvas and reaching right up and over the thighs, they were the most awful uncomfortable things imaginable and, needless to say, eventually were useless.

Along with Sister 'Tommy' Thomas (Mrs McGregor), Jessie Higgins went to join the staff of 61 MFH, who gathered to begin experiencing life under canvas in a remote area of Essex. 'Getting used to this kind of life was not easy, especially trying to bath in a large canvas bowl . . . We still had no idea where we were going. Rumours ran riot, but we never considered the Far East and knew nothing then of the 14th Army in Burma.'

The Med reopens

With the Allies in command of the Mediterranean, the Suez route to the Far East again became safe for trooping and cargo vessels. The first convoy through, in August 1943, carried with it four mobile field hospitals (Nos 60, 61, 62 and 63), each with two PMs on its staff – the first RAF nursing sisters to go to India.

The call came suddenly. One evening the CO of 61 MFH informed his staff that they were to dismantle their unit, pack up and be ready to leave by midnight. 'Panic stations!' is how Jessie Higgins recalls it. They boarded a train and next morning found themselves at Liverpool. The ship was full, with five of the PMs sharing a one-berth cabin, but Jessie Higgins thought this 'terribly lucky, as we had a shower and loo of our own!' The former cruise liner had been stripped of all comforts, 'no chairs anywhere so we had to use our life-jackets as cushions . . . We sailed that night not knowing to where. Seasickness was bad . . . The sea seemed to be so huge and rough. We were in a very large convoy escorted by destroyers . . . quite exciting as depth charges were frequently dropped into the ocean, hopefully to keep away the German submarines . . .'

For Rona Black, it seemed 'A pioneer expedition! I'd always wanted to be a pioneer so this was just up my street! . . . Setting out from England we zigzagged across the Bay of Biscay. (The second convoy was not so lucky.) I was so seasick all I wanted for my birthday on the eighteenth of August was a torpedo amidships.'

The eight PMs, along with a few other servicewomen, including army nursing sisters and VADs, formed a small female contingent among thousands of men. One of those men was Fred 'Blondie' Payne, whom we last met during the bombing of Torquay; like Rona Black and her friend Jay Gardner, he was attached to 62 MFH.

Rona's letters reveal that she 'had thought of writing a little every day, but the writing of diaries is not permitted as it would give away valuable information . . . I feel rather like Granma sitting on the leeside with great-coat on and a net over my hair – my knitting is the only thing I haven't got, and that's in my cabin.' One big anxiety was the mail, whether hers was getting to her family at home and why none was coming in. However, women being in a minority on board ship, she and the other sisters had plenty of 'dates', many admirers, even some proposals. 'It's amazing being so popular, we have had a laugh out of it ourselves. The chaps congratulate themselves on getting a word in or a seat beside us, so we are rather tending to be monopolised – at least, three of us are.'

After a week or so, having sailed through the Suez Canal watched by crowds of Egyptians curious to see this first convoy in three years, they reached Port Said and had to change ships, transferring from their cruise liner to a small Atlantic steamer, 'which was dreadful!' Jessie Higgins recalls. 'The heat and discomfort through the Red Sea were awful – and the drinking water so chlorinated that it became a nightmare to keep ourselves hydrated.'

Rona Black, writing soon after the event, remembers:

We had to change ships at one stage . . . You have no idea what that entailed. It was a boiling hot day with not a breath of air and a haze hung all around. We were to have trans-shipped at 6 a.m., everyone was up and ready to go. At 8 a.m. we were all browned-off, so we started a pontoon school. They didn't get moving until 11 a.m. But the new ship is much more comfortable, except for the bread, which always tastes bad. We have 100% better food including melons, dates, grapes, bananas, really lovely! Fruit salads are superb.

We got a fresh supply of water at the last port of call, which tastes simply awful . . . We are lucky to have an open bar . . . the great drink is brandy squash, which goes down very nicely, in moderation . . . Though the sky is blue the sea ain't so good and I have felt a bit under the weather. I'm taking belladonna after meals, which is making quite a difference, and a drop of scotch before meals is just keeping my head above water. I don't think pleasure cruising is at all in my line.

When they reached Aden and turned east they must have suspected where they were heading, and as they approached Bombay the smell of the land – the spices, the dust, the amazing aroma that is peculiarly India – came wafting to meet them. Lists of postings went up, finally, twenty-four hours out.

First impressions of the Orient

The staff of the four MFHs arrived in Bombay on 15 September 1943 eager to begin their work. However, to their dismay their equipment had been delayed leaving England and, since for some reason it went round via the Cape, it did not reach its destination at Calcutta until mid-December. In the meantime other duties were assigned to the MFH's personnel.

Bombay proved 'interesting, certainly a shock after UK in wartime!' as Tommy Thomas comments, but the transit camp at Worli just outside the city was even more of a revelation. Jessie Higgins describes how they had been told to dress up for their arrival in

> . . . special white tricoline dresses and white Dicks [thick silky cotton-poplin dresses, worn with smart tropical quatrecorns] only to find ourselves being helped up into lorries for the drive out to the transit camp at Worli. Never will I forget it. The camp was for hundreds and I think we were some of the first women to arrive there. The huts were of wood and very dark, and had charpoy beds . . . every door and drawer one opened, huge cockroaches ran everywhere, and the chairs and mattresses were full of bugs.

She hated bugs. Having waited at Worli for about ten days, they were sent by train to Calcutta.

> 4 days and 3 nights of dirt, dust, sweat and tears, four of us to a compartment, which fortunately had a loo and hand basin en suite. Food was arranged whenever we stopped at a large station and it was brought to the train – mostly greasy fried eggs and bread, and fizzy drinks and tea . . . We left the train at Calcutta, where the troop Officer informed us we were not expected! No one knew what to do with us, so another transit camp for a short stay.

Eventually the PMs were attached to the army hospital in Calcutta, which was crowded with patients. At that time the army provided most medical services for the RAF in India. The PMs looked forward to rectifying that state of affairs – as did the airmen: 'If we appeared in a ward when there were RAF chaps we received a big cheer!'

They stayed in Calcutta until December, when their equipment arrived. At last something was happening. At last they were going to establish their own mobile hospital encampments. Or were they? Rona Black tells the story:

Christmas Eve, 1943. We were told to be ready early in the morning. We set off by river and train for Chittagong, arriving early the next day. We sang carols on the boat, convinced that the 'big push' was beginning, only to discover we'd had to travel then because no-one else would! There was no-one to meet us. Our hopes were dashed. Once again we were seconded to the army . . .

She and Jay Gardner were supposed to be with 62 MFH, but one delay after another kept them from fulfilling the role they had been assigned. The frustration of it all comes vividly to life in one of Rona's letters to her mother, written on 29 December 1943 from 61 MFH, at Chittagong:

We have moved again as you will see, but unfortunately this is not the last move. There has been such an awful upheaval, I have felt so browned off I have not dared write home. I see from my book it's 13 days since I wrote. As far as my health is concerned, I'm fine, but the bloody RAF has let us down badly. We all planned Xmas, as you know, and on the 21st they said we were to move at 5 a.m. Xmas Eve, arriving here at 5 a.m. Xmas Day. That we did. The others went to a party on the 23rd and didn't go to bed . . . 3 a.m. I was wakened, dressed, had eggs and bacon and off we went. The train journey wasn't too bad. Then at mid-day we went in a boat, and then back on the train . . .

When we got here, no one to meet us and eventually, when the CO arrived, we found we were re-posted to another army hospital. We were mad! The next bombshell, Gardner and I, not belonging here, were put to work the next day on the wards. We found when we got here we really weren't expected . . . our patience is exhausted and we all let everyone know who mattered, from Air Cmdres to S/Ldrs (we don't deal in anything less). Of course we were all terribly tired after the journey, so after a drink of rum I went to bed and slept solidly until 3.30 p.m. When I woke I felt like I used to on night duty – rather sick and really stupid . . .

What's more, when we got here we discovered they had no idea where we were going to live . . . they expected us to sit down quite cheerfully and live here with the QAs. That, of course, is a damn lot of nonsense and we aren't going to do it . . . Today I'm recovering from the blow of being uprooted for Xmas unnecessarily, and the thought we are annexed by the b— army medical corps . . .

Anyway, we have a flat now, very nice room each and every comfort. We have tin pots for lavs and canvas baths . . . We are moving in on Monday, after the place is clean.

Having let off steam, she soon calmed down, writing in January:

We're settling down here now and have practically recovered from our depression and gloom that settled over us at Xmas . . . our living quarters are wizard now, we have had the whole place painted and we have acquired furniture, rugs and curtains, and really it's going to look wizard. Six rooms in the top flat of a house. It isn't very large but it gives us a room for a lounge . . . We are hoping to join our unit very soon. Work is very plentiful here. We are certainly seeing life . . . My dress at the various parties from now on, unless specially informed, will be bush shirt and khaki slacks. The mosquitoes are bad and it's more comfortable not being bitten.

It took courage for a young woman raised in Britain to travel at short notice out to snake-ridden jungles where she was obliged to live and work in primitive, makeshift conditions. Faced with downright squalor, she rolled up her sleeves, swapped her white ward dress for khaki slacks and shirt, and by sheer hard work brought a semblance of home comfort to cheer her patients' blackest hours as they fought the effects of dengue fever, dysentery, typhus, hepatitis, and – always and above all – malaria.

The smallest enemy

Hundreds of hastily built airfields, landing strips and RAF stations had spread across India and Ceylon. Unfortunately, owing to the speed of their construction, not enough attention was paid to proper siting or to using building materials suited to the climate and conditions; so huts leaked in the monsoon, camps flooded and many personnel found themselves living next to mosquito breeding-grounds. Dysentery and malaria became the two arch-enemies, engaging everyone in a never-ending war against the ubiquitous mosquito.

The worst problem with malaria was its ability to lodge in the human system; an apparent cure would be effected, only for the disease to break out again weeks later. Prevention being preferable, items for malarial control were issued: metal gauze screening for doors and windows; camouflage netting, khaki or green, for beds and sundry openings; protective clothing – slacks and long sleeves to be worn from sundown, also the hated mosquito boots for the PMs; insect repellents, though these were unpopular and not very effective; and drugs – when quinine became scarce, mepacrine hydrochloride, which turned skin yellow and irritated the human stomach, was introduced. The most effective malaria preventative was discipline – taking the proper precautions – but many men couldn't be bothered with all that.

Given the benefit of hindsight, the liberal use of DDT, sprayed not only on stagnant ponds and vegetation but in living quarters and kitchens, sometimes on skin, or sewn into the seams of clothes, looks horrifyingly ill-advised. The *History of the RAFMS* (published in 1954) speaks casually of 'Paris green', DDT and pyrethrum solutions being 'spread by hand-held sprayers of poor workmanship, cheap material and parts liable to corrosion in the hot, moist atmosphere of the tropics'. Official anti-malarial control units were generally efficient and well organized, but all too often these spraying devices were in the hands of squads of untrained service personnel or 'mechanically unskilled coolies', who merrily squirted gallons of poisonous insecticide, directly and daily, virtually everywhere their sprays would reach. But such was the threat of malaria and other diseases carried by insects that eradicating them was of paramount importance and, at the time, DDT and its cousins provided the best weapon.

Some relief and relaxation came from sunbathing and, if your unit was near the coast, sea bathing provided a popular form of recreation and did wonders for morale. The benefits far outweighed the possible dangers of sunburn, jellyfish and sharks. But inland lakes and rivers were often forbidden because of the ever-present risks of infection.

This miniature war, with the need for constant vigilance, twenty-four-hour precautions, and personal hygiene – with clean water in desperately short supply – provided an added trial for everyone involved.

Chittagong

By the end of 1943, all four of the MFHs had settled in what was then East Bengal and Assam, which remained the main location for RAF units at this stage of the war. For a while, personnel of 61 and 62 MFHs combined to establish a hospital in the village of Chittagong. The CO and doctors went to look for a suitable site while Jessie Higgins, being the senior nurse, took charge of the nursing team of sisters and male orderlies. They took over a derelict girls' school and for extra wards built *basha* huts, described by Jessie Higgins as 'bamboo buildings with just a roof of bamboo, no windows or doors, but better than canvas tents as at least we had a little breeze. Latrines and a washing area were built for the men.'

> The equipment we had was nothing! Because, of course, every-thing that was supposed to arrive in the Far East never did, they were torpedoed so much. We had one set of so-called theatre instruments, and we had to sterilise with methylated spirit lamps to heat the water. As a field hospital, of course, we only used the operating theatre for emergencies – tiny little room at the end of this old school that we took over . . . and of course we had the snakes, scorpions, every sort of creepy crawly.

Snakes and bugs became the bane of Higgie's life.

No sooner had they set up the hospital than patients came in, soon filling the 150 beds. 'So much sickness,' is what Jessie Higgins remembers.

... dysentery, malaria, jaundice, typhoid, and even smallpox ... very few surgical cases ... mostly abscesses – very common – appendix, leg fractures, and occasionally a real casualty such as gunshot wounds, flying accidents and crashes ...

One thing that brought it home to us was ... we had an air-raid and [Japanese pilots] were shot down. They brought two of these Jap boys in to us. Neither of them were badly wounded, just broken legs and things, but they had to be guarded ... We only had charpoy beds. Exactly the width of a body between the beds, and all these damn mosquito nets and of course the two guards had to sit either side of the bed ...

We had awful problems getting ill boys to eat and drink because the food was absolutely ghastly and of course you couldn't get any oranges or lemons, the only thing you could get was limes. We used to barter them for pilchards in tomato juice ... We had a lot of boys with minor heart conditions, a result of dysentery or typhoid.

They used the precious limes to make squash to add vitamin C to the diet of the very ill patients, but since the two Japanese pilots were not seriously ill they had only plain water. One evening, as Sister Thomas poured drinks by the light of hurricane lamps, one of the Japanese reared up and threw his water into her face.

Of course the two guards jumped on him, and I think even the illest patients in those wards were out of bed. How he wasn't lynched ... It was the most frightening thing! I was on the other side, doing something in the surgical ward, and heard all this noise. Fortunately one of the MOs was around so I shouted for him and we ran across ... it was terrifying ... Very next morning, they were off and we never saw them again.

Jessie Higgins especially remembers working with surgeon Peter Greening, who was not much older than she but a wonderful surgeon. The Far East didn't offer much for a surgeon beyond very basic work, but one particular patient presented an unusual challenge. Flight Lieutenant Mike Bush, a South African pilot with the RAF, had been out on a mission to the jungle in one of the little aircraft which, says Higgie, could land on a sixpence. Having brought back a patient for the hospital, Mike Bush went to hand in his revolver, but somehow the gun went off and shot him in the stomach.

He had twenty-two holes in his intestines! And we couldn't find the bullet! All night! It was dreadful. This dreadful theatre and this silly light . . . Finally, we closed him up, tied up all the holes in the intestines – Peter did, and me giving him the anaesthetic – and of course we didn't dare move him, because we didn't know where the bullet was. We never did find out, until he was finally flown to Calcutta – we had no proper X-ray or anything – and there it was, lodged in between his vertebrae. Another quarter of an inch and he'd have been paralysed.

Anyway . . . he was flown home to England, went to the spinal and head injuries place at Wheatley . . . they couldn't operate. He had that bullet inside him to the day he died – he died last January [1998].

She always wrote to the mothers or wives of patients who couldn't write for themselves and she struck up a friendship with Mike Bush's mother, staying in touch for over fifty years.

Higgie also remembers being permanently wet – either from sweat or from monsoon rains. 'The rain was unbelievable! It would rain for five days at a time and it never stopped POURING down!' Hospital staff were drenched going from *basha* hut to *basha* hut, 'and of course we had those latrines, all in a row, with palm-woven walls between . . . boys from the dysentery ward always out there. I remember going out one day and . . . a terrific blow of wind, and both the walls . . . and there were all these lads . . . I just walked past, thinking, Oh God, Higgins, don't go purple . . .'

A visiting senior matron 'was astounded at the conditions under which we were working'.

Snakes of all types and sizes, bed-bugs galore, cockroaches, ants . . . rats and snakes in the roofs of the huts, and iguanas very active . . . At the monsoon time everywhere was soaking wet, roads and paths all mud, and snakes very obvious . . . [Since] we only had lamps – and electric light if the generator worked – the dark wards were not very welcoming to a sick man . . . We had no pillows and patients had to use their kit-bags . . . Most patients lay in a blanket (no mattress) and possibly a blanket and a sheet in the cooler weather in December and January. Linen was a nightmare as we did not have the facilities for laundering. Lack of so many comforts was heartbreaking.

She need not have worried – her patients found the hospital a haven of comfort. C.E.Beale, of the RAF Regiment, fondly remembers the PMs he met at Chittagong. 'I shall never forget their kindness to me and many others. It was wonderful to find oneself in a very comfortable bed with sparkling white sheets after months of no bed, a groundsheet and a rough blanket.'

An unexpected reunion took place one day. Jessie Higgins 'was walking across the grounds of the hospital when a voice behind me said, "Miss Higgins, I presume?" – and it was my brother!' Her brother was in the army, stationed then in Burma. Her sister Joan was in the navy, seconded to Lord Mountbatten's personal staff. When Mountbatten became C-in-C Far East, the three Higgins siblings managed to meet, 'for one single day! I managed to get across to Calcutta, my brother had just come back from the jungle, and Joan . . . don't know whether she got a flight up, but we all met in Calcutta – so broke, we had about five shillings between us! It was lovely to see them . . . And my mother had no idea where any of us were!'

A visit from the Viceroy

When Lord Wavell visited Chittagong in his role as Viceroy of India, Senior Sister Higgins attended a dinner party in his honour, held at the local United Services Officers' Club.

It was an experience . . . That so-called 'Club' had been one of the tea-planters' clubs – it just had a bar! Every CO of every unit within miles was invited. The matron from the Indian Medical Service hospital, and I, were the only two women, other than Lady Wavell and a lady-in-waiting of some sort. *We* had to turn up in our khaki trousers, khaki kerchief round our neck, khaki bush shirts, and *she* walks in with a tiara, a beautiful grey chiffon dress, with a train, and diamonds . . . talk about feeling like Barnardo's girls!

It was all so *official*! They had a hundred staff. They came on the train. All these waiters . . . it was unbelievable, because we had nothing, no knives and forks, and they brought *everything* – and all the staff with their white gloves on! We were presented to them when they arrived, and then after dinner they had these four little tables with chairs round . . . and everybody that was an official guest was taken round and sat for five minutes at each table and chatted . . . and there's us feeling like nothing, our khakis all perspiration . . . And then, of course, they got on the train and disappeared, went back to Calcutta.

That was the beginning of '44. Lord Mountbatten wasn't in charge then. What a difference when he came. It was like turning a page! Things began to arrive – things we'd been waiting forever for. People came alive. That was when the fun really began, because Mountbatten decided there was no coming out of the jungle in the monsoon.

Until then, when the monsoon came the troops had been withdrawn and fighting virtually ceased until the rains cleared.

62 MFH

After a while, Rona Black and her colleague Jay Gardner rejoined their own unit and moved to a place named Cox's Bazaar, nearer to Calcutta. Rona reported to her mother:

Life here is primitive. We're blessed with electric light but . . . bare wires sticking out of the bamboo, with no sockets and no bulbs . . . We have no furniture at present except our camp kit which we brought from England, and a carpet each . . . Tonight we have a turned-up packing case to write on – in the *basha* – an oil hurricane lamp each, and a glass of rum. We are quite happy, thank you.

The hospital is getting ship-shape at last under our auspices. We think we are a little more appreciated by the orderlies as they see we are here to help, not only to order. We're taking mepacrine now, to try and suppress malaria. We're getting a great number [of malaria cases] in already, so I hate to think of what we shall have when the season is in full swing . . .

The camp is in two small valleys, one taking the medical unit and tents for convalescents, the other the surgical unit and officers. The bamboo huts we live in are most intriguing. The bamboo is split down in narrow strips, opened out quite flat and interwoven with hundreds of others . . . so there's plenty of daylight between the cracks. The door is the same material with the odd bamboo pole to strengthen it and a piece of bamboo strip bound round to make it fast at one side. The windows are the strips of bamboo put criss-cross. There's no glass anywhere for about 300 miles, so the air just blows in and we're thankful for it. The roof is just bamboo criss-crossed with rushes laid on top like thatch, and more bamboo to keep them on.

Sanitary arrangement is very pukka. We have a very deep pit about thirty feet deep and two feet wide, surmounted by a round petrol tin and a pukka wooden seat with lid. The bath is the inevitable canvas square type, just big enough for me to sit cross-legged in, cold water, and a slant in the mud floor to the trench . . .

We are about a quarter of a mile from the 'road', which is a good thing as the dust is frightful. Women and children are employed along a stretch of about 130 miles of road, to throw water . . . to keep the dust down. Our little 'lane' doesn't get watered under this scheme, as we built it, so clouds of dust come sweeping up the valley daily and into the wards . . . All day aircraft buzz overhead. It's very cheering because we feel the Japs are really getting what they deserve. The lads down here are grand, they are doing a wonderful job.

Imphal

In February 1943 a guerilla force of British, Gurkha and Burmese soldiers – the 'Chindits' – marched into the Japanese-occupied jungles of northern Burma, supported by elephants, mules and bullocks, with a few supplies dropped by air. Their successes alarmed and mystified the Japanese, and galvanized morale among the dispirited Allied armies in India, but the main value of the expedition was the lessons learned for the later airborne expedition, which began in late December 1943. It coincided with a fierce Japanese offensive and by the time it ended the myth of Japanese invincibility had been dispelled.

For three months during this long engagement, British and Indian forces were besieged in Imphal, the chief town of the remote Indian border district of Manipur. The steep, jungle-clad hillsides surrounding the town saw some of the most desperate fighting of the war. For both sides, defeat was unthinkable. The RAF made the difference – along with the US Air Force they flew a continuous shuttle service, bringing in supplies and reinforcements and taking out casualties and civilians. For the Japanese besiegers, at the end of an over-extended supply chain, reserves slowly ran out.

Later that year, after the siege was lifted, a New Zealand pilot, hero of eighty-eight dog-fights and with 500 flying hours to his credit, crashed near Imphal and became seriously ill with tetanus. Squadron Leader Doran, the RAF doctor attending him, decided he might benefit from expert nursing, so radioed for nurses and special drugs. As an *Evening Standard* correspondent reported:

> Two Royal Air Force nurses have been flown to Imphal in an old bomber, to help save the life of a New Zealand airman . . . They are Sister Barbara McDonald, of Calne, Wiltshire, and Sister Patricia Dawson, of Leigh-on-Sea, Essex . . . The girls are the first European women to re-enter Manipur since the fighting of five months ago . . . When [they] arrived, Sqn Ldr Doran took them to the patient and said, 'Look what I've brought you.' The airman opened his eyes and said one word: 'Popsies!'

Jungle conditions

An idea of the dangers faced by troops in the Far East may be gleaned from the contents of 'jungle packs', which contained tubes of aspirin (to alleviate pain and fever) and quinine or mepacrine (against malaria); tablets for sterilizing water; a snake-bite outfit; needles and thread, safety pins, and a fishing line with hook and float.

For everyone, supplies were scarce. Rona Black told her mother:

We have room for about 100 patients and are equipped for fifty . . . you can put up a bed here and there but the equipment doesn't arrive. The linen problem is quite acute – no sheets or pyjamas. We have mostly malaria, dysentery and jaundice. We haven't had many very ill patients, but we are thankful as the staff is inadequate.

I long for a comfortable chair, a good film, a decent table to do my writing, a cool refreshing wood of primroses, and our home. We wear khaki, no caps, no stockings, and heavy shoes. I have a pair of native sandals . . .

March 1944: I had a lad in with malaria. He had been out 14 days trying to escape from the Japs. He was in a bad state when he came in here. We tried every kind of treatment, but he died about six days later. It really upset me and that evening I had a quiet weep to myself. Yesterday we had another busy day, admitted 15 new cases of malaria, so we now have topped the 100 mark . . . Half my staff have malaria. The sun is so hot I have to wear a hat now, and sunglasses. We work hard in the morning, sweat in the afternoon, and work in the evening . . .

In the early hours of the morning we admitted a cerebral haemorrhage, another serious case. Tonight I went over at 8.30 p.m. to see how the lad was and the whole way was lit by fireflies darting about – really lovely. The orderlies are wonderful, and would do anything for me. I had more volunteers than I wanted for duty tonight with that sick lad. I give them a great deal of freedom, smoking on duty, etc., and they thoroughly appreciate it . . .

My underclothes have been wrecked by the washerwoman, so I'm living in rags, but no-one cares as we are both the same. We just wash them ourselves now, and wear them rough-dried . . . Jay and I are wearing our oldest clothes and my pants at the moment are the flowery voile ones we bought years ago, with a little vest to match, remember? at Dickens and J. They are, needless to say, falling to pieces . . . I'm wearing my 'Dick' at the moment but we have put in for 'Terri' hats – rather like a girl guide's hat, khaki with a stiff brim and RAF ribbon on one side, very snappy. It's RAF issue.

Three of the four MOs are off sick with malaria, that leaves the CO, the Dental Officer, the other sister and myself to cope. We've had about half the orderlies off with malaria, too, so it's great fun! . . . You are lucky to have fish as we live on hammerhead shark. It's usually done up in batter. It's very tough and tastes bloody awful, putting it mildly . . . We are expecting to move when the monsoon comes, so we shall get away from the malarious area.

Before this could happen, the unit's surgeon, suffering from a third bout of malaria in three months, killed himself with a bullet through the head; then Sister Jay Gardner also went down with malaria and had to be flown to Chittagong.

I flew up with her, in a Moth . . . We were transported by ambulance to the other hospital. I stayed there two days and lazed about. I really was nearly passing out with exhaustion as I had had Jay to nurse and cook for, and the whole hospital to supervise. However, at the end of two days I contacted a Wg Cdr down here who flew up to Calcutta and took me back to the 'drome in the Gp Capt's Chrysler, and so home in his private plane and jeep. We flew along the shore and round the islands, then made inland, circled over the hospital and landed in a paddy field. I felt a little sick going, but the return was superb. I've been on my own for ten days now.

Relief in the hills

Because of these troubles, 62 MFH moved to the hill depot at Shillong, a much cooler spot which offered a better social life, with lots of dances and parties at various local units. Occasionally the medical team swapped places with staff from 61 and 63 MFHs so that the others too might have some relief from the heat.

From Shillong in May 1944, Rona writes:

It's cool, even cold, at night especially. I've had four blankets and a hot water bottle. We have been so energetic, it has been a treat. The orderlies have bucked up their ideas. The first few days they were awful but it nearly always takes a week for them to settle down and get into running order. They called us the 'binding sisters' and so we were, but now they reap the benefit and it's so much easier to be organized. We've had nearly all malaria and dysentery . . . very little nursing except routine. So we have plenty of time for making the hospital interesting, and the diet appetizing.

It's the most lovely country around here – hills, pines, lakes. A lot of rain, but it's so marvellously cool it doesn't really matter. There are also some very good shops – though not as you would imagine them. It's different from Cox's Bazaar, which was very much in the jungle.

On 7 June 1944, she reports: 'I was feeling ropey last night – rather sick, but with the *news of the second front* and a few sherries I changed and went to the dance!' News of the Normandy landings took only a few hours to reach this far corner of the Empire.

FIVE

Towards a second front

At the Casablanca conference of January 1943, the Allied warlords agreed that after they had pushed the enemy out of North Africa the next step must be an invasion of mainland Europe. Such an enormous undertaking needed long and careful planning: they anticipated it would take around eighteen months.

Over the next year, England witnessed a great gathering of troops and materials. American servicemen poured in to charm the female populace, and the accents and uniforms of many other friendly nations became familiar in the streets and pubs. Whole swathes of southern downland sprouted a thick coating of armour – tanks, aircraft, lorries, armoured cars, field guns. People joked that the only thing keeping the laden island from sinking was the support of hundreds of tethered barrage balloons. An elaborate deception was taking place, designed to make the enemy think that the coming invasion would strike near Calais. In fact, the objective was Normandy.

Since 'Operation Overlord' could not succeed without great human cost, the authorities made plans to cope with casualties. RAFH Wroughton was designated the main casualty clearing station (CCS) for wounded troops flown home from Europe. Its available beds would expand to over a thousand, with eighteen extra nursing sisters ready to serve as required. Other sisters were posted to airfields at Down Ampney, Blakehill Farm and Broadhill, all within easy reach of Wroughton and all preparing to act as reception centres for the incoming wounded. Most fortunate of all, in their own estimation, were four PMs who received orders to join the new mobile field hospitals which would follow the troops into occupied Europe.

Under starter's orders

Monica Railton Jones (Mrs Chandler) had the impression that the male staff of 55 MFH felt 'very dubious' when she and her colleague Pam Renton arrived to join them at a large house in Weybridge, in Surrey. The transport sergeant immediately put Monica behind the wheel of a truck and gave her a lesson in driving, through the busy streets of the town. 'The following evening I had to drive a 3-tonner on a night convoy using only reflectors for light – a gruelling experience.' She slowly worked her way through every vehicle with the MFH – every member of the team had to be versatile.

Early in January 1944 the unit moved to Fontwell racecourse, near Bognor Regis, where they erected their tented hospital for the first time and began to practise: pack the equipment, load up the twenty-eight trucks, travel in convoy to a new site, unload, unpack and set up the tents; then pack again, load, convoy . . .

'Fluffy' Ogilvie, who had survived the bombing of both St Athan and Torquay, was working at the RAF Medical Rehabilitation Unit at Loughborough. She was now a war widow – Squadron Leader Donald Ogilvie's bomber had been shot down over Holland, with no survivors, a few months after their wedding. In response, feeling that she 'wanted desperately to make some contribution', Fluffy had asked for permission to serve with one of the mobile field hospitals. She joined 50 MFH, whose winter quarters, like those of 55, were at Fontwell racecourse.

She too found her welcome less than ecstatic. 'We don't want any bloody women in this outfit!' was the general opinion among the medical orderlies. But the sunny Sister Fluffy soon won them round. 'We lived in fields, woods, sunshine and mud, but the wonderful spirit of comradeship . . . made everything worthwhile.'

Based at Fontwell, the MFH teams went on practising mobility. They travelled with their own generators, field telephones, water supplies, kitchens, signals unit, operating theatre, X-ray equipment, dental unit and, of course, all available medical supplies. They knew they were to be part of the coming invasion. The question was, when would it be? While they waited, they enjoyed some fun and laughter – one particular incident left Sister Ogilvie blushing to the roots of her fluffy blonde curls: 'Our unit was visited . . . by some VIPs, including the Air Marshal, Director General of the RAF Medical Service. I was walking towards my tent when I saw them all standing stiffly to attention, saluting my 'smalls' hanging on a line. One of them turned to me and said, "I'm certain they will bring us luck!" '

D minus 30 and counting

At RAFH Halton one bright spring day, twenty-two-year-old WAAF clerk Con Smith (Mrs Gilbert) was summoned to Ward 10 to take dictation from an officer who had been admitted with a minor skin complaint. She was amazed to find herself sitting beside Group Captain Frank Whittle, inventor of the jet engine. She still has his autograph, dated 3 May 1944, to prove it. But she often wishes she had kept the shorthand notes, too. They concerned 'something mysterious called Operation Overlord'. That enigmatic title became far more meaningful a month later, on 6 June 1944 – D-Day.

As spring turned to summer, the RAF and the USAF combined to prepare the way. Attacks on German oil installations virtually stopped production of enemy armaments; in France, to interrupt transport and communications systems, the Allied air forces knocked out such places as marshalling yards and big railway junctions; and finally on the night of 5 June they concentrated on German batteries guarding the Channel coast.

The 'sausage machine'

Fluffy Ogilvie writes:

> I sat in silence in my battle dress and tin hat, with a Red Cross armband prominently on my left arm. Straight ahead, jeeps, trucks and ambulances could be seen mounting the hill in the distance. In spite of the familiar sound of the convoy making its progress, it seemed incredibly still, almost unreal. The memorable day was the fifth of June 1944 and I was setting out on what was to be the greatest adventure of my life.

She and colleague Mollie Giles were the only women in the massive host that day (55 MFH, with Sisters Railton Jones and Renton, was to follow some ten days later). They were heading into the 'sausage-machine', whose funnel lay at Old Sarum, Wiltshire, and whose nozzle lay at the south coast, pointing towards France. The vast concentration area had hard standing for 1,650 lorries, and enough tents to accommodate 8,500 personnel at any one time. The rows of canvas seemed to stretch for miles. Once there, troops were sealed off from the world, behind barbed wire and armed guards. The success of 'Overlord' depended on surprise.

Just after midnight on 6 June, a fleet of landing craft laden with men, guns, tanks, transport and armoured cars, all protected by navy warships, set out to cross the gale-tossed Channel. During the hours of darkness advance troops flying by glider and parachute opened the way, and as daylight came fighter aircraft of the RAF and the USAF went in to protect the first sea landings. Within hours, though at terrible cost in life and hardware, the Allies established several beach-heads, and on the first evening the advance party of four doctors from 50 MFH arrived on the Normandy beaches. One of them, Squadron Leader Grant, was killed during the landing. It was to be some days before his colleagues back at Old Sarum heard the news.

The MFH remained at the concentration area for a few days, during which time Fluffy Ogilvie and Mollie Giles stayed in the WAAF officers' mess, where it was assumed their purpose was to tend the sick among the encamped troops. This caused some puzzlement: 'Do you find much work to do? The chaps must all be pretty fit.' Until the last moment none of the WAAFs knew that the two PMs were actually 'going over' with the troops.

At the MFH one day they were handed emergency packs whose contents included concentrated porridge, some chocolate, a piece of chewing gum, and a tiny box containing a collar stud with a compass at one end. Fluffy thought that if she had to depend on that she would probably end up in Germany! Aware that the 'off' was not far away, that night in her quarters she made sure her back-pack contained everything she might need – tin plate and 'eating irons', with a tin mug dangling from a strap, and, 'very important as far as I was concerned, a little waterproof bag with my Elizabeth Arden make-up ... I wasn't going to land in

Normandy looking a sight! Bright red lipstick did wonders to pull one's face together.'

She and Mollie lay on their beds waiting, in full battle dress, with Red Cross arm bands on their left arms. It was just before midnight when the dispatch rider came to call them, much to the astonishment of one of the WAAF officers who saw them leave.

In pitch darkness, with only reflectors for lights, Fluffy Ogilvie clambered to her familiar seat beside the driver of one of the trucks and they were off, making for the marshalling area at Fareham. Years later, one of the officers told her that he owed her a debt of gratitude: 'I used to say to myself, if she can go, I can go!'

After two days at Fareham, on 11 June they travelled the final few miles towards the 'hards' at Gosport – the beach where they would embark. Just after dawn they paused in the town and housewives brought the troops tea, and hot water for a refreshing shave. Some of the men accepted invitations to breakfast in homely kitchens. A woman gave Fluffy a tin of peaches, 'such a treasured possession in the war. I sat on the pavement and ate the contents of the tin with relish. Morale was tremendous . . . the generosity and kindness of the people did so much . . .'

Finally, as the sea-borne convoy continued to move slowly out into the Solent, they boarded their landing craft. 'In addition to all the tanks and vehicles, it carried hundreds of troops . . . It seemed enormous to me . . .' What struck Fluffy most was the silence maintained by nearly everyone: the enormity of the undertaking held them in thrall. But she does not remember being afraid. 'A couple of men started counting the vessels aloud, they reached two hundred . . . I felt strangely elated as there came a roar of aircraft . . .'

All day Allied aircraft came and went overhead. The landing craft's commander offered the two women use of his cabin, but mostly they remained with the men. Then night, and silence, descended. 'There was an eerie darkness filled with differing sounds from nearby vessels. Troops sat on the deck, in every available space . . . In the comfort of the cabin I slept soundly for a few hours – I remember crawling into the bunk in full battle dress, thinking, I'm going to sleep if it kills me . . .' Somehow she did manage to sleep.

Next morning they were near the Normandy coast, with the sky full of Allied aircraft, fighters taking off from a strip near the shore, and navy warships firing their guns to answer enemy shore batteries. The landing craft with the two nursing sisters on board waited for hours for the tide to allow them in close enough to land; but the first lorry down the ramp tipped into a vast mine-hole in the shingle, blocking the way. They had to wait again, while more hours passed, and darkness came. And still the guns kept firing.

> At some stage we became aware that disembarkation had started again. I remember standing next to Mollie in the dark, on the left side of the lower deck, facing the ramp. The inside towered above us. I felt as though I was inside a monstrous whale. I couldn't see what was happening in the darkness but I was very aware of the noisy vehicles and personnel dashing about. I felt No emotion, nothing at all, just standing there with my pack on my back looking down towards the ramp . . . We didn't speak a word. Suddenly we were told to go. We scrambled down the ramp and the next thing I remember was feeling sand under my feet. I had landed on Juno/Red Beach, in pitch darkness, on June 12th 1944.

They stepped into history, being the first women to land with 'Overlord', several days ahead of any others.

Into battle

Fluffy and Mollie spent a short while in an underground bunker with some appreciative troops. The men had prided themselves on being among the first to enter France; now to their amazement they found two slender RAF nursing sisters along with them! One of the men joked, 'Watch out, Adolf, you've had it now!' Amid confusion, under night skies filled with the boom and glare of gunfire and the glow of red-hot shells that the men called 'flaming onions', the two PMs accepted a lift in a lorry going to the assembly area, where they rejoined their colleagues.

The area was so closely packed with men, vehicles, ammunition dumps and anti-aircraft guns that attacking enemy planes could hardly fail to hit something. The waiting slit trenches – short ditches dug into the ground and covered by a tent – looked very inviting to Fluffy and Mollie, who took off their packs and occupied a trench each. Exhaustion did the rest: 'I put my tin hat over my face and fell fast asleep.'

Next day the MFH in convoy moved slowly amid active tanks and firing guns, past signs bearing a skull and crossbones with the words *Achtung Minen* (Beware mines). The battle went on, guns booming both in front and behind, shells whistling overhead. But a cleared track, denoted by white markers, led them to their allocated site, in a field where they erected their hospital tents in tidy lines, dug slit trenches beneath the canvas, and laid out a huge flag, red cross on white ground. As the first of the wounded came in they sprang to work, saddened by the need but relieved that at last they could do the work for which they had been training for so long. 'Ambulances arrived in a long convoy. There were just over two hundred surgical cases to be evacuated, and many in poor shape. Some had to remain for immediate surgery . . .' Fluffy found herself changing field dressings, preparing intravenous infusions and giving injections of morphine and precious penicillin. She and Mollie distributed gallons of hot tea, fed those who could eat, handed out urinals and bed-pans and lit cigarettes for men too wounded to do it themselves. Most of all they talked to the men, trying to keep up their spirits, rewarded by smiles on bloodied faces and warmth in weary eyes.

More ambulances took the men on, some to return home by sea, more urgent cases to fly from the improvised airstrip nearby. The two PMs took it in turns to accompany casualties to where, amid clouds of white dust, trusty Dakotas came and went on a runway that was no more than a stretch of ground flattened by the Royal Engineers and covered with wire meshing. In the nearby woods tank battles continued, while Allied warships fired from the shore and German guns answered from inland.

When she reached the first Dakota, Fluffy was surprised to see WAAF nursing orderlies on board, the first WAAF to take part in the air evacuation. Nursing of casualties in transit was a risky business: the airstrips came under fire on occasion; the transport aircraft wore no guardian red cross; and, as WAAF Corporal Biddy Spencer (Mrs Wilson) recalls, the air ambulance nursing orderlies went into service 'without 'chutes because their stretcher patients couldn't have 'chutes; and there were casualties. The ones I knew were Leading Aircraftwomen, probably being paid around 24/6d [£1.22] per week.'

Within six days of their arrival in Normandy, the staff of 50 MFH had seen 1,023 casualties safely aboard flights for home. One of the Dakotas was struck by flak as it flew out and Fluffy Ogilvie later heard that it had seventy holes in its fuselage, but by some miracle no one had been hurt.

A vicious storm blew up on 18 June and lasted for five days, delaying the Allied build-up and destroying or stranding 800 ships. The hiatus also allowed the Germans time to redeploy. Torrential rain poured down, along with shrapnel, churning the ground into mud and preventing aircraft from flying close-support missions, which included air-ambulance evacuation. All the time casualties kept arriving to await the return of the Dakotas. Fluffy Ogilvie noted worriedly:

> Some of the injured were in a poor state. One night was particularly noisy, due to the gunfire and shelling and we were all busy . . . I stopped by one of the lads, who was very poorly, lapsing into periods of unconsciousness . . . This time he had his eyes wide open and said in a perfectly clear voice, 'Where's your tin hat? Who do you think you are, a blinking fairy?' . . . I went to find my hat and hurriedly put it on. I returned to reassure him, to find he had just died. It was an incident that shook me greatly and that I could never forget.

They were followed into Europe by 52 MFH, staffed by the Royal Canadian Air Force, which erected its tents near Caen. Then, in early July, 55 MFH also went through the 'sausage machine' and set up in what Monica Railton Jones describes as 'an orchard two miles inland at a small place called Banville next to the airfield . . . We received casualties immediately from the forward Field Dressing Stations . . . Air Evacuation was very successful . . . We also had quite a number of German PoWs . . . many of them were young arrogant Nazi youth, and although badly wounded were very aggressive.'

A more grateful patient that July was Lieutenant Eric Brown of the Royal Artillery.

> Having been burned and wounded as a result of a direct hit on my Mobile A/Tk Gun (Tank Destroyer), I had been rescued from the battlefield and taken in by the Canadian Field

Hospital near Caen. Swathed in bandages and plaster from head to foot, I was taken to Mulberry Harbour by an RAF ambulance. For hours and hours we waited to be embarked and during all that time the two RAF nurses took the greatest care of me . . . the courage they gave me to soldier on was absolutely vital . . . PMRAFNS were a really VITAL LINK in my preservation. Thank God.

Casevac procedure

As soon as a new landing strip opened, transport aircraft brought in urgent stores or extra troops and went out laden with casualties. Fighter planes gave them cover. As the fighting front moved away, the airstrip would be extended to an airfield, with a casevac unit capable of tending up to 200 patients as they waited for the next air ambulances. Wounded men from any nearby medical unit, whether RAF, army or civilian, would be examined, fed, treated, and operated on if necessary, or, if not considered well enough to be flown out, would be sent back to a field hospital.

The forward air shuttle service removed thousands of casualties from under the noses of the enemy, taking them straight to Britain at first and later to temporary base hospitals in France, Holland and Belgium. The same aircraft returned again to the front bringing stores, equipment, and medical supplies, including around 162 lb of blood and 700 lb of drugs, every day.

Back in Britain, RAF Down Ampney was one of three airfields which served as 'feeders' to the casualty clearing station at Wroughton. The other two chosen airfields closed down before the end of 1944 after problems with flooding, leaving Down Ampney to cope. More of the ubiquitous and endlessly useful wooden huts, erected near the airfield, formed emergency sick quarters manned by RAF doctors, PMs and members of the medical service.

A dozen or so WAAF drivers worked at Down Ampney. Among them, Kay Chamant (Mrs Watts) drove 'one of the fleet of small standard ambulances, all of which were fitted up inside with supports and rails to receive four stretchers, two on either side'. As the laden Dakotas came winging in, she and the other drivers revved up their engines, forgot missed meals and headed for the aerodrome.

About three-quarters of all patients were stretcher cases. They would be transferred from aircraft to ambulance by trainee aircrew and Italian prisoners of war drafted in as bearers. Kay Chamant drove her wounded passengers slowly and carefully back to the emergency medical huts, where, 'seeing the Princess Mary's Sisters always looking so neat and fresh in their blue and white uniforms I often wondered how they managed this, working as they did among battle-soiled boots and uniforms and the bodies of men on stretchers in confined spaces of little huts as they arrived off planes, before they had been examined, washed, shaved and fed.'

Some patients came fresh from battle, with only field dressings on their wounds; some arrived with the letters 'M' or 'T' written on their foreheads to indicate that morphine had been given or a tourniquet applied. Medical staff graded them as: A (immediate emergency treatment), B (less urgent) or C (suitable for transfer straight to other units). Most of them went first to Wroughton RAF hospital, which took patients in every other night. They stayed two nights before being transferred to other hospitals, freeing the beds for a fresh intake.

As Winifred Gardner (Mrs Penman) recalls, a prisoner-of-war camp was situated 'at the far end of the hospital's vast grounds, occupied originally by Germans, then by Italians. They made a valuable contribution to the work force. Some made efficient ward orderlies, others cleaners and gardeners.'

For Joan White (Mrs Cool), her 'first patient after D-Day was a Canadian soldier from the Regina Regiment, still in his uniform with field dressings ...' After Arnhem (17 September 1944), patients down one side of the ward all had fans playing over their legs 'to see how far their circulation was reaching down their limbs in order to decide how extensive an amputation was necessary'.

The flow of casualties through Down Ampney and Wroughton steadily reduced as the Allied armies moved on into Germany and in their wake more permanent hospitals, RAF and army, opened across western Europe.

European hospitals

That summer, Matron Helen W. Cargill, in charge of nurses at the convalescent hospital at Matlock, was summoned to London where

she learned that France was to be her next posting. Just as she was
leaving the Air Ministry a flying bomb exploded nearby. Though
shaken she was unharmed and, after a few moments, continued her
journey to Austin Reed of Oxford Street, to order more uniform
dresses. Only as she bent over to write her cheque did she realize
how narrow an escape she had had – showers of splintered glass fell
from the 'Dick Turpin' hat which had acted as her shield.

Her new unit, No. 8 RAFGH, formed at RAF Aston Down in
Gloucestershire. Its convoy of trucks and equipment, with some
staff, went through the 'sausage machine' and opened temporarily
in Bayeux, France, on 30 August 1944. Its contingent of twenty-two
PMs went by air, in an RAF Dakota, flying from Northolt. Helen
Cargill comments, 'Never before had so many "Dick Turpins" been
seen on any airfield and we caused quite a stir . . . The sun was shin-
ing and it was a perfect day for our flight, which took two hours.'

Christina Watson (Mrs Hunter), one of the sisters travelling to
join No. 8 RAFGH, remembers wearing battledress and sitting on
her camp kit on the floor of the Dakota. She too writes of the
sunlight, which showed up 'many wrecked ships and plenty of
debris floating', in the Channel below. When they reached the
airstrip near Bayeux, she heard a sergeant exclaim, 'Heavens,
they've sent women!'

No. 8 RAFGH, despite its impressive title, turned out to be six
marquees in an orchard, with sisters accommodated in smaller tents
in an adjoining field. Christina Watson says, 'water was in short
supply, a tanker came twice a day and filled our buckets. Food was
mainly white bread (so white it looked bleached – and was supplied
by the Americans) – and corned beef just as it came from the tin, or
fried.'

The hospital had ten wards, each with twenty beds. All of them
were soon filled by patients 'pleased to have proper beds and sheets.
We had started to use penicillin – what a wonder drug that was!'

As they soon discovered, some of their sleeping tents were less
than waterproof – the occupants came to breakfast looking as if
they'd just washed their hair: they remedied the problem by sleeping with towels for turbans. They also resorted to wellington boots
to combat the mud. They did their own washing, while a mobile
laundry dealt with hospital linen and patients' clothing.

Helen Cargill felt the people of Normandy were 'not at first amicably disposed towards the British'. This was partly because of the heavy bombing they had endured, and partly because the Germans had treated them well, had plenty of money to spend and gave sweets to children – largesse which the impecunious, sweet-rationed Brits could not match.

One night Helen woke to hear peculiar noises which turned out to be a horse sniffing round her tent – farm animals shared the orchard. Apples and mushrooms grew there too, a welcome addi-tion to the dreary diet of bread and bully beef, and farmers' wives sometimes gave flowers to brighten the hospital. Though social life was minimal, off duty one could walk in fields and country lanes, and another small blessing was a generator which powered both lights and sterilizer – and an iron! It did not, however, supply heat and when the nights grew cold paraffin stoves warmed the marquee wards. A bucket of water placed on top of each stove by night sisters as they came on duty provided a mug of hot water for each patient's shave next morning.

The cold prevented Christina Watson from sleeping, but 'my "great treat" came when the theatre instruments were unwrapped – they came in large sacks, padded with shavings and straw. I thought this the best bed I ever had, and so warm!'

No. 8 RAFGH had been near Bayeux for six weeks when the PMs heard the exciting news of the liberation of Brussels and the unit prepared for a move to a proper hospital in Belgium. Matron Cargill and her nurses travelled to Brussels by air, at first sharing a hospital with an MFH and an army general hospital. However, the number of army casualties far exceeded those of the RAF, so in October the PMs 'quite cheerfully packed up their wards for the second time', and moved to L'Hôpital St Gilles on the outskirts of the city – the same hospital where nurse Edith Cavell had hidden prisoners during the Great War. In the Second World War it had been used by the *Luftwaffe* and some of the beds still displayed the names of captured British pilots. The Germans' haste to evacuate had caused them to abandon much of their equipment – the oper-ating theatre still bore evidence of the last operation to be performed, and bottles of three-star French brandy displayed labels stamped 'German Army Stores. Commercial sale forbidden'. Sister Eve Loxston (Mrs Hall) took one of these bottles home with her when she flew back for some Christmas leave.

She adds, 'One of the sisters always called out "Hello darlings" when she came on duty. When an air raid was on and the flying bombs started coming over, the patients would say, "We can't have these darlings frightened by the doodlebugs!" They would then break into song so that the sisters, busy with the dressings, would not hear the sound of the bombing outside.' To this day whenever she hears the voice of Edith Piaf singing 'La Vie en Rose' it reminds her of those times.

Living under the path of the V1s and, later, the V2s could be nerve-wracking. The sisters knew very well where the missiles were heading and every now and then one of the rockets failed and came down over Belgium or Holland. One of those 'noisy nights' was 21 December 1944, when a flying bomb landed on a tenement block not far from St Gilles and No. 8 RAFGH took in many of the casualties. They themselves escaped with only slight injury to two sisters, plus the shattering of several windows – a nuisance in midwinter, with glass hard to come by in war-torn Europe.

At 50 MFH, Fluffy Ogilvie and Mollie Giles had been joined by Ellen Robison and Mary Griffiths. During the long and terrible battle for Caen they had been at Camilly, close enough to hear the noise of guns, rockets and aircraft, and at night the skies seemed on fire. Many severe burns cases came in. 'Part of the treatment was to cover the areas, after initial cleansing, with a very thick application of Tulle Gras, impregnated with an antibiotic, then the limbs and body, if necessary, encased in a loose plaster. This was more efficient than anything else in our field conditions for their subsequent journey by air . . .'

When thunderstorms kept air ambulances away, burns patients encased in plaster lay waiting in the tents for days. One day, to their horror, the nurses saw maggots crawling from the plaster on a man's leg. They decided to remove the plaster and reapply the dressings, but to their surprise the healing process was well begun. It continued so after the patient returned to hospital in Britain.

At the end of August they moved through the 'liberated' city of Caen, where bulldozers had cleared a route through the rubble left by the bombing. Whole streets lay in shattered mounds littered with the charred remains of German equipment and dead pets. The human dead had been removed by burial squads before the convoys went through, but, Fluffy recalls, 'the stench of death was still heavy in the air'. Further on, in Paris, three days after General de Gaulle had led in the Allied forces, liberation celebrations were still in full swing. She and the other nurses enjoyed being greeted, kissed and fêted by so many friendly, happy people, laughing through tears of joy and relief.

They pushed on, heading north in stages, opening up their hospital to deal with casualties, speeding them on their way and then packing up to move again. At Eindhoven, in Holland, the MFH housed itself for the first time in a proper building – St Joseph's Hospital, one of the most modern civilian hospitals in Europe, where they were joined by the Canadian-staffed 52 MFH. The two units had been leap-frogging each other across France and now, to their mutual pleasure, they were to work in close harmony. The building had been untouched by the bombing and street fighting, and the MFH remained there over the winter.

Before long, local nurses and VADs swelled the strength. One of the Dutch nurses spoke fluent German, which was a great help in dealing with the fifty-five German patients who had become prisoners of war and were kept under guard. Fluffy Ogilvie enjoyed being back in a proper hospital, walking along solid corridors and tending patients in clean, well-equipped wards – and sleeping in a real bed again. They made friends with the Dutch people and at times they took in Dutch patients, including two boys peppered with burns that glowed in the dark – they had been playing near a sulphur bomb when it exploded.

One of the Dutch helpers, an attractive young person who spoke perfect English, told of escaping through the German lines with only the clothes she stood up in. She made many friends among the Allied personnel – until the day she was uncovered as a German spy. A complete PMRAFNS uniform had gone missing and when the girl was arrested the military police found a quantity of money in different currencies hidden in her mattress.

Over that winter, while the battle front advanced ever deeper into Germany, nursing staff had time to relax at the RAF Club. Celebrities paid morale-boosting visits. There was even skating on a frozen lake. And at Christmas the two MFHs threw a party for 200 Dutch children, saving rations for weeks to supply them all with sacks bulging with toys, chocolate, wooden clogs and rosy apples. St Nicholas and his traditional assistant 'Black Peter' gave out the gifts; then the young guests enjoyed a Mickey Mouse film show before going down to the dining room for a feast.

Last salute from the Luftwaffe

On New Year's Day 1945, horror returned to both Brussels and Eindhoven when the *Luftwaffe* staged their last vengeful raids on nearby airfields.

In Brussels many of the PMs from No. 8 RAFGH had attended a New Year's party at the Regent's Palace, Headquarters of 2nd Tactical Air Force. To Christina Watson it seemed 'a very splendid place – and food likewise, and plenty of champagne – Air Marshal Cunningham made a speech where he likened it to the grand ball given on the eve of Waterloo'. The likeness deepened when the *Luftwaffe* struck before dawn next morning.

By that time Monica Railton Jones was working with No. 1 Casualty Air Evacuation Unit, sited near the airfield at Evere in Brussels. 'On New Year's morning we had a surprise raid by German Junkers 88, who strafed the airfield just as we were entering the mess for breakfast. We had no breakfast that day but all got rapidly into the vehicles and went to the airfield . . .'

At the hospital in the city, Christina Watson and her colleagues 'worked all day and into the night in both theatres [while] minor injuries were treated in the corridor, like a casualty department. The *Luftwaffe* did not return again.' Similarly, the airborne attack on Eindhoven caused an influx of casualties at St Joseph's Hospital – eighty-two of them within the first hour; the chapel which was used to receive them soon filled with stretchers and Fluffy Ogilvie walked with the surgeon as he made quick decisions on who to treat first, who could wait, and who, sadly, had to be passed by. 'Everyone gave a hand. The aircraftmen who were not medical orderlies were a tremendous help . . . One of my most vivid memories was seeing them continuously mopping up blood . . .'

To their amazement, on 2 January Fluffy Ogilvie and Mollie Giles learned that their names had appeared in the New Year's Honours List. Both of them had been awarded the MBE for their work in Normandy. Soon afterwards, VIPs including Air Marshal Sir Harold Whittingham, Director General of RAF Medical Services, with Matron-in-Chief of the PMRAFNS Miss Gladys

Taylor, arrived at the hospital. Fluffy was not impressed: 'We didn't take too kindly to officialdom after all we had been through. Red tape in our lives had gone by the board. However, we were determined to put on a dignified performance.' After months in battle dress while under canvas, they dressed up in their smartest white uniforms with their blue capes and flowing white head-dresses with RAF wings at the back. The visit went well but, as the VIPs were leaving, a huge truck went by carrying some Canadian aircrew who called out, 'Hiya, Fluffy!' Matron-in-Chief was not amused!

Endgame in Europe

Inexorably, the Allies marched on towards the Rhine and beyond, while from the east the Russians advanced, both forces closing in on Berlin and the bunker where Hitler lurked. Following the troops, 50 MFH convoyed deeper and deeper into Germany. Fluffy Ogilvie enjoyed being under canvas again: 'We began to see columns of civilians, mostly just walking with their belongings, but some had various forms of transport. This time there were no waves or smiles . . .' At the Rhine their means of crossing was a pontoon bridge, but they had to wait as a long column of German PoWs trudged over the river, making towards them. 'We stood by the ambulance in complete silence. I seemed to be witnessing inevitable despair. We waited until the last prisoner and their guards were over [then] our convoy started moving . . . it was quite an historic moment, crossing this famous river . . .' On they drove, past burnt-out German vehicles and gutted buildings. Numbed by so much devastation, they reached their next intended site and once again set up their unit. They found their workload lighter than expected – by that time the Allies were making good headway and, with victory near, the human toll had lessened.

The next advance took the MFH to Celle, twenty miles north of Hanover and near to Belsen. The PMs themselves did not visit the detention camp, but the medical officers did. Just four days after liberation the scene was horrendous: 'The dead were still being buried and hundreds of emaciated victims were near death. Dirt and excreta everywhere . . . stench overpowering . . .' Accustomed as they were to witnessing horror, the MOs came back physically sickened.

The strongest of Belsen's former prisoners were to be flown to hospital in Belgium. They arrived at the airstrip in ambulances and orderlies carefully set the stretchers on the grass near the runway. That was when Fluffy became aware of the overpowering stench and remembered how pilots had said the stink of Belsen sometimes got into their planes if they flew low over the camp. She felt stunned. These tragic people looked like old men. Their eyes haunted her, staring and almost lifeless, without emotion. She wasn't even sure whether they knew what was happening. She did give them the odd drink and saw to their comfort, but what she now finds very sad is that she didn't smile at any of them. Perhaps she was, this time, just too shocked to react in her usual cheery way. When the last of them had been loaded, she and the others simply stood and watched until the plane took off. They were deeply affected, feeling helpless.

While they stayed in Celle, the war ended. A corporal rushed past the tent shouting 'It's all over!' and everyone became very emotional. But after all they had seen and experienced it was hard to take in the reality of peace at last.

No. 50 MFH moved on again to Luneberg Heath, to Kreussen, near Fassberg. While working there, Fluffy was able to return by air to Holland and visit Flushing, where her husband Donald had died. The area had been deliberately flooded as a defence against the German takeover and they were taken in a little motor-boat along drowned streets to the hill where the cemetery lay like an island. She placed some flowers 'on the grave we had come to find'.

After only two weeks at Fassberg they moved to Schleswig, on the Baltic. The date was 1 June 1945, a few days under a year since they landed in Normandy.

No. 50 MFH finally disbanded in April 1946 and Fluffy Ogilvie flew home to her next posting, at RAFH Cosford. Weeks later she was off to Palestine, then Egypt and Aden. It was in Egypt that she met Major Bower, the man who was to become her second husband and the cause of her leaving the PMRAFNS in 1949.

Matron Helen Cargill returned to Ely from Brussels in May 1945 and her career continued. In 1948 she became the Service's fifth matron-in-chief.

As for No. 8 RAFGH, it left Brussels in September 1945 and settled to care for post-war RAF personnel from a base in Rinteln –

in the valley of the River Weser, not far from the Pied Piper town of Hamelin (which, happily, was untouched by bombs).

In the eleven months between D-Day, 6 June 1944, and VE Day, 8 May 1945, the RAF evacuated 77,348 patients to the UK from the Continent. Figures for 1944, the busiest casevac year, show that across all the theatres of war almost 300,000 patients were evacuated by the RAF, all without a single flying accident.

The war with Germany was over. In the Far East, the war against Japan had still some months to go.

SIX

Dressing down

In January 1945 the Nursing Advisory Board proposed a new beret-type hat instead of the unpopular 'storm-cap', and on the wards button-through coat-dresses were to replace the old, gathered-waist style. However, PMs in the Far East had already made their own, unauthorized, adjustments.

In 1944, the new chief principal matron (the first to hold that post) had arrived at Chittagong to be shown around by Senior Sister Jessie Higgins: 'We'd all got into khaki trousers and kerchiefs and what have you, and she was appalled to see nursing officers dressed like that.' The visitor particularly wanted to know why no sister was wearing mosquito boots. Higgie had tried them and 'they left you red raw – they came right up your thighs! . . . So I said, "Well, ma'am, I'd like *you* to try those boots." (Cheeky, really, other girls were saying, "Don't you say a word!") But of course she couldn't even wear them for one night, so that was forgotten.'

Rona Black had had a visitor, too. Writing again to her mother, she enclosed copies of some photos, saying, 'If you are half as amused as I am about this, you'll be sure to have a good laugh.' A certain Wing Commander Webb, of the Inter-Service Research and Development Section (Clothing and Equipment), faced with accoutring some Canadian army nurses for the Far East, visited 62 MFH to observe conditions and ascertain what the well-dressed nursing sister should wear while in India. He took three pictures as examples – Rona holding up a scuffed mosquito boot, a pair of khaki slacks and a crumpled khaki dress. She herself is wearing an unironed khaki drill dress, with huge black buttons and four bulging patch pockets, fetchingly accessorized with puttees and black lace-up shoes! (See illustration number 14.)

Calcutta

A signal dated December 1944 ordered Jessie Higgins to report to the principal medical officer (PMO) at Calcutta. She flew down to the city, where the RAF had taken over

> . . . this huge old Indian school. Huge ceilings, went up for ever . . . there wasn't a bed, wasn't a chair, wasn't a sheet . . . The PMO said to me, 'It's all yours. If you go to the accounts department, they'll give you the money and you just go down to the souk, the market, and buy all the things you want.' I had to employ all the domestic staff; I had to get the nursing officers' mess ready . . . I don't know how I did it.

No. 9 RAFGH Calcutta, as it became, took over from an army transit hospital sited in La Martinière School. This one-time palace, inevitably filthy and impossible to clean, had wards opening off each other and some lavatories could be reached only via the tiny kitchen. One sphygmomanometer (for measuring blood pressure) and one inaccurate weighing machine totalled its clinical equipment, while laboratory facilities comprised one small room – sink, water tap, and partitioned shelter containing bucket latrines. The carefully locked 'cholera cabinet' held nothing but button-cleaning materials. And this hospital was due to take all RAF patients from nearby units on New Year's Day! Undaunted, Jessie Higgins set about the task.

In the midst of her labours, still in her working khaki, she had to hurry to the station to meet a contingent of eighty sisters arriving from Bombay. They had been four days cooped up on a train, wearing their heavy white tricoline. Higgie 'knew exactly what they'd all been through'.

> But no matron with them. And no letter from Air Ministry saying, 'You're to take over and do the best you can, Miss Higgins,' not a word . . . I gave them the first day off, but said, 'The next day it's sleeves up and just see what you've got to

do.' But they were marvellous! Every one of them. There they were up to their eyebrows in soap-suds, and making up beds, and there was every Tom, Dick and Harry from the market bringing in all the stuff . . .

Meantime . . . the doctors and ancillary staff, quartermaster . . . they all came out in a bunch. Fortunately I knew the physician very well, I'd been his ward sister for a couple of years, and the other chap – a VD man!

With Christmas only a few days away and the hospital due to open at New Year, members of the Aircrew Club in Calcutta asked permission to invite all the sisters to a dance on Boxing Night. Senior Sister Higgins replied, 'If they can get the hospital ready they can come.'

Well, they worked like Trojans, so that by Christmas Day we could have taken people in, all the beds were made . . . mind you, they only had sheets on them, no blankets or anything . . . Must have been over three hundred patients we actually took in on New Year's Day, from all the different army hospitals – there was the Indian Army Service, and the Army Nursing Service, and a lot of ratings, naval people . . . they came from all these odd hospitals all round Calcutta . . . by five o'clock that night there they all were. The doctors had never nursed anyone with dysentery in their lives . . . And of course the sisters, most of them, had never been out of England before, let alone the Far East. All went down with snips and snows and tummy ache . . .

RAF hospitals, South East Asia Command

As the Allies pushed the enemy back through Burma, new casualties demanded attention and longer-term cases needed beds. Apart from Calcutta, three more RAF general hospitals opened in 1945: No. 11 settled in Allahabad, No. 12 in Cawnpore, with No. 10 at Karachi, surrounded by the Sind Desert. As the only European hospital for some hundred miles, No. 10 boasted a female wing, including a maternity ward, for servicewomen and families.

More nursing sisters came to augment the staffs of all three units. Among a large party who arrived aboard *Orontes* was Maureen Lumley. 'We had three Matrons with us. One went with about 45 sisters to Karachi; another took a similar number to Cawnpore; the rest of us went to Calcutta, by train.'

Jessie Higgins was still acting matron in Calcutta. She never did discover what had delayed the new matron and sisters, 'whether they'd been held up, or torpedoed'.

> The hospital had been open about five weeks before they arrived . . . and she gave me hell because she had been told that *she* was going to open No. 9 RAF Hospital. She really was unkind to all of us – all the girls that were there then. Then she brought this whole bunch more out with her. All the girls that were there with me were intended for all the field hospitals, not for the general hospital . . . PMO was furious about it all. He asked me if I'd be happier going back to Chittagong and I said, 'Oh, yes, please, let me go back to the jungle!' So he said, 'I think we'll just inform matron that you're being posted.' The joke was . . . news got back to Air Ministry that the hospital had been opened by a very junior sister . . . Nothing to do with me, I'd been posted there to do it . . .

Good news from Europe

In a letter dated May 1945, Rona Black tells her mother of reaction to the victory in Europe:

> Everyone went quite mad. But the war out here means so much more we couldn't be over-enthusiastic – and we don't see an early settlement, either . . . What relieves us most is the fact that all those who are left are safe. It must be grand to be at home at this time.

Another MFH – No. 67 – had settled at Kyaukpyu on Ramree Island, just off the west coast of Burma. One of the sisters who served with it (now Mrs Joy Knowles, of New Zealand) remembers they were miles away from the fighting but 'close enough to feel the earth rumble and see the explosion into the sky of flaming mud'.

RAF Corporal Denis Winstone, a patient stricken with a tropical wasting disease, took away more lyrical memories:

One of the nursing sisters arranged for a dozen or so stretcher cases to be taken down to the nearby beach and placed in a circle on the sand. On that warm moonlit tropical night we lay beneath the stars with land crabs scurrying around us and fireflies and other insects flitting round the hurricane lamp. In the centre of the circle the nursing sister sat with her portable gramophone, winding the handle ... I can only remember one of the 78 rpm records she played. It was 'The Dance of the Sugar Plum Fairy' ...

Meanwhile, No. 61 MFH, still in Chittagong, now had the benefit of eight PMs on its staff. Jessie Higgins was relieved to be back with them, though the food was awful: 'Corned beef came squelching out of tins ... I lived on mangoes.' Her friend 'Tommy' Thomas (Mrs McGregor) remembers a night when 'the makeshift cookhouse went up in flames, after which the cook managed with two sheets of corrugated iron over the stove – he really did wonders with bully beef every day, no fresh vegetables and very little fresh fruit'. She has never forgotten the wonderful boys whom she met and nursed, especially those who were never to return to their distant homes. 'We did have some very ill boys,' Jessie Higgins agrees. 'Jaundice was one of the main things. And typhoid. We even had smallpox. I don't know how many times I was vaccinated in those two years.'

Into Burma

With the war front moving ever southward, clearing Burma of its occupying enemy, the MFH expected to be moved any day. The signal came in July 1945, summoning Jessie Higgins and surgeon Peter Greening to Rangoon.

That was the first time we realised the war was nearly over, because Rangoon had been absolutely saturated with Japs. Off we went, in an old Dakota, sitting on the floor of the aircraft, sliding about. It took about three hours, and we had to land on Mingaladon, which we had been bombing for months. Poor aircraft came down, in and out of pot-holes ...

We arrived and, of course, nobody expected us – every-

where you went, nobody expected you. Peter and I didn't
know one end of Rangoon from another, but we were told,
just go out and find a building, suitable for a hospital. We
finally settled for a building without a roof, but it had water
and electricity.

When the rest of the unit arrived, they needed accommodation:

We found four beautiful houses out on Lake Victoria, which
had belonged to the Directors and local Chairman of the
Burmese Oil Company, but they'd all been stripped. No bolts,
no locks, no taps, no toilet seats . . . Hadn't been there more
than a month when a new Commander-in-Chief was posted
out and he liked our house, so we had to go into horrible little
places, like cheap four-roomed bungalows, nothing in them.
Just snakes. [How she detested snakes!] Oh, snakes until they
came out of your ears . . . so bad in Rangoon, mainly because
of the monsoon drains . . . So it was decided we'd have to
have a crew of coolies to come and catch them. They had to
chop their heads off, lay out the rest of the body and at night
the sergeant or whoever would go round and count them all
and pay them whatever it was – about 1/3d [6p] a head.
    And then we had the trouble with the dacoits [robbers] . . .
looting was terrible. There was never any glass anywhere, just
iron bars across the windows. You'd lie in your bed at night,
four or five to a room . . . and all these mosquito nets and
wretched camp beds and things . . . You'd lie in bed and you'd
see these poles coming through the window, with a knife, and
a hook, and they'd pinch anything they could pick up. We
never attempted to move. It really was not funny.

War's end

In the closing stages of the war, two new MFHs formed part of the
allied 'Tiger Force', preparing to invade Japan. However, as their
convoy reached the Admiralty Islands, news came of the atom
bomb strikes on Hiroshima and Nagasaki. Japan's subsequent
capitulation ended the need for invasion and Tiger Force separated
back into its individual units. The two MFHs, Nos. 80 and 81, were

diverted, one to Hong Kong, the other to Singapore, to give medical aid to released prisoners of war and to the forces who were mopping up the last of the Japanese stragglers.

No. 81 MFH was the first RAF hospital in Singapore, the embryo for the later SSQ at RAF Seletar. No. 80, with two nursing sisters on its ration strength, took over the Central British School in Hong Kong. The school building was relatively clean (with 'only slight insect infestation'), but stripped of all but its basic fabric. Looters had removed all fixtures, including floor tiles – they had even taken the plaster off the walls. Apart from that, writes Squadron Leader (Rtd) Cedric Rosenvinge, who was deputy CO of 5358 Wing, RAF Airfield Construction Branch, the place was in 'a fairly clean condition'.

Somehow, No. 80 MFH swiftly opened adequate wards for all ranks of air personnel, but the senior of the two sisters

> . . . was not entirely satisfied with the feat and asked the Chief Executive Officer for some white sheets, only to be curtly informed that there weren't any, but she could have as many service-issue blankets as she wished. That was not good enough for the lady and her powers of persuasion prevailed! . . . The Senior Administration Officer somehow or another produced, within 24 hrs, enough lily white sheets to complete bedding arrangements to the Senior Nursing Officer's satisfaction!

Troops in Burma rejoiced at the announcement of victory over Japan, as Jessie Higgins remembers well. With thousands of drunken men out celebrating, she and the other PMs in Rangoon thought it prudent to lock themselves in! Later, though, they experienced the other side of the coin, 'the joy and heartbreak of nursing returned prisoners of war. They were flown in from all camps and were examined to decide if they were fit to travel on to Calcutta . . . I hope never to see such a thing again as one could never forget such wickedness and cruelty to human beings.'

For some ex-prisoners the long sea voyage home proved curative; for others it added torment. Fran Keech (Mrs Judson), who was stationed in Aden on VJ Day, went aboard

> . . . the first hospital ship bringing home the very sick servicemen, many of whom had suffered so cruelly under the

Japanese ... These men were too ill to be flown home and needed time to readjust to normal living again. The mental strain [they] had endured was plainly evident and quite a number had to be warded in our hospital ... Normal diet was impossible after so many months of near starvation ...

When the MFH in Rangoon disbanded in the closing months of 1945, Jessie Higgins was posted to Karachi. Care of RAF patients in Burma devolved upon a new unit, RAFH Mingaladon, where Matron Collie Knox and eight sisters led a nursing team which included Japanese prisoners of war acting as orderlies. Posted in from Calcutta in January 1946, Maureen Lumley found the Japanese orderlies strange, especially one named 'Son of Heaven': 'It was odd to call, "Son of Heaven, come here!"' She asked him to wash a patient and returned to find Son of Heaven washing the floor. When she tried gestures, he started to wash the bedstead – he couldn't seem to understand that a human being might need cleaning!

With little or no electricity, the PMs often worked by the feeble light of hurricane lamps. In the monsoon their rain capes came in handy as drapes across window openings and they went 'improperly dressed' – in all the humidity starched white caps ended up drooping comically round one's ears, so they were discarded except during panic moments when a senior matron loomed. In a quiet period, Maureen and her friend Elsie Lay planned a treat for the patients: 'Elsie made peppermint creams with sugar and peppermint oil, dipped into melted ration chocolate. These were moderately edible, but when I attempted to make toffee it set hard on the plate ... in trying to break it, the plate smashed before the toffee!' However, a large mango tree grew outside their mess, bearing fruit 'so lush and juicy that the only way to enjoy eating them with decorum was in the bath! ... We were really very happy there,' Maureen adds. 'I wrote glowing letters home, apparently. It was all quite an adventure. When you think back on it, we were very lucky.'

Early the following year, the two confectionery-makers went to Singapore where they helped to open a sick quarters beside Changi jail, the notorious former prison camp. Together with 63 MFH they formed the nucleus of what became RAF Hospital Changi. The arrival of a matron and a team of sisters allowed Maureen Lumley and Elsie Lay to return to England.

Today, the Second World War cemetery at Chittagong contains the graves of over 700 soldiers from Commonwealth countries and Japan, while near Kohima, north of Imphal, stands the monument which reads, 'When you go home, tell them of us and say: For your tomorrow, we gave our today'.

Land of the rising sun

Immediately the war ended, British Commonwealth forces arrived in Japan to oversee demilitarization and to repatriate prisoners of war. Air force personnel from Britain, Australia, India and New Zealand formed BCAir – British Commonwealth (Air) – with squadrons stationed at Miho, Bofu and Iwakuni. The main BCAir hospital, at Iwakuni on Honshu Island (only a few miles from Hiroshima), was staffed by all ranks of the RAF Medical Service, including a strong contingent of PMs. A Royal Australia Air Force (RAAF) base at American-controlled Okinawa provided a stopping point for medical teams flying ex-prisoners of war to Changi hospital, where they would be assessed and, wherever possible, put on hospital ships.

The BCAir hospital dealt with accident victims, too. On a Saturday in June 1946, a military jeep crashed on the north-western side of Honshu Island, badly injuring an army officer. He was taken to the SSQ at RAF Miho and signals went out for an aircraft and medical escort to convey him to the BCAir hospital. The aircrew assigned to this duty had just completed a long flying day. Instead of enjoying a good meal, they had to make do with a few sandwiches rushed to them when they briefly landed at Iwakuni to pick up Sister L.M. 'Sally' Blaen and an RAAF surgeon. During the flight to Miho, Sally Blaen was invited to take the co-pilot's seat, where she became acquainted with the pilot, Flight Lieutenant Bill Drinkell. He recalls: 'I don't think she was much impressed by the dishevelled appearance of the crew, nor by the answer to her enquiry as to when we would arrive – "The sandwiches are finished, so we must be almost there".' He, however, admired both her aplomb as they landed in the dark on a poorly equipped airfield, and the calm, efficient way she handled her patient. Their friendship developed from that beginning and on Easter Sunday 1947 Sally Blaen became Mrs Drinkell.

Matron 'Tilly' Tillbrook and Sisters Pat O'Kelly, Beryl Irving and Doris Stanford (Mrs Kent), were in the China seas aboard the troopship *Dilwara* when a typhoon struck. The storm hurled the PMs out of their bunks but fortunately caused few casualties. At Iwakuni they discovered that the sisters' mess had not been completed; so they stayed in the officers' mess, with Japanese 'room girls' to tend them. Doris Stanford was particularly impressed by the baths – 'miniature swimming pools . . . We were rinsed clean by the room girls, with additional uncontaminated water'. She found the devastated Hiroshima an awe-inspiring sight, but elsewhere Japan remained a tourist paradise. Off duty the PMs went skiing, toured beauty spots and temples, enjoyed a sukiyaki party and marvelled at Mount Fuji's 'glistening white snow cap on a spring morning with a profusion of cherry blossom surrounding the lake . . . unbelievably beautiful'. These highlights remain vivid, though 'the more mundane routine of night duty and hard work on the wards is a fading memory.'

In May 1947, eight more PMs bound for Japan shared a cabin aboard the *Empress of Scotland*. Mary Williams (Mrs Hancock) recounts how she and Angela O'Brien were later detached from Iwakuni to RAF Miho, where the young pilots christened her 'Mary the Matron of Miho'. Male orderlies did the routine work while the sisters 'gave injections, did dressings and other advanced treatments, plus all the administrative work . . . The busiest time was when we had an outbreak of Japanese encephalitis, caused by a special type of mosquito. The patients were very ill and needed a great deal of nursing, though thankfully most of them survived . . .' During a party to mark the departure of one of the squadrons, the Indian officers' mess caught fire and the PMs 'had to return to sick quarters to deal with very merry smoke-inhalers'.

Hundreds of Japanese worked on the station as personal servants and if Mary Williams rested on her bed in an afternoon she would wake to find her own little Japanese maid fanning her very gently. This treasure also 'invisibly-mended everything within sight'.

The BCAir hospital at Iwakuni closed in March 1948, but during the Korean War both the hospital and the RAF base were reactivated from October 1951 to March 1955.

Loose ends

The letters that have flowed in as contributions to this present book bear witness that, fifty years on, many patients still gratefully remember the care and kindness they received in RAF hospitals during the war years. One of those patients, John P. Soltau, tells of a lengthy stay in Halton after he was shot down over the Channel in August 1943. One of his enduring memories is of being taken out in an oversized wicker 'pram': 'These vehicles enabled relations, friends and staff to take out bed-ridden patients for "walks" in the fresh air. The destination was either a café in Wendover or the nearby woods, depending who was taking the patient out!'

Later, Mr Soltau spent some while at the RAF rehabilitation unit at Hoylake.

In the spring of 1944 some wounded exchange prisoners of war came back to the UK through a scheme arranged by the Red Cross. Most were amputees and it was amazing to note the quality of some home-made artificial limbs . . . made by DIY enthusiasts in the prisoner of war camps, using bits of scrap metal, beds, bedsprings, Red Cross parcel cases, odd nails, etc . . . They included intricate knee-locking and other devices . . . some of the patients were not too happy when they received the Roehampton standard issue limbs!

The RAF considered rehabilitation one of the most important factors in effecting a patient's swift return to health and duty. A rehab centre at Blackpool dealt with airmen; Hoylake looked after airmen aircrew; Cosford took in technicians and, after Torquay was bombed in 1942, the Officers' Medical Rehabilitation Unit (MRU) transferred to Loughborough College. This former PT centre had excellent facilities, remembered by WAAF nursing orderly Corporal Louisa 'Pat' Hill, who worked with physiotherapists in the early mobilization room. She recalls some famous sportsmen who acted as instructors: 'Raich Carter, the footballer, took groups of "leg patients" for walking and leg movements and Dan Maskell, the tennis coach, was in charge of arms and shoulders when the patients were ready to progress on to more advanced movements.'

When Loughborough reverted to civilian use in 1947 another

MRU, at Collaton Cross, took over its work; then in 1949 Headley Court opened. In its early days, it too boasted tennis ace Dan Maskell on its staff.

The RAF's skill in treating burns had borne fine fruit. At the end of the war a network of specialized units existed across the UK, to which RAF specialists flew from Halton airfield to teach others the new skills and techniques. In his short history of PMRAFH Halton, Squadron Leader Richard Laurence retells some of the stories of those days:

> Patients were flown into Halton from all over the world . . . One DC3, laden with cargo, crashed in the woods behind the hospital. Staff rushed out to see the pilot, unharmed, dangling from a tree. What really drew their attention, however, was the cargo – several tons of then-rare oranges scattered around. Clear-up was achieved in record time . . . When stores of olive oil (used in the treatment of scars) ran dry, fresh supplies were flown in by Mosquito bombers over the Atlantic Ocean from Canada . . . One extraordinary story is told, of a young USAF airman who was admitted with a live anti-aircraft cannon-shell embedded in his chest. The bomb disposal squad, duly called, could only offer soon-to-be-dispensed-with lead shielding. The patient survived and the defused cannon-shell became a memento for the brave surgeon.

The war hastened and improved diagnostic techniques for many diseases and conditions, especially the use of mass X-ray, which, in the closing stages of the war, vastly increased the detection-rate for tuberculosis (TB). The disease proved rife among returning PoWs and in May 1945 RAFH St Athan made available sixty beds for TB cases, beginning a new speciality which lasted long after the war ended. When demand exceeded bed-space, further TB wards briefly opened at RAFH Church Village in Glamorgan. Such advances, accelerated by the demands the war had made on doctors, nurses and scientists, continued to bring benefits to humankind long after the peace was signed.

But not all wartime memories were of sickness, sadness and horror. Many nurses write of happier times – singing Christmas carols by lamplight, amid falling snow – magical even in wartime; others tell of tennis parties in the jungle, dances in the desert, and romance flourishing everywhere. Another theme is clothing – the difficulties of remaining starched and ladylike (as Matron required) while scrubbing filthy rooms, coming under fire or facing freak weather conditions; and let us not forget the problematical hats – the storm caps, the bush hats, the fur-trimmed hoods for Iceland, the broad-brimmed white tropical felt with the RAF ribbon and, always, the cherished black four-cornered 'Dick'.

Following a party, Beryl Chadney was forced to order a new quatrecorn as a matter of urgency because her own had been 'confiscated by air crew to drop over Germany'! Fran Keech's friend Jean heartily hated her 'Dick Turpin' and 'instead of wearing it square with the badge to view over the forehead, she had cut at least one inch off . . . to enable her to wear it on the back of her head.' As Fran and Jean sat on the train which would take them back to Yatesbury after leave, they were joined in the carriage by Matron-in-Chief Gladys Taylor, who was horrified by the sight of this mutilated and non-King's Regulation headgear. She leaned forward and adjusted it to sit on Jean's head 'in the correct manner, resulting in the two side tricorns resembling wings'. Poor Jean was confined to the mess until she had bought a new hat. 'You can well imagine the embarrassment she suffered,' says Fran, 'but the hilarity amongst the rest of us lasted for days.'

Jessie Higgins finally returned to England in January 1946, accompanying 'a very ill soldier with a cerebral tumour . . . Everyone looked grey, everything drab. And there was me, yellow as a guinea, having been on mepacrine for two and a half years!'

Left behind at Karachi, Rona Black heard that she had been awarded the ARRC – the equivalent of the DSO. She wrote home:

Phew! I've been sitting up in bed thinking, this a.m., wondering if it's really me . . . The award has been given to all of us who came out and stood the test . . . Higgie and Lawford got theirs last time . . . I hadn't dared tell you that Higgie flew home ten days ago . . . I pictured you making your way to Air Ministry to ask why your daughter hadn't been included . . . Anyway, I'm off tomorrow.

Jessie Higgins and Rona Black had both joined the PMRAFNS as regular members: 'Higgie' was to make the service her lifelong career; Rona chose to leave after the war 'because there are so many other things which interest me.' As for the wartime reserve sisters, they were gradually demobilized and allowed to resume their interrupted lives. Beryl Chadney, demobbed in 1947, took away a gratuity of £39 – £1 for each month of her war service as a sister with PMRAFNS(R).

For those who like statistics, the official history of the RAFMS during the Second World War records that, at home in the UK, seven general hospitals and seventeen station hospitals offered over 6,000 beds. Most patients belonged to the RAF, next came the WAAF, but RAF hospitals also treated personnel from the Dominions and Allied nations, as well as those from the British Army and the Royal Navy. To take only one year and one hospital, Halton's records for 1945 reveal a total of 11,311 admissions, all but eight of them being air force personnel – the exceptions were a VAD and seven civilians!

For their wartime service, 145 members of the PMRAFNS won official honours and awards. 'No human praise can do justice to the debt we all owe to the nurses . . . Their skill, their care and their compassion for the sick and wounded, often under fire from the enemy and in conditions of great danger and hardship, were a real inspiration to the men and women they tended and worked with . . .' So wrote Britain's great war leader, Winston S. Churchill.

SEVEN

Empires' end

The war had brought a pause in the rising desire for independence among colonial countries. Now, nationalist feelings resurfaced, sometimes with violent results. On a few days' leave from RAFGH Allahabad, Joyce Kellow (Mrs Wyatt) and Dot Ashley flew to Calcutta, where they visited the bazaar and had lunch at the then-famous Firpo's Hotel. As they left, they were confronted by the sight of thousands of angry Hindus

> . . . all shouting *Jai Hind!*' ('Quit India!') and waving sticks . . . I said to Dot, 'Come on, we must fight our way through this mob . . .' We stepped out from Firpo's and walked through the moving wall of natives, waving our arms in a breast-stroke motion to force our way back to the YWCA . . . we were through before they had time to realise what was happening.

Having seen the appalling slums of the city, where people riddled with disease starved in hovels, the two PMs understood the anger they had witnessed.

That same mood caused native workers to strike, closing the airfield at Dumdum, so Joyce and Dot decided to take the train back to Allahabad – an eighteen-hour journey. That evening, in uniform, they went to the station in an open taxi.

> We were surrounded by a violent mob of rioting Hindus. Shouting *Jai Hind*', they stood on the running board of our taxi and spat on us . . . we were hit by stones . . . we lay face

down on the floor of the taxi and thought we would be killed. I screamed at the driver of our taxi '*Jeldi Jao, Jeldi Jao!*' which means 'Go quickly'. When the car moved, the rioting mob stepped back for fear of being run over. The taxi drove through the seething mass . . .

The train for Allahabad was due to leave at 10 p.m., so we went to the ticket office – and found only enough money between us for one ticket! This was a minor problem I felt, having escaped with our lives. All night we travelled in the train, dozing fitfully. Next day, with no food or drink, we were silent and apprehensive. At midday a ticket collector approached our carriage. Dot locked herself in the latrine and I showed our one and only ticket! He nodded and departed. Later, when he returned, I hid in the latrine and Dot showed the same ticket! Thus we had yet another escape.

They arrived in Allahabad at 4 p.m., twenty-four hours absent without leave. Joyce envisaged being sent home in disgrace, or court-martialled. Instead, 'we saw Matron, Miss Minchin, running towards us . . . she hugged us with tears streaming down her face . . . they had heard about the riots in Calcutta and were certain that we were amongst those British who were murdered.'

Demobilization called home all nursing sisters of the reserve, necessitating their replacement with members of the regular PMRAFNS. Thus, when on 12 August 1946 the MV *Georgic*, of the Cunard White Star line, departed Liverpool, she carried around 2,000 troops, officers, civilian workers and families, plus twenty PM sisters. One of them was Winifred Gardner (Mrs Penman), whose first impression was of the food aboard ship: 'luxury to have *white* bread rolls after years of eating wholesome (no doubt) but monotonous "utility" bread.'

They reached Bombay on 29 August and spent a night at Worli transit camp before setting off on the four-day rail journey to Karachi, four sisters and two armed escorts to each compartment, self-contained with toilet and washing facilities. They stopped at stations for most meals – fried eggs, bacon, chips and tea seemed to be the staple fare, be it breakfast, lunch or dinner – and they slept in bed-rolls while the train chugged on through the night. Winifred Gardner was fascinated by the changing scenery and the local fauna: 'water buffalo, kingfishers, peacocks, many strange and brightly coloured birds, but always the sweet cheeky sparrows ... cows, goats and camels ... primitive wells, waterwheels turned by yoked oxen, ancient wooden ploughs, washerwomen at the water's edge ...' At the Braganza Hotel in Lahore they enjoyed 'the longest, most welcome shandy ever, followed by a BATH (pure joy!) and a good meal. 2nd Sept: Woke early to the sound of bells from passing bullock carts ...'

Entrained once again that evening, with two armed sergeants for escort, they found the compartment filthy, so:

> We 'Dettol-ed' it from top to bottom before sitting down ... Woke to find ourselves surrounded by grey sand, inside as well as outside! Everything was covered with a thin layer of it, and when we looked at one another we dissolved into hysterics! The sand had stuck to our moist faces and little rivers of sweat ran down ... This was the Sind desert, which is always crossed in daylight, *never* at night for fear of raiding tribesmen ...

Winifred thought the sisters' mess at No. 10 RAFGH delightful. The PMs lived in eight-room bungalows, each room having a bed with mosquito net and its own bathroom – stone floor, cold tap, tin bath, basin and wash-stand, plus 'thunder-box'. Bearers, dhobi-wallahs and sweepers looked after the practicalities, and armed guards patrolled at night. The hospital spread over a wide, sandy area, each ward fringed by a verandah; the families' ward and maternity unit stood a few hundred yards away, near the main road. Patients came from nearby RAF units, the Black Watch (the garrison regiment at the time), and the Indian Army, with some Royal Navy officers, plus service families and British, French and Dutch civilians.

RAF men John Barrow and Reg Wheeler, six months apart, underwent serious mastoid operations in RAFGH Karachi. Both write with high praise for the care they received. 'Sisters and nurses did a wonderful job in the conditions, always cheerful and always had time for a chat,' says Reg Wheeler, while John Barrow remembers an occasion when two intrepid sisters accepted a dare and, 'took a bike ride to a small village called Mango-Pir. There a pit of sacred crocodiles existed and each day a goat was killed, skinned and thrown to the crocodiles.' He adds warm thanks for the 'dedication, high standard and professionalism which made it possible for me to be writing this letter today,' though in fact his wife wrote the letter for him since Mr Barrow is now registered blind.

In those days, says Evelyn Addison (Mrs Glen), despite

> . . . the awful disease, lack of hygiene, flies and incessant heat, we sisters were really able to nurse the patients, 'sponging' to get high temperatures down . . . There was very little air conditioning and few antibiotics, and so many snakes in the grass at night that on night duty we had to be escorted across the gardens with a torch light. We wore long white stockings, a white overall and big RAF cap.

While at Karachi, Evelyn met and fell in love with a pilot who had earlier flown many missions over Germany. 'I had barely finished my first year in India and had to ask the Matron for permission to marry . . . She said, "Do you realize you are going to marry a man who has the highest bar bill in the Officers' Mess?!" However, the marriage lasted fifty-one years . . .'

One by one, the RAF hospitals in India closed. MFHs dispersed as soon as their last patients were transferred to one of the general hospitals. In turn, the hospitals in Allahabad, Calcutta and Cawnpore gradually emptied their beds, posted their RAF staffs elsewhere, and handed over to Indian control during 1946. That left only No. 10 RAFGH, Karachi. But Pakistan Independence Day came on 15 August 1947 and by the end of the year British withdrawal was well under way. 'We were privileged to see history in the making – the end of the British Raj and the birth of a new nation – Pakistan,' says Winifred Gardner (Mrs Penman). She and fellow PMs Mary Coffey and 'Greg' Gregory, left Karachi on 5 January 1948 and sailed for home aboard the *El Nil* (a yacht once owned by King Fuad of Egypt).

This was not the end of the RAF in India, however. The sick quarters at RAF Mauripur, near Karachi, became an invaluable staging post on the long-haul aeromedical flights which were soon to send PMs winging round the world.

The Promised Land

For half a century Palestine had been troubled by unrest between resident Arabs and the Jews who wished to be allowed to return to their historic homeland. While the country remained under British mandate, strenuous efforts to reconcile the two sides all ended in failure. From 1945 the revelation of the horrors of the German death camps caused fresh demands for the creation of a Jewish homeland, and when the area erupted once again into violence Britain asked the United Nations to find a solution.

The original RAF hospital in Palestine had closed in 1940 but a new unit, transferring from Tripoli, opened at Tel Litwinsky, near Jaffa, in February 1944. One of its wartime patients, Geoffrey Hobbs, had been taken to the army hospital at Nicosia, in Cyprus, after his 'two-fan, two-place harasser ship' crashed in flames. He was badly burned while rescuing his pilot and, after a couple of weeks in an army hospital at Nicosia was scheduled to be transferred to Tel Litwinsky, which had a special burns unit complete with saline baths. 'Came the day and I was put on a Dakota accompanied by an elderly [army] nurse who, shaking, asked me if I was all right whilst four soldiers held my stretcher down as we took off . . .' Travelling via Beirut, he eventually reached No. 3 RAFGH Tel Litwinsky, where he was transferred to a stretcher trolley.

> Running along the path between Nissen hut wards, one of the front wheels left the path, the trolley tipped over and shot me off into the bushes. The orderlies were very concerned . . . but despite my initial groan I took it in good humour. Why not? In a few minutes I was to be at the Burns Centre with its soothing facilities . . . [but] pinned to the door was a notice 'Closed for re-decoration'.

Despite this bad start, Mr Hobbs evinces his lifelong admiration for the treatment he received from 'those angels of mercy' of the PMRAFNS.

Airman L.A. Murray was still in his teens when, stationed in Palestine in 1946, he became dangerously ill with jaundice. During his five-month stay in Tel Litwinsky he came to know several members of the PMRAFNS, including a 'lovely matron who sat by my bed and wrote a letter to my parents and girlfriend (now my wife) telling them that I was "making it". Because I tried to grow a moustache she referred to me as "Murray – you shocker" – but what a lady.' There was also 'Sister Flowers, face of an angel and everyone's favourite', and, 'a nurse called "Dot" . . . so attentive to me, doing things I couldn't do for myself . . . Although I said thank you at the time, if any of them could know how valuable their efforts were, wouldn't it be grand?'

Those days are still vivid to Sister Dulcie Flower (Mrs Wright): 'We could not leave the camp without an armed escort, but the hospital was on the same camp as the 6th Parachute Division, so there was no problem there! I can well remember climbing into an armoured car in cocktail frocks to attend a cocktail party at HQ in Jerusalem!'

Susan Armistead (Mrs Sutcliffe) had started with the Service in 1943, at RAFH Weeton, where after D-Day she helped to nurse many very sick ex-prisoners of war. In 1945 she was posted to No. 5 RAFGH at Cairo, in time for a typhoid epidemic, and the following year saw her at Tel Litwinsky, where she nursed the first British officer to be shot by terrorists – 'He was desperately ill, but I am pleased to say that he recovered.'

A brief glimpse of Tel Litwinsky awaited Doreen Francis. Posted to Cairo, she and her friend Mary Spink joined other sisters waiting at a transit camp at Burtonwood, from where, 'after five wet days trekking backwards and forwards to the ablutions hut across the strategically-placed paving stones, about sixteen of us embarked at Liverpool on SS *Britannic*.' Arriving at Cairo, Doreen and colleague Eileen King discovered they were posted on yet again, to Habbaniya. They were taken to Heliopolis airport and rushed by jeep to an aircraft waiting on the runway. Too late, they discovered it was the wrong plane – though bound eventually for Habbaniya, it was at the disposal of a group captain on an inspection tour. 'He did not speak to us,' says Doreen, 'he thought we were cadging a lift.' Eileen King's tin trunk 'hand luggage' came in useful as a passenger seat.

The group captain decided to spend the night at Lydda, which had no accommodation for women and so, because of the terrorist troubles in Palestine, 'one of the officers collected a pistol and ammunition and escorted us to the RAF hospital at Tel Litwinsky, where Miss Williamson was the Matron, and we were given beds for the night. The following morning we were taken back to Lydda early, before the roads were checked, to resume our journey.'

Their Anson was overloaded and the pilot 'had to nose between the mountains to get to Iraq. We also needed to refuel and landed at H3, an oil station on the pipe-line. The personnel there were intrigued to see "skirts" and drove over to investigate. As a result, we were all treated to an excellent lunch.'

When they finally arrived in Habbaniya they were greeted with relief by colleagues who had thought them lost. It was February, but Doreen Francis thought she had arrived in Eden: 'The mess was surrounded by parma violets – the scent glorious – [and] between the sleeping blocks, where we had bedroom, bathroom and boxroom, were apricot trees in full blossom.'

RAFH Tel Litwinsky closed on 1 January 1948, anticipating the end of the British mandate and the creation of the Jewish state of Israel.

Casevac to aeromed

Although the Second World War had ended, equally bloody conflicts – in Malaya and then Korea – soon called for air evacuation of yet more casualties. Much had been learned during the wider war, and as early as January 1945 plans had been laid for an extended service, to be known in peacetime as aeromedical evacuation. These flights would bring patients back from the Far East in five or six days, flying eight or nine hours each day and resting overnight at RAF staging posts. Nursing orderlies would accompany the patients in flight, but nursing sisters were to be posted to each of the stops *en route*, to care for in-transit patients in SSQs overnight. (In practice, from around 1950 PMs did start to accompany patients aboard air ambulances, much to the delight of the ladies involved.)

Pioneering the Far East aeromed

Anne Caird (Mrs Austin) borrowed her flying gear from WAAF supplies when she and an orderly boarded one of the Dakotas doing the 'casevac run' during the Korean war. The Australian air force brought the patients from Korea to the BCAir hospital in Japan, from where the RAF ferried them back to Changi. They flew out from their base at RAF Kai Tak, Hong Kong, to the USAF base at Okinawa, where they refuelled, then on to BCAir Hospital Iwakuni. The patients they collected were a mix of Britons, Turks, Greeks, Australians and New Zealanders, some on stretchers, some able to use passenger seats. One group whom Anne Caird remembers with

affection were Turks 'who spoke no English, so we communicated
by using a board containing basic English-Turkish phrases, primitive
but effective . . . Onboard conditions were very cramped . . .
moving about was an exercise in agility! No one had a clue how the
stretcher harness fitted to the fuselage, but fit it we did – and prayed
it would not collapse.'

Returning by the same long, slow route, they stayed overnight in
RAF sick quarters in Hong Kong before reloading the Dakota for
the onward flight, first to Saigon for refuelling, then on to
Singapore. Anne Caird usually spent two days at Changi before
returning to Hong Kong to begin again. It was 'a tiring schedule,
but a real challenge and the most gratifying experience of my nursing career'.

Monica Railton Jones (Mrs Chandler) says the sturdy Dakotas
they used 'had been swiftly adapted to carry casualties, having
recently been taking part in the Berlin airlift, carrying coal!'

Joy Harris did only one trip, but 'it took quite a long time'.

> We did it in a Valetta, which meant we came down in Borneo
> for refuelling, spent the night in the Philippines, came down
> in Okinawa . . . that was where the chaps had to pee into the
> hydraulics to get the wheels down! . . . The Australians were
> so welcoming . . . I felt I'd gone home when I landed there.
> We got up at four a.m. every morning, to take off, and every
> morning the aircraft was still u/s [unserviceable], so they did
> something with me for the day. I was sent off round the sacred
> islands in a boat. I was sent on a train to Hiroshima . . . there
> I was, not long after the war, walking round in uniform. No-
> one thought anything about it, there was a great acceptance
> . . . I even managed to spend the day in a Sunderland [flying
> boat], which I certainly shouldn't have done . . . They took
> me up for the day and we did sweeps round the islands . . .

Eventually the Valetta was ready for take-off. 'I think there were
only about ten patients. One was on a "striker frame". He'd injured
his spine, so he was on something like a stretcher and you could
screw another stretcher on to him, so you could tip him over – we
just had one orderly with us.' They returned as they had come,
stopping at Okinawa, then in the Philippines, then on to Borneo for

refuelling.

They off-loaded the boys each time – they used to be off-loaded for refuelling in those days. And they'd all get back on again, or be carried on, with cartons of cigarettes and gum. But they never did anything in these medical centres about their dressings – changing them, or making them comfortable . . . Anyway, when we stopped at Borneo . . . the boys were all out on the rough grass near the airfield and the planters' wives came along and sat down with them, and they'd brought a tin of boiled sweets with them, and they handed these round . . . and when we got back on the aircraft the chaps thought this was wonderful . . . people who had spoken to *them*, interested in them, human beings again, not just being passed through. They were terribly impressed with these planters' wives and their boiled sweets – and hadn't thought very much of the Americans.

An unusual air evacuation took place in April 1953 when an aeromed team, including PM Jean Weir, went to Moscow to bring home seven civilian ex-prisoners of war who had reached the Russian capital by the Trans-Siberian Railway. The RAF team flew via Berlin, where a Russian navigator and signaller boarded their plane to escort them through Soviet airspace. Their patients included a former British minister from the Embassy in Seoul, and an Irish missionary who turned out to be related to one of the seven flight sisters waiting on standby at Wroughton!

The Korean War armistice was signed at Panmunjon in July 1953. Soon afterwards, to her delight, Tessa Lawless, stationed at Changi, was chosen as a last-minute replacement for a casevac from Japan. The rush to prepare included having two pairs of khaki trousers made (in two hours flat!) by a tailor in Changi village. Trousers were still non-regulation, but necessary 'for climbing steep and narrow steps into the aircraft, and when nursing patients at floor level in cramped conditions'.

The old, unpressurized aircraft lumbered along at low altitude, on piston engines, for stretches of seven or eight hours at a time, taking its usual overnight stop in the Philippines. Next morning as they waited on the tarmac some technical trouble with the aircraft became apparent. The crew asked Tessa if she had a hair-clip: 'I didn't use hair-clips, but by some miracle I had one in my make-up case – just in case!' The clip helped the pilot to effect repairs and off they went.

At the Australian air force base at Iwakuni, Tessa Lawless learned that, rather than returning to Changi next day, she was to wait two weeks for the first batch of PoWs released from Korea. In the meantime she had a house to herself, and a car with a driver who showed her the sights. These included Hiroshima, rebuilt into the most modern city in Japan. But the legacy of the atom bomb remained in the burned and limbless casualties Tessa met, and in the stories told: '22,000 bodies had floated down the river and the whole place was gutted except for one skeleton of a dome-shaped building.' Elsewhere she found shops full of the latest technological gadgets, and she loved the scenery of tiered mountains with every inch of land under cultivation, and 'pagodas, bridges and small streams, sacred gateways and cherry blossom'. The fortnight of waiting flew by.

She brought back thirty-three patients, including eight stretcher cases, loaded in tiers, all needing feeding and close nursing. Some of the sick men had beriberi, and two of these cases, mentally affected by the disease, were placed at the front of the aircraft, where the crew and some of the fitter patients could keep an eye on them. 'My lasting impression,' says Tessa, 'is of total commitment . . . the crew and the walking patients were co-operative and helpful, to me and to each other . . .'

The final leg to Singapore ended with a landing in monsoon rain. Tessa had a glimpse of a crowd of VIPs – including Matron! – waiting under umbrellas to greet these very first returning prisoners of the Korean War. A team of RAF men swiftly took the patients to waiting ambulances and transported them away while Tessa, very aware of her non-regulation trousers, 'went down the stairway feeling very scruffy, only to be greeted by flashing cameras . . . within seconds I found myself facing Matron amidst this crowd of people, and the crew, with the Press bombarding me for my name . . . Rather than upset RAF protocol, I declined . . .'

The return of the PoWs made world headlines, on TV, radio, in the papers and on *Pathe News* in cinemas. The Korean War was over. Perhaps an era of real peace had arrived at last.

PART IV

The Best of Times?

ONE

The bombs that fell on Hiroshima and Nagasaki starkly announced the opening of the nuclear age. But devastated cities rose again, transformed into utopias of modernity, and as production lines restarted, bringing more employment and better wages, so new consumer goods began to reach the shops – refrigerators, washing machines, Coca Cola ... At the same time, with the doctrine of Communism spreading, the Great Powers braced themselves for the stand-off that became known as the Cold War. And in the field of medicine a more subtle enemy, called infantile paralysis (poliomyelitis), posed a fresh challenge for doctors and nurses.

The RAF's temporary war-time hospitals, at home and overseas, had closed. In Britain, the remaining five general hospitals (Cosford, Ely, Halton, Nocton Hall and Wroughton) and another five station hospitals (Padgate, St Athan, Weeton, West Kirby and Wilmslow) adjusted themselves to meet the needs of a peacetime air force. Abroad, RAF hospitals in Aden, Egypt and Iraq were joined by new ones in West Germany and Singapore, and staging posts on the transport and aeromed route from the Far East to the UK all opened sick quarters or small hospitals. These new units offered exciting postings for PMs such as young Joy Harris, who was on leave when a telegram came to inform her she had been posted – to Greece! She was thrilled! Then she reread the telegram – not 'Athens' in golden Greece but 'St Athan' in wet Wales. Even so, for Joy it was 'the furthest I'd been from home in those days'!

Olympic event

When crowds of athletes arrived in London to take part in the 1948 Olympic Games, Sister Pam Love (Mrs Batchelar) was stationed at Uxbridge. The small hospital lay in the grounds of the RAF station, whose CO 'did the weekly round with matron, which caused a lot of tension; hospitals with sick people are, after all, most unlike barrack blocks'. That summer, the Uxbridge barrack blocks served as billets for teams of Olympic athletes. At the hospital, Pam Love recalls, 'duties varied from giving enemas to overweight boxers to dressing injuries, and even comforting some athletes who were panicking and overstressed.'

> On one notable occasion a dinner was held at the Mess for VIP Olympic people as well as many RAF VIPs. Curried chicken was on the menu, but sadly the day was hot and the chicken was off. There was no mean panic when our beds quickly filled up with very sick men suffering from food poisoning. I was the only sister on night duty then and my big problem was to keep the story from the press; reporters phoned in all manner of guises . . . The *Daily Express* some-how got hold of it and splashed it on their front page the next day . . .

One of the men badly affected by the bug was the station CO, with whom Pam Love 'had crossed swords over a ward inspection. It may sound callous but . . . when I literally caught him with his trousers down I felt somehow that justice had been done.'

Parachuting PMs

A different kind of athletic challenge occurred when seven PMs became the first British nurses to undertake a parachute-jumping course identical to that used in training paratroops. This training was intended to cover any future emergency in some remote and inaccessible area where medical teams might literally have to leap to the rescue. At Wroughton, in the spring of 1948, a notice in the sisters' mess called for volunteers to undertake a 'parachute medic' course (not to be confused with 'paramedic' as we now understand it). When no names appeared on the form, it became a case of 'You, you, and . . .'

Vi Craig (Mrs Gibbons), one of the chosen few, accepted the challenge with wry humour: 'Life had seemed a little dull after two and a half years in India, the weather was lovely and Upper Heyford was in a nice part of the country . . .' She went along to No. 1 Parachute and Glider Training School, at RAF Upper Heyford in Oxfordshire, where she joined the rest of the experimental group – Senior Sister Joan Maffey; Sisters Margery Bradley and Molly Savage; four male nursing orderlies and a doctor, all of the RAFMS; and Audrey Penfold, OC WAAF of Upper Heyford. They spent their first day in a hangar, 'swinging around, learning to roll', under the eye of RAF instructors and other interested observers.

One of those instructors, Mr T. Wilson, remembers being 'surprised to receive these ladies'. A few women had parachuted into France during the war, as wireless operators or resistance leaders, but nurses were an innovation. What was more, safety rules decreed that no one over thirty-five should parachute on to land, and 'these Sisters were obviously over this age, so we looked after them with care'.

The standard course involved eight jumps, three from a balloon and five from a Dakota, including one jump by night, using parachutes of the old 'X' type, with no reserve 'chutes. Trainees wore overalls, heavy military boots and rather fetching protective 'helmets' filled with Sorbo rubber. They also avoided late nights in the bar.

Before they could jump down they had to climb up – 'first a perpendicular ladder attached to a wall . . . to reach a platform 30 ft from the ground . . . next a 90 ft tower . . .' Vi Craig found the next stage, from a barrage balloon tethered 800 feet up, 'a bit of an ordeal', but when they finally came to jump out of a real aircraft 'there was so much engine noise and hustle and bustle . . . you jumped on your number, with no hesitation'.

A former CO of Halton, J.G. Kingan, recalls that on a later course, as the plane took off for their first real drop, tension reigned among the group of male and female embryo parachutists. Then one of the PMs took out a mirror and nonchalantly checked her make-up. Tension evaporated – if she was so relaxed, what was worrying all those husky males?

In 1950 the PMRAFNS Advisory Board commented that nursing sisters had done excellent work in 'demonstrating the capacity of women to undertake arduous and unique duties'. However, after a year or two when no need for emergency medical teams arose, parachuting disappeared from the PMs' curriculum.

Ranking officers – at last

On 1 February 1949, long-awaited changes confirmed the vital role performed by all women in the modern air force. The WAAF ceased being a mere auxiliary service and regained its original 1918 title of the Women's Royal Air Force (WRAF); its members, along with members of the PMRAFNS, achieved full integration into the RAF. At last PMs became recognized holders of the King's Commission: where before they had held only 'emergency' wartime commissions, they could now apply for permanent or short-service commissions, on salaries commensurate with other service scales of pay, and, although on the wards they would continue to be addressed as 'Sister' and 'Matron', officially they held officer rank titles equivalent to the WRAF:

PMRAFNS	WRAF	RAF
Matron-in-Chief	Air Commandant	Air Commodore
Principal Matron	Group Officer	Group Captain
Senior Matron	Wing Officer	Wing Commander
Matron	Squadron Officer	Squadron Leader
Senior Sister	Flight Officer	Flight Lieutenant
Sister	Flying Officer	Flying Officer

King George V later approved the appointment of the Princess Royal as Air Chief Commandant of the PMRAFNS.

A changing role

To proclaim the advantages of a career in the PMRAFNS, Matron-in-Chief Helen Cargill instigated a new recruiting drive. She had observed that while many nurses enquired about joining the PMs, few returned their application forms, partly because of false rumours that no acute nursing was done in service hospitals. In fact, recent changes meant that the work of RAF hospitals was as vital and varied as that of any civilian hospital.

After the National Health Service began, on 5 July 1948, the ten RAF hospitals accepted patients from local civilian communities and also offered extended care for service families. Midwifery was becoming a speciality: until 1948 only one RAF maternity unit had existed, at St Athan, but two years later both Halton and Cosford had opened 'midder' wards, and other hospitals followed suit. The PMRAFNS established a first-class midwifery organization and, since babies rapidly grow, soon introduced children's wards too.

Wherever possible, PMs were appointed to work in their field of preference, be it theatre nursing, midwifery, orthopaedics, paediatrics, oncology, plastic surgery . . . Such a comprehensive choice – allied with postings across the world, the chance to work aboard troopships and on aeromed flights, good prospects for promotion, plus decent pay and an attractive uniform – ensured that a career as a nursing officer in the peacetime PMRAFNS offered an excellent future for any SRN. New recruiting literature was to spread this message far and wide.

Five PMs then stationed at Uxbridge, including Pam Love (Mrs Batchelar), were summoned to Matron's office, where 'we were inspected by an arty gent in a velvet cap'.

> He looked at us from every angle and announced that there was only one possible choice, though she was far from ideal – that possible one was me. I had to spend a day in a dusty studio having my photo taken, with the deputy matron-in-chief as chaperone. This arty chap produced tea in jam jars for his refreshment and mine, but nothing for the deputy matron, which was most embarrassing . . .

The new posters and booklet encouraged a steady stream of trained nurses to apply for membership of the PMRAFNS.

New girls

Pam Love had joined the service in 1947. She arrived for her first day at Wroughton 'feeling very odd in my uniform with its wretched tricorn hat which clipped over the eyes when one stood to attention. I had no square-bashing training, nor did I know how to salute, so panic set in when I passed the guard room. I vaguely raised my right hand and hoped for the best . . .' (Many PMs refer to the hat as a tricorn, though it has always had four corners to its brim, not three.)

'Our tricorn-shaped hat,' says Margaret Crombie (Mrs Price), 'had a badge at the front. We used to wear it on the back of our heads, at which Matron observed that the badge "had to be seen by pedestrians, *not* by oncoming aircraft!"' This witticism has been borrowed by so many matrons down the years that no one is sure who first uttered it.

A few years later, new member April Reed bought her uniform from Boyd Cooper's, as instructed, but forgot to include white shoes. For her first day on the ward another nurse lent her some shoes, but they were half a size too small and by coffee break next morning, April's feet were 'ghastly'. She changed into black shoes with her ward whites, much to Ward Sister's horror: 'Matron's about to come round! You'd better hide in the sluice!' Being a junior sister was never easy.

What was more, as full ranking officers in 'the big air force', PMs had to do more than know their jobs – they had to learn service procedures, how to fill in official forms, how (and whom) to salute correctly and, of all things, how to march!

After joining in 1951, Margaret Kingston went on the first-ever Nursing Officers' Course, held at RAF Hawkinge, near Folkestone: 'I'd only been in the Service six weeks and I hadn't a clue what they were talking about – all this F Med 12s and 50s and all these numbers and things – so one of the girls on the same course every evening used to translate it into English for me.'

The ladies also learned 'square bashing on the cliff-tops at Folkestone'.

We had to take it in turns, seven of us, taking the squad, marching, and Flight Sergeant Pomeroy – I can see him now with his pacing stick, you could see your face in his boots . . . It was my turn to command this little gathering of PMs. And he stopped them and he came up to me and he said, "Scuse me, ma'am. Permission to touch?' and with that he put his hand on my tummy and he said, 'From *there*, ma'am!'

The drill instructor was a vocal coach, too!

Another course of six trainees went on parade in their new best blues. It was raining and one of the innocents turned up holding a red umbrella – she didn't want to get her nice new uniform wet!

Most PMs were not called upon to march very often, but a few proudly remember taking part in one of the annual Festivals of Remembrance at the Albert Hall. Olive Kirkham and eleven other PMs gathered at RAF Uxbridge.

> Each morning we were taken to the Hall where we met Ralph Reader, who was the organizer . . . As part of the large muster we practised marching up and down these wretched stairs and across the arena for hours on end . . . When the great day dawned, we dressed in the whitest of our uniforms, starched sleeves and caps and shining white shoes . . . I shall never forget waiting at the top of those dreaded stairs . . .

But the most poignant moment, then as now, was the floating down of the millions of poppy petals.

Another year, at a similar event, Margaret Kingston represented the PMs:

> When we went up on the stage, Chelsea Pensioners were next to me, and this old boy sat next to me – must have been well in his eighties – and he nudged me and said, 'Duckie, would you mind if I took my teeth out?' So he took his teeth out and put them under the chair. Well, the whole service, I was terrified that he'd go off without his teeth!

In due time, prospective PMs undertook courses at the female Officer Cadet Training Unit (OCTU) at Henlow, and later they joined the men at the OCTU at Cranwell. But in the interim, in the late fifties and early sixties, training in RAF ways became an integral part of the first few weeks of a PM's service – usually at the 'home base' hospital, PMRAFH Halton, Bucks.

Doreen Smedley recalls that when she first went to Halton in 1955, every morning new sisters had half an hour's training with a deputy matron. Doreen kept a notebook, in which she wrote copies of the various formal letters she might need: 'You had to write a letter if you wanted leave; when you came back from overseas you had to write to MOD and go for an interview; if you wanted to get married, of course, you had to write a letter . . . there was even one if you had to write on behalf of the mess to thank Princess Mary for her annual Christmas card!'

A little later, Liz Sandison spent her introductory month at Halton, 'before OCTU at Henlow or Cranwell and all those goodly things'. She learned to march behind Halton's garages, where 'on the last day there was this great cheering and hullabaloo and here were the kitchen staff, holding up score cards as if it were *Come Dancing*'.

Thérèse Saunders (Mrs Ayres) also had a memorable introduction to the service. On her first night at Halton – a winter night, with ice and snow on the ground outside – she stood on a chair in order to draw the curtains in her allocated room. The chair collapsed. She clutched the curtains to save herself but the curtain rail came away from the wall. Rail and curtains landed in a heap on top of her. Wondering if it was worth even unpacking after such a disastrous start, she decided to go across to dinner. Stepping outside the main door, she slipped on some ice, fell flat on her back and gashed her head open. 'I arrived at the Sisters' Mess with blood everywhere . . . I shall never forget the look on their faces! I'm sure they thought me a very weird addition to their number!'

The Fifties

For those PMs who remember them, the two decades following the war were the best. It was the heyday of sea-trooping and of the long-haul aeromed flights which suddenly became much faster with the introduction of jet engines. It was also the era which offered the widest range of postings. And, in those halcyon days, national servicemen added their own sly humour to the wards. Though everyone worked hard, they also had time for fun. Sisters wafted down the wards in high starched head-dresses, white dresses and short blue capes (with officers' rank markings proudly displayed on epaulettes), looking like 'graceful and compassionate commissioned angels' – at least, that is how they appeared to bronchitis-stricken J.M. Pettigrew's eighteen-year-old eyes. The only item that seemed to detract from the overall effect was 'rather clompy white ward shoes – which nevertheless served to warn our illicit smokers of the approach of authority'.

Kathleen Hird (Mrs Bion) sums up the feelings of many PMs who served during those post-war days:

> How very lucky we were. We had trained during the war [when] life really didn't consist of anything else but hospital – no social life or excitement. Suddenly there I was in beautiful Buckinghamshire being treated as an officer and all the perks, and then overseas ... In the days when holidays or travel didn't exist for the average public, we were spoilt, and I'll always be grateful for the memories.

By the time the fifties ended, however, several of the RAF's overseas hospitals would be defunct.

South of Suez

In Cairo, the wartime No. 5 RAFGH had closed in 1947 and was due to be replaced by a new unit on the shores of the Great Bitter Lake, south of the Suez Canal, an area where several RAF stations then existed. An officers' club by the lake provided a base where personnel could swim, sunbathe and socialize.

Dulcie Flower (Mrs Wright) had been at RAFH Tel Litwinsky in Palestine, but ...

> In 1947 a couple of us were posted with four other PMs to open a hospital in the Canal Zone. As nothing was known about us or the hospital, we did not know what to do, so we took ourselves down to the Great Bitter Lake most afternoons. Then more officers arrived who got on with building the hospital and the sisters' quarters (up until then we had been housed in appalling conditions in a disused NAAFI hut). In the meantime, the wives of the troops serving in the Canal Zone were arriving from the UK, so it was decided to open a Families Hospital at Abyad, just up the road ...

While this hospital was being prepared, the two midwives and the obstetrician all went on leave to Cyprus, confident that no babies were expected before they returned. However, Dulcie Flower was on duty one night when the wardmaster rang to warn her of the imminent arrival of a maternity patient. 'Having only Part One Midwifery Certificate, I was not allowed to do a delivery without a doctor in attendance, so I dragged a sleepy Duty MO out of his bed . . .' The patient arrived, in advanced labour – she had been at a cocktail party at the officers' mess in Ismailia and what with the gin and the heat . . . Happily, she produced her baby without problems, but the puzzled MO asked, 'Was there any question of you having twins, Mrs Evans?' She replied, 'No, that was the other Mrs Evans.' X-rays had got muddled! Just as doctor and sister were relaxing and congratulating themselves, another expectant mother turned up, also well into labour. She too had been drinking gin cocktails at that party in Ismailia!

With both mothers and babies comfortably settled, Dulcie set off across the desert taking the linen to the sluice room. 'I knew that the electric light had not been fixed yet, but it never occurred to me that the rest of the building would be unfinished because the water was laid on. When I started the sluicing, I found to my horror that my feet were getting wet. With typical Egyptian (in)efficiency, the pipes had not been connected!'

The Fayid/Abyad hospital opened officially on 1 January 1948, when it was joined by all staff from the defunct hospital at Tel Litwinsky, which was now in the new state of Israel. Later that year, Doris Stanford (Mrs Kent) was sent to Fayid from Habbaniya to help nurse an epidemic of typhoid which affected two hundred RAF and army patients. With the temperature outside up to 100°F, no air conditioning, and few, if any, antibiotics, the sisters relied on good nursing and tepid sponging. It was back-aching work with patients on low iron bedsteads, but it paid off – they didn't lose a patient.

Margaret Kingston and her friend Meg Goulbourne had

> . . . only been in the service about six months when, to our amazement, we were told we were going overseas. 1951, November – you can imagine, trying to get summer clothing in November . . . We were called by the Wing Officer matron to say goodbye . . . [Her] last words to us were, 'I do hope you enjoy Germany'. We were off to Egypt!
>
> We eventually got to Fayid . . . and were met by the Wing

Officer, Margaret Ashworth, with an enormous Alsatian dog
– we felt very honoured to be met by the Wing Officer. We
learned afterwards she'd come to the plane to see if they'd
brought the dog food for her Alsatian! And another sister, a
very beautiful Irish girl, Kay, had come to meet us, which was
very sweet, but when she turned round . . . the back seam of
her white dress – with all the washing, the cotton had given.
A belt held the top, the hem held the bottom, and there was
her backside with these white panties . . . Tropical kit!

A military coup in 1952 overthrew Egypt's King Farouk and
launched a strongly pro-Arab republic, providing a focus for anti-
Israeli feeling. Britain held on to control of the Canal Zone, but as
political tensions grew, at RAF Fayid dissidents blew up some
ammunition dumps. For security reasons most local mess servants
were barred from camp.

To Margaret Kingston, however,

Egypt was a nice posting, although we were confined to camp
because of the Suez trouble, and the mess servants had gone
. . . Off-duty in the afternoon we could go swimming, in the
Bitter Lake, but we had to have an armed escort. There was
an open garry [truck], and four airmen with guns at each
corner, and the sisters on deck-chairs – you can imagine,
bumping over the open desert . . .

Two of the bearers, who had been security-vetted and allowed to
stay, decorated the mess for Christmas while off-duty staff went to
church. 'When we got back . . . all our bras and pants, and any old
cotton dresses we'd thrown out during the year, were chopped up
in bits and all on strings . . . We had to be very tactful, but the CO
was coming over for coffee and we had to do a very quick removal!'

Theatre sister Eileen Adams (Mrs Knapper) remembers
Christmas fun when she and the surgeon swapped uniforms and did
a full ward round – 'It went down well with the patients!' She had
specifically asked to be posted to Fayid, so that she might visit the
grave of her brother, an airman who died with two others in a road
accident while serving in Egypt. This she was able to do. She recalls
having plenty of work: during a severe outbreak of dysentery, tents

had to be erected to take extra beds, a flying officer was brought in from the desert, having had to bail out of his aircraft; and a surgical team remained 'on standby, with equipment packed and ready. Early in the morning we were called to a sick airman at RAF El Adem, a staging post inland from Tobruk.' Having nursed the airman for two days, they flew him back to Fayid for an operation.

The desert outpost of El Adem (described by one PM as 'two camels and a sand-dune') found itself short of women in 1953, so 'an aircraft known as the Sisters' Special was laid on to take some of us over for their Summer Ball,' says Eileen. She also met her future husband while stationed at Fayid: 'When I informed Matron Miller that I was getting engaged to Flt Lt Knapper, within 48 hours I was sent to the RAF Hospital Aden. Then on marriage I had to resign my commission – what a waste!'

In July 1956, when Egyptian President Nasser nationalized the Suez Canal, Britain withdrew all her personnel from the area. Joan Metcalfe was aboard the troopship *Devonshire* at a historic moment at Port Said when 'we brought out the last troops of the Grenadier Guards, who had been the first troops into Egypt after Napoleon had left.' When RAFH Fayid – the last RAF hospital in Egypt – closed, its staff moved to the newly opened hospital at Akrotiri, Cyprus.

Sea trooping

In those days of slow aeroplanes with limited passenger space, British troops and their families moved around the world by sea. Nursing and medical officers, with a full sick quarters staff, went with them to look after their health on the long voyages.

Jessie Higgins sailed aboard the famous troopship *Devonshire*, 'backwards and forwards to Singapore and it used to take thirty or thirty-one days'.

> Went through the Med, down the Canal and through the Red Sea, to Aden, then straight across to Colombo, in Ceylon . . . *Devonshire* had 120 hospital beds on it. We had all the families, umpteen wives and children . . . Coming back, we used to bring all the sick . . . It was before the days when antibiotics were being used properly, and a lot of people being given

penicillin couldn't take it. People with prickly-heat, penicillin made it ten times worse . . . We had to put them up the top where it was airy. We got to the stage where we'd say, right, we're going up the Canal tomorrow, turn left into the Med, and they'll all be better in a day – and they were!

The ill-advised Anglo-French invasion of the Canal Zone early in November 1956 ended in humiliation, mostly because of pressure from America, but Nasser retaliated by sinking forty-nine ships to block the canal. The seaway remained closed for five months.

During the closure of the Suez Canal, troopships faced extra-long voyages. When the civilian-run *Orwell* called in at Singapore, on the way home from Japan, Joy Harris was one of the medical team who were asked to bring home 'a tremendous number of psychiatric patients'.

In those days, the aeromeds only ever carried one, or two, psychiatric patients – they weren't very happy about having a lot, because they were slow aircraft . . . Both the doctor and myself were worried about this, neither of us had any psychiatric training at all. So, the psychiatrist at Singapore came on board and said, 'They'll be all right. Just humour them. Let them do more or less what they want.' The ship's captain wasn't too pleased about that [but] we all got on very well until we came into port, when one of the sergeants on board, being evacuated home because he had ideas of grandeur and went around selling everything – he tried to sell the Raffles Hotel in Singapore – he kept going ashore and we thought he might try to sell the ship while he was gone! . . . They didn't come to any harm, they all got home safely. It was a marvellous trip . . . when we got to Cape Town the South Africans were so hospitable. They all turned up on the quayside and every passenger on board, being trooped home, was taken off for the day, and we were 'sung out' [by] the 'lady in white'. She used to sing as the troopships went round in the war. She had a beautiful voice.

On the doughty *Devonshire* again, in summer 1957 Joan Metcalfe and Christine Bramley (Mrs Bull) sailed, with men of all three services, out to Christmas Island for 'Operation Grapple' – the first British hydrogen bomb tests. Calling in at Singapore, they picked up the Fijian Regiment, who had been serving in Malaya, and took them home, anchoring in Suva harbour for three days while welcoming ceremonies took place. Then they sailed to Christmas Island, where most of the British troops disembarked to prepare for the coming tests. Christine says:

> With an almost empty ship, we sailed on to Honolulu, where a small army team was to set up a staging post for troops flying out to Christmas Island via the States. Before any of us could go ashore we had to be interviewed by US immigration officers, who were amazed to find females on a troopship. Not only that but the ship was not 'dry' like the US troop ships!

Because of currency restrictions they went ashore with an allowance of $3 a day so, 'being short of ready cash, we took our packets of *Devonshire* sandwiches and bottles of Merseyside lemonade and went off to Waikiki beach to surf and swim'.

The three-week voyage back to Singapore, on an 'empty' ship, seemed like a leisure cruise, with interesting fish swimming by and spectacular sunsets blazing across ocean and sky. 'I kept saying, "This is the best Pacific tour",' recalls Joan Metcalfe, 'just lounging around – we had nothing to do.'

They made up for it later, coming home from Singapore with a full complement of men, wives and families, via Colombo, Mombasa in Kenya, Cape Town, Dakar, and finally north through the Atlantic. Hitting rough weather in the Bay of Biscay reminded Christine Bramley of the story of another PM encountering terrible weather, which had *Devonshire*'s treatment room 'awash with gentian violet and liquid paraffin . . . She hadn't been able to decide which to save if they were told to abandon ship – her fur coat or her jewels!'

HMT *Devonshire* made many voyages with PMs on duty in her sick bay. Doreen Smedley was aboard when they took Irish Fusiliers out to Tripoli and brought the King's Royal Rifles back. EOKA terrorists were active in Cyprus at the time, so the ship stayed in the harbour and everything was brought out to them, including the station band, on a float, to play for them. On another trip they had

200 children aboard: 'The first measle appeared as we sailed down Southampton Water . . . But generally', says Doreen, 'for the wives and families it was like taking a six-week holiday.'

However, Kathy Mogg (Mrs Ostler), sailing with a shipload of soldiers and their families, recalls ill-feeling because of

> . . . insufficient cabin space for corporals and below to share with families . . . [and despite] talks on living in a hot climate, health advice and lists of necessary clothing, many of the young wives were out of their depth. Young children were dressed in non-absorbent materials, resulting in skin problems. The general overcrowding . . . for the third class passengers added to the misery.

And of course there was seasickness.

> I had it! I remember attempting to give a bedbath to a patient in sickbay when I was feeling terrible. After two days I was told to pull myself together and get on with it . . . I was given some special ground-up powder to take, which cured me! . . . Meanwhile one was expected to enter into the social whirl . . . bingo, dancing, talent night, a raffle, and film shows. Later, when the weather improved, we had a fancy dress ball . . .

But sea-trooping was coming to an end. *Devonshire*'s last trooping voyage was in December 1961, when on leaving Malta the ship received a rousing send-off – she was a favourite visitor at Mediterranean bases. But all the troopships are fondly remembered by the many PMs who served aboard them. They provided a means by which single girls could get away from home and see the world – an opportunity not to be missed in those pre-feminist days.

Long-haul aeromeds

Two-year postings to overseas hospitals provided a more in-depth method of sampling foreign climes for some PMs. Others saw the world in fleeting glimpses, as they escorted patients on the aeromedical evacuation flights which, more and more, became a vital part of a nursing sister's career.

The object of post-war aeromeds was to bring back to England
any ill or injured service personnel, members of their families, and
British government employees (such as teachers and diplomats)
who, while working abroad, might require specialist or urgent
treatment not available locally. Other patients might benefit from
the service if circumstance warranted. At first, any nursing officer
might be plucked from her ward and sent to escort an aeromed
patient half across the world. She learned, perforce, by doing the
job.

For a while Dakotas and Valettas continued in use for medium-
length flights, but from 1948 the Handley Page Hastings became
the RAF's standard long-range transport aircraft. It could be fitted
out to carry between twenty-eight and thirty-two patients, with
stretchers fitted in tiers down each side of the central aisle.
However, flying aeromed aboard a Hastings was not ideal: being
unpressurized and unable to fly above 10,000 feet, the aircraft
encountered a good deal of turbulence. Respiratory distress among
patients, allied with cramped working conditions, and the need to
shout to be heard (while sometimes wearing ear-protectors against
the deafening noise of those slow old piston engines) caused added
problems for nurses, especially on those long, long flights to and
from the Far East. The minimum time for a flight to Singapore was
five days, including stops for refuelling and overnight rest breaks
when patients would be unloaded and taken to the hospital or sick
quarters attached to each staging post. In practice, journeys often
took longer than scheduled – many stories of early aeromeds
include the words '. . . the aircraft went u/s [unserviceable] and we
were delayed.' The delay could last hours or days.

Some flights were one-off specials, others more routine – for
instance, once a month, in the early fifties, flight sisters based at
Wroughton packed their medical panniers and flew from RAF
Lyneham to Wildenrath in Germany, bringing back mainly TB
patients. While airborne, the nursing sister would *not* be sitting, like
a tourist, with her feet up, snoozing, reading a book and/or enjoying 'duty-frees'; she had too much to do keeping her patients
comfortable, seeing they were fed and watered, supplying them
with bottles and bedpans, ensuring comfortable respiration at altitude . . . the list varied with the needs of each particular patient.

Many sisters spent the night prior to take-off at the 'rather bleak spot' known as Clyffe Pypard, a village near RAF Lyneham. Joy Harris remembers it well.

I flew out to Singapore in 1951, on my first posting, in my first aeroplane, from Clyffe Pypard . . . I remember going into this room, with a coke stove . . . red-hot! I got into bed, next thing I knew, the chap who was driving the coach down to the aircraft was saying, 'You've been called, ma'am, you should be on the coach now!' I hadn't been called at all, although somebody produced a thing that I'd 'signed' – it was only a squiggle. I think I got dressed and was on the coach in two minutes – and when you consider those were the days of suspender belts, full uniform, collar with studs in it, tie, and greatcoat – I don't know how I did it . . . Nobody told you that the stuff you wanted on your trip had to be in a small bag. So all my tropical uniform, to change into halfway out, was going in the hold . . . One of the fellows who'd met me the night before helped me out – he must have been the Movements Officer, because he took me up to where all the stuff was and got my case out . . . He took a liking to me, probably had his eye on the main chance – you learn these things very quickly – he'd got me a bacon and egg sandwich . . . well, I was surprised to have my breakfast in a sandwich, but I'd have been even more astounded not to have had breakfast. You always had a cooked breakfast.

Doreen Smedley was posted to Wroughton to do aeromed though, unusually, she had not volunteered for it. At some stops there was no relief sister, as there was later; you did the whole trip on your own and the saying was that 'you walked all the way back from the Far East'. She was not too enamoured of aeromed duty, but adds, 'I will never forget the sight of the night sky at Idris. It was blue-black, and studded with diamonds – a wonderful sight!'

Ann Tickle (Mrs Waters) spent three and a half incident-full years on aeromed duty at Wroughton. She specialized in nursing polio victims and escorted one lady back from Egypt in an iron lung. In Cyprus during the EOKA terrorist troubles, she and her colleagues drove with an armed guard in their car, escorted by an ambulance with a gun pointing out of the window.

Any flight might run into unexpected situations, as Julia Inkpen (Mrs Jenkins) found out. Her aircraft, with twenty French typists as passengers, made a forced landing at Sharjah, where the men hadn't seen a woman for five months. The CO spirited his female visitors to a fort on the base complete with double locks and armed guards!

Despite the security, we had a great time in the 24 hours we were there. Men appeared from all directions. One doctor insisted that we visit his hospital and two locust control officers took us off over the desert to Dubai where we met other European officials who laid on a party. We were quite embarrassed by the flimsy state of our cotton dresses as the local women were in deepest purdah with only their eyes showing . . .

Joy Harris tells of a stop-over at Car Nicobar, in the Nicobar Islands, Indian Ocean, which provided a staging post before the island of Gan came into RAF use.

They had one very young officer – it was just a refuelling base, no doctors – they didn't wear any clothes at all unless there was an aircraft with some women on, and then they'd put shorts on . . . When I got there the cook had a most terrible rash – he'd cut himself and the local 'witch-doctor' had shoved some paste on it.

They'd seen on the manifest that there would be a nursing officer on board, so they thought they'd wait until we got there and ask our opinions. I asked if they'd got any medical supplies – 'Oh, in the safe' – so they opened the safe, and all they'd got was some codeine, some morphia, and a pistol! I think we told them to get on to Singapore to ask the next aircraft to bring them some anti-histamines.

PMs on parade! Ready for the Queen's coronation, June 1953. *Second from right on back row:* Maureen Lumley and *centre front* Matron-in-Chief Dame Veronica Ashworth (© British Crown Copyright/MOD)

Aerial view of RAFH Changi, Singapore, 1950 (© British Crown Copyright/MOD)

Dame Joanna Cruickshank's last appearance at a PMRAFNS
tennis tournament, 1957

Dinghy drill during aeromed training, 1960s
(© British Crown Copyright/MOD)

Sir Winston Churchill brought home by RAF aeromed team, including
Flight Officer 'Penny' Penrose, after breaking his leg in Monaco, 1962

TWO

As PMs flew more and more aeromeds, sisters assigned to this duty underwent special flight-nursing courses at RAF Lyneham. At first the course was fairly basic, lectures and demonstrations with a session in what Sally Donovan (Mrs Pullan) calls 'the dreaded decompression chamber'. In this test, because of euphoria caused by lack of oxygen,

> . . . we were quite sure we could survive everything, and then you looked at the paper afterwards – you'd written awful rubbish. And the most cocky amongst us was the one who passed out, of course . . . You did all the bits of airworthiness . . . when you were chucked around everywhere in those awful old Hastings – lovely old Hastings – to see whether you could cope . . .

Adult patients, whether mobile or strapped in stretchers, presented problems enough: for younger patients, ingenuity helped. 'You had a little crèche made up of four boxes – huge wooden crates with a red cross. You used to put three in a row and a rug on the floor, and the children all sat in there – obviously they weren't going to be pinned in a seat.'

As an illustration of the kind of workload flight sisters experienced, Sister Elizabeth E. Chalton (Mrs Walker) kept a detailed record of one of her missions, flown in a Hastings in August 1956:

Date	From	Flying time	Destination
2/8	Lyneham	6hrs 20 mins	Idris, N.Africa (via El Adem)
3/8	Idris	8hrs 5 mins	Habbaniya, Iraq
4/8	Habbaniya	7hrs 10 mins	Mauripur, Pakistan
5/8	Mauripur	6hrs 35 mins	Negombo, Ceylon (Sri Lanka)
6/8	Negombo	8hrs 35 mins	Changi, Singapore
7/8 free day			
8/8	Changi	8hrs 35 mins	Negombo, Ceylon
9/8	Negombo	7hrs 30 mins	Mauripur, Pakistan
10/8 free day			
11/8	Mauripur	7hrs 30 mins	Habbaniya, Iraq
12/8	Habbaniya	7hrs 50 mins	Luqa, Malta
13/8	Luqa	7hrs 30 mins	Lyneham, UK

Since in practice a 'free day' *en route* was often spent helping out at the local RAF hospital, these journeys were no rest cure.

Staging posts at El Adem, Idris, Mauripur and Luqa all had large sick quarters, most of which eventually claimed PMs on their staff; at the others, non-commissioned male SRNs of the RAFMS supervised the orderlies. These experienced male nurses also worked side by side with female nursing officers of the PMRAFNS at hospitals at Habbaniya in Iraq, Negombo in Ceylon, and Changi in Singapore. But in Iraq and Ceylon the flags of the RAF were soon to be hauled down for the last time.

'Lido of the East'

By the late forties, RAF Habbaniya had grown into a huge sprawl, 'the second largest town in Iraq, after Baghdad', according to those who knew it. Its airfield had an extra runway on the plateau above to take the huge new transport planes. The camp included quarters for families, churches of several denominations, shopping centres, well-tended gardens with trees and flowers, sports facilities (including grassed football pitches), clubs of all kinds, various messes, a riding school, a civil cantonment, a race track and even a taxi service to get people around the enormous 28 square miles of the camp. It was the 'Lido of the East', an oasis with permanent stone buildings and an elusive perfume of Arabia – gardens and football pitches stayed green by nightly flooding from irrigation ditches fed by the pungent waters of the Euphrates!

Doris Stanford (Mrs Kent) arrived in Habbaniya by air, in a York aircraft: 'I'll never forget that, because we were flying low and we hit a dust storm. We were all frightfully sick and we arrived feeling and looking like nothing on earth.' A team of twenty sisters, led by Matron Tisdale, staffed the large hospital. Sisters' rooms lay apart from the mess, beyond gardens full of oleander bushes and eucalyptus trees where 'coming back from a dance or from a club at night with our escorts, we might linger a little bit. Suddenly out of the bushes these men would appear – "Halt, who goes there?!" They knew who we were but they would always jump out . . .' On occasion the guards were less vigilant. One sister was alone in her room when two men burst in and threatened her with knives while they stole all her possessions.

Most of the local people appreciated the work brought by the RAF station. Iraqi women helped in the hospital and Iraqi men did labouring work, or acted as personal bearers. But cultural differences caused misunderstandings, as Margaret Kingston points out: 'My bearer knew that I *loved* Marmite and Bovril – in the mess I often used to ask for it at tea-time. So, every morning, when he brought my cup of tea, I had a jar of Marmite and a cup of tea! What he thought I was going to do with a whole jar I don't know! *Every* day . . .'

On the occasion of the coronation of Queen Elizabeth II, Habbaniya staged a military tattoo. Margaret Kingston says:

We had to go in our mess kit, which in those days was like a white nightie. We had our rankings up on our shoulders, and brass buttons, and sleeves with pointed bits over our hands, and then a big white hat turned up at the side, with the RAF cockade at the side – we used to call it our bowling team outfit! And white court shoes, from Moss Bros. Well, we got to the arena and everything stopped – they didn't know what had arrived – the matron with her ten ducklings parading behind . . . It was a very good spectacle they put on, but like a fool I took my shoes off and, of course, come time to leave, I could *not* get them on. My escort very nobly put one in each pocket and I had to walk back in my stocking feet . . . They had solid toes, these shoes. We used to fill them with water and bang them on the handle of a broom, to soften them – they were really impossible.

The rest and leave centre at Ser Amadia, up in the Kurdistan hills, still required sisters to stay on short attachments. During her sojourn, Joan Metcalfe 'used to go out into the villages; you'd get a message somebody was ill, out you went on mules . . . In Kurdistan they were all so nice, so friendly – but primitive – they had swinging electric light bulbs down the main street, with hovels either side.' Margaret Kingston also rode out on a mule to treat the tribespeople, some of whom still had stocks of old-style powdered penicillin, long past its sell-by date. 'You had to put sterile water in it and shake it . . . So, diplomatically, we used to take some fresh penicillin and treat their children . . .'

An adventurous incident recalled by Doreen Elston (Mrs Curston) began at Habbaniya when a signal came from Ser Amadia requesting urgent medical assistance for a member of the WRAF who was dangerously ill with a fractured dislocation of the neck. A team consisting of Sister Elston, a surgeon and a theatre technician, flew to the nearest Iraqi airfield, at Mosul. They were still forty-five mountainous, roadless miles from Ser Amadia. They spied a helicopter 'but we were told it was just for the use of King Faisal II.' However, by pulling a few diplomatic strings they obtained permission to borrow the helicopter and its pilot. 'We were sitting in luxuriously upholstered seats when the pilot informed us it was not safe for him to fly at more than 6,000 feet. The only compensation . . . was that we flew over some of the most beautiful mountain ranges and gorges we had ever seen . . .' Ser Amadia lay too high in the mountains for the helicopter to reach and, seeing the terrain ahead, they began to wonder how on earth they would bring the girl safely down the mountain. Landing at a local levies' camp, they had tea while the Iraqi soldiers saddled mules for the final leg.

It was at this point that we learnt that the injury to our patient had occurred due to her falling from a mule . . .

We set off on the final lap, the mules insisting on walking at the very edge of each precipice, with thousands of feet drop below, only stopping for the call of nature, after which they would take off at enormous speed to catch up with the others . . .

At Ser Amadia they found the patient in reasonable condition.

She had a fracture dislocation of the cervical spine with, fortunately, no cord involvement, and a fractured humerus. We
immediately set to work reducing the dislocation by traction
and immobilising her in plaster ... Next morning we
enclosed her in a Neil Robertson stretcher and general service
stretcher for transportation, and again with the help of the
levy troops, we transported her down the mountain. The
descent was a more gentle slope ... but still very hazardous.

At the bottom of the mountain a pickup waited to transfer them
along 'an unbelievably bad road full of pot-holes' to an airstrip
where an Anson waited, piloted by the senior wing commander
from Habbaniya. They managed 'to squeeze the patient into the
plane and strapped her in firmly ... Mountain sides flashed
perilously close as we banked and climbed steeply ... our last view
of the airfield was the adjutant of Ser Amadia down on his knees
praying for us ...'

The RAF's position in Iraq was, however, no longer secure. In
July 1956 the status of Habbaniya hospital was reduced, with a
sister-in-charge instead of a matron. Two years later, the assassina-
tion of King Faisal II ushered in a pro-USSR republic with a deter-
minedly neutral foreign policy. At this point, all British forces withdrew from Iraq.

Ceylon

Another exotic staging-point provided a posting for PMs from 1950
to 1960. This was Ceylon (now Sri Lanka), island of shady palms
and coconut groves, warm western beaches and jungles where
elephant and crimson butterfly roam free. From Biblical times,
merchants and invaders came here seeking spices and gems:
Solomon sent for Singhalese jewels to impress the Queen of Sheba,
and later the Romans, the Moors, the Portuguese and the Dutch
came, wanting cinnamon, rubies, topaz and moonstones; and
planters settled to grow coffee and tap rubber. From 1815, Britain
controlled the island. Plantations of coffee, which brought a
seasonal influx of Indian pickers, were replaced by tea, which
required picking year-round by Indian incomers – the Tamils.

During the Second World War the island acted as a springboard for Allied operations. Naval and army bases grew up, with the RAF at Katunayake and an MFH nearby. The airfield, some four miles south of Negombo, would eventually become Colombo International airport.

On Ceylon's assumption of independence in 1948, the British military hospital at Colombo closed, but the flight staging post at RAF Katunayake remained in operation. In order to provide medical cover both for RAF personnel on the island and for patients brought through on air evacuation flights, Flight Officer Kathleen Hird (Mrs Bion) and Squadron Officer (Matron) Gwen Jones trooped out on the *Orduna* in 1950 to help open a new RAFH at Negombo.

What Kathleen Hird considered 'a lovely single storey hospital in the middle of the vast coconut plantation' was still in the building process when the nursing officers sailed in that February. They accepted their first patients in March, when Sisters Robertson and Boutland arrived – as did the first baby, born before the paint was dry! The PMs lived in the officers' mess, which made for pleasant off-duty hours with

> ... long nights on the verandah with the chaps and visiting Hastings crews doing the supply routes, and many G&Ts. No swimming pool for us but a wonderful lagoon a couple of miles away with superb empty beaches and curry in the Rest House ... Quite a few cases of poliomyelitis – someone found an old iron lung in Colombo and brought it back to us.

Over the ten years of the hospital's existence, Ceylon left different impressions on all the PMs who saw it. On leave from Aden, Margaret Kingston enjoyed a holiday there. She had visited the island before, staging through while on casevacs, but never for long enough to get used to the frogs: 'They never stop all night. This awful croak-croak-croak-croak-croak-croak ... it goes on and on.'

Tessa Lawless recalls the beauty of the harbour lights at night as she arrived by ship, the dancing elephants at a zoo, and the brilliant colours of sunset fading to the paler glory of moonrise.

On the last Comet to stage through Negombo, Rosie Partington and a friend arrived from RAFH Changi to spend ten days' leave in Ceylon. They toured the island by taxi, the cheapest way, and the driver, asking if they were interested in 'stones', took them to the back of a wood, to a little shed where they saw all manner of gems in screw-top jars – opals, aquamarines, garnets . . . 'Afterwards,' says Rosie, 'we wished we'd known more about them.' The little man left them to pick out what stones they wanted and later he came back to fix a very reasonable price. Rosie only wished she had bought more while she was about it!

Jessie Higgins (who had hated the bugs and snakes in Burma) spent six months in Ceylon. She remembers 'a horrible little hospital'.

Absolutely open. No windows, just balconies. We were about 25 miles from Colombo and, with casevac, they were in and out twice a week, very hard work when they'd come in . . . I was terrified there, because . . . I'm one who sees snakes – or so I was told by an old boy in Ceylon: 'Missie see snake, Missie see snake.' We had maternity there, and we had a 'caesar' one night . . . I went over, being a midwife, and was bringing the baby back when suddenly I realised something was going across my legs – I had the baby in my arms, so I couldn't see down – I looked round and there was about ten feet of snake . . . How I didn't drop that baby, I'll never know. I could not move! I just stood and let the snake go. It was terrifying.

The joke was, when I reported it in the morning they all said, 'Oh, go on, Higgie – you see snakes everywhere,' and I said, 'I saw snake!' Then about two days later . . . we had those great big iron lungs in those days and I went and pulled the lid back – and there's a snake in the iron lung! I worried about them getting into babies' cots. I would have died if any baby had been hurt . . . I must say, I hated Ceylon.

Jean King (Mrs Flower) writes of 'the heat which hit us as we left the aircraft. Having left England in mid-winter wearing our blues, we changed into KDs [khaki drill] in Karachi, but even in lighter uniform we still wore stockings and regulation black shoes . . .' RAF Katunayake had a capacious officers' mess designed to accommodate crew and passengers on unexpected stopovers, from aircraft needing repair or otherwise delayed.

I remember coming off night duty one morning and walking into our large mess dining room to find it full of American soldiers grounded from their u/s troop carrier – unfortunately repaired very quickly.

The situation with the Tamils was in its very early stages but there was an incident during 1958 which resulted in us being confined to camp for six weeks . . . The station cinema was our salvation . . . the programme was changed every night!

Jean was one of six nursing officers stationed in Ceylon in 1958, of whom four were midwives; the 'midder' unit was kept very busy. It and the families' ward had Sinhalese women as orderlies, but the airmen's ward had national servicemen. 'There were many long-haul flights in the '50s and the same crews dropped in . . . Casevac sisters came through quite often, and the girls coming to Ceylon on leave from Changi often spent a night with us on the way.' PMs and pilots shared balmy evenings on the verandah under the palms 'with a long cool gin and fresh lime in my hand [or] in the ante room listening to music . . . Records were few and precious, easily broken, so that the oft-repeated music from those days does stick around in my memory . . .'

The darker side

The happy, social side of casualty evacuation lingers in many memories. But there were dangers, too.

In March 1953 an aeromed flight with Julia Inkpen (Mrs Jenkins) as flight sister approached Lyneham in thick fog. 'A dreadful crash and rending sound convinced us that our last moment had come, but then, with a roar, we climbed into the blue sky again.' They had hit the tops of trees and were told to divert to RAF Tangmere, near Chichester, flying no higher than 1,000 feet. After a safe landing,

> . . . we were horrified to see that the wings were ripped to pieces, propellers bent, and the tail almost severed. Everyone at Tangmere was on the runway. I heard one officer remark, 'If I hadn't seen it with my own eyes I wouldn't have believed

that an aircraft could fly in such a condition.' Getting the stretchers off was quite a problem (Lyneham had ambulances with opening roofs). It was achieved by backing three-tonners up to the door of the aircraft, unloading the stretchers onto the roofs, thence lowering them into other vehicles. I think we all suffered from delayed shock. The pilot's last comment was 'We must have had angels on the wingtips.'

In 1956 Kay Burrows (Mrs Bennett) was 'escorting a small party of patients from Kai Tak [Hong Kong] to the RAF hospital at Changi, in a Valetta'.

We had just left Saigon when we lost one engine, then lost height. The pilot decided to put down in a paddy field, which was also a Chinese cemetery, so we hit a grave! We evacuated quickly for fear of fire. Nobody was injured except the pilot, whom we feared might have broken his spine (not the case, in the event). We put him on an aircraft door and tied him firmly. A crowd of curious Vietnamese arrived and brought up a car. We put the poor pilot in the back – at an angle with his feet sticking out – and I went in the front with the driver, and a marvellous Scots lad, a patient, ran as long as he could supporting the pilot's head.

On the main road an open truck met them and they loaded the pilot into the back of it. 'By then he was complaining of his eyes, which he feared had glass in them. The friendly villagers were still round us [so] I asked for water and one produced a bottle of lemonade – I washed his eyes out with that. We eventually reached the French hospital in Saigon . . .' Kay found accommodation with an American family, who drove her round to visit and distribute sedatives to her various patients, scattered among host families, but 'most particularly I was able to thank that marvellous Scottish boy who ran beside the pilot . . . The pilot made a full recovery.'

She adds modestly, 'This small incident was, I fear, exaggerated, but it brought a small measure of recognition of the PMs. I am very proud to have been a member.' For her part in this 'small incident', Kay was awarded the Royal Humane Society Bronze Medal – the first award of its kind to be made in a peacetime incident.

An even more terrible accident occurred on 4 March 1956, when an Anson aircraft on a casualty evacuation flight over Germany lost oil pressure at 4,000 feet, obliging the pilot to feather the engine. Unable to maintain height, and with the ground below obscured by cloud, he decided to make a forced landing, but on breaking through the cloud he found himself low over a heavily wooded area. He tried to turn to avoid the trees, but caught his starboard wing. The plane crashed. Flight Officer Daphne Jane Budgen of the PMRAFNS and SAC R. Flint of the RAFMS were both killed; the pilot and another nurse, Sergeant J.P. Moynan, suffered serious injuries.

Steamer Point, Aden

Aden's RAF hospital, set high on its hill above the busy port, took in all service personnel, their wives and families, merchant seamen of all races, and personnel from the BP oil refinery which, in the fifties, was still under construction. Everyone who worked at Steamer Point mentions the heat and the impossibility of staying crisply starched. Matron and her twelve ward sisters had to change clothes at least twice a day to stay comfortable.

Margaret Kingston remembers the problems caused by having a families' ward on two floors, 'children down below where it was impossible to see them without going up and down outside steps'. However, one blessedly air-conditioned room provided a respite for certain very ill patients. One patient was resting there under Margaret Kingston's supervision when the air-conditioning machine, 'a large noisy tractor-like affair outside on the verandah' stopped working. Unable to persuade anyone from 'Works and Bricks' to come to her aid, Margaret 'rang the CO, Group Captain "Kiwi" Corbett'.

> He immediately gathered up his tool bag and in his baggy KD shorts appeared on the scene. He had the thing in bits on the verandah when Matron came to do her round. Kiwi kept his head down and continued banging. 'Sister!' says Matron, 'Stop that man making such a noise when I'm doing my round!' With that, Kiwi looked up and laughed. Blushes all round.

Later, on a morning when a staff photograph was to be taken, nursing sisters and MOs, dressed in immaculate whites, stood around waiting for Kiwi Corbett to arrive. They heard his old banger chugging up the hill, and, 'at that very moment, a vulture flew overhead, having gathered a sheep's entrails from the village slaughter below the rocks . . . it dropped the mess bang onto the head of one of the sisters . . . she had to retreat for a quick shower and change of uniform.'

A genuine life-or-death emergency called Barbara Millar (Mrs Wight) into action when, in 1952, Flight Lieutenant Percy Henry Mason was accidentally shot – in the heart – while hunting baboons out in the *bundu*. On theatre night call, Sister Millar was woken at 1 a.m. with orders to be ready to fly at first light from RAF Khormaksar to Dhala, a primitive state sixty-five miles away in the protectorate. With the help of the corporal theatre technician and an Arab orderly she had to prepare and pack the necessary equipment which, with no pre-packed trays in those days, meant that 'instruments had to be selected, rinsed, arranged in the trays wrapped in dressing towels and autoclaved [steam-sterilized]. This included all drums with dressing gowns, towels, etc – sutures, needles, lotions . . . I prepared a general set, and specialized instruments such as bone cutters, large retractors, etc, and the corporal prepared the anaesthetic trolley.' Time was of the essence. They only hoped they had remembered everything.

Two Ansons waited for them at Khormaksar. The first flew with surgeon Squadron Leader Dickie Prior and his anaesthetist brother Derek; the second carried Sister Millar, the corporal technician and the equipment. After an hour's flight they landed at the airstrip in remote and mountainous Dhala. Local Arabs had gathered to watch proceedings and the emir's young son arrived on a donkey, with his bodyguard alongside. Having assessed the situation, the surgeon decided it was too risky to perform heart surgery out in the rocky desert; they must fly the patient back to Aden. Barbara says 'Dickie, Derek and myself . . . took it in turns to hold up the drip with the left hand and give slight pressure with swabs on his chest with the right hand, to stop the oozing.'

From the airfield at Khormaksar an ambulance took them the ten miles back to the RAF hospital at Steamer Point, where the theatre team waited. Twenty-two donors from the RAF and WRAF each

gave a pint of blood. Using a technique practised only once before
by a British doctor (patients with perforated hearts did not usually
survive long enough to reach the operating table) the team trans-
fused blood via the patient's artery instead of a vein. Almost
instantly his pulse revived and his blood pressure rose. Barbara
Millar adds, 'Nursing care was excellent, bearing in mind that we
did not have the facilities of an Intensive Care Ward . . . Flt Lt
Mason recovered, with a slight enlargement of the liver.'

Changi

Much further east, Singapore lies at the southern tip of the Malay
Peninsula, a cosmopolitan whirl of different tongues, religions, ritu-
als and customs. At the eastern tip of the island, Changi village
looks northward across the Straits of Johore, a vista of flowering
trees and blue seas, with two or three miles away the deep green
forests of the Malay Peninsula. The RAF hospital, opened in 1947,
stood on a hill and was originally two large blocks of buildings
separated by a famous flight of ninety steps.

Joy Harris arrived in Changi in 1951.

> On your first day there, you were sent down to the village to
> buy a packet of starch and some washing powder for the amah
> – oh, and an umbrella, because it poured with rain every day.
> And the amah starched *everything*. You had cotton dresses in
> those days – they'd stand up without you in them. And you
> had to wear stockings, and she'd starch those too, and your
> knickers and everything – awfully uncomfortable.

For Olive Kirkham, a visit to a leper colony at nearby Seletar
proved thought-provoking. 'How sad it was to see these poor disfigured patients sitting cross-legged on their beds, which were so close
together . . . some of them were suffering also from dementia . . . They
had living quarters for families, so they could all live together . . .' A
happier memory for Olive and her friend Meg McPherson is of being
guests at the first day of a Malay wedding – a three-day feast at which
one of the ward boys was married. Olive and Meg were the only
Christians to join in the procession to the bride's house, where they
saw the bridal couple 'beautifully dressed and surrounded by flowers'.

As always romance was never far away. Joy Harris found herself 'having a difficult time ending a friendship, and he persuaded me to have one last evening out . . .' They ended up, inevitably, at a local beauty spot named Paradise Beach, where 'a discreet survey of the scene revealed friends with their own chaps . . . I was upset, and finally reduced to tears . . . He never knew the tears were not due to him but to a rare moment of home sickness – I could hear the Grand National commentary on a car radio parked nearby!'

The busy maternity unit at Changi Hospital, as remembered by Jan Smith (Mrs Campbell), had a main ward with fourteen or so beds; a side ward and a first-stage room, both with two beds; plus a delivery room just large enough for 'a bed, a delivery trolley, a sink, a stool and a bucket with a lid. It was half-tiled for easy cleaning and, biggest bonus of all, it was air conditioned.' In the nursery a table for changing nappies stood against one wall, with cots packed round two other walls, and against the fourth a sterilizer and a trolley for making up feeds – a duty accomplished by passing kettles of boiling water through a hatch from the kitchen. Baby baths, too, were filled each morning in the kitchen before being carted through to the delivery room 'which, in the heat and hurry, was no mean task . . . One sister bathed and a nurse dried and applied a nappy. It was like piece work on a production line . . .'

Shelagh Glenn (Mrs Barber) worked in theatre, which was in the upper building, connected with the lower hospital and the wards by the famous steps. Many days, when on call, Shelagh would be left alone in theatre when everybody else had gone. 'I used to think, This is a bit silly, sitting here doing nothing, so I'd finish what I had to do and nip down, fifty or sixty steps, to the back entrance of the mess. I'd been doing this for ages.' One day, she was halfway down when she saw Matron Jessie Higgins on her way up. 'So, well, fair cop, I'd been doing it for ages and hadn't been caught . . . as she walked past me she looked at her watch said, "Oh, you're late today, Glenn, it's usually about ten past when you come down" – she'd been watching me all the time!'

Shelagh remembers a new operating theatre being built, which made life easier.

When people came up to theatre they went into a ward, stayed there for twenty-four hours, and were carted down by ambulance, to the place at the bottom – three quarters of a mile round by road! – from there they were carried by porters up the stairs, into the various wards . . . It was quite hysterical when they were building. A chap came into the surgical ward and said, 'We're having problems, can I bring my cement mixer through the corridor in the ward?' so the sister said, 'I suppose so, if it helps.' She thought he meant literally a cement mixer, but of course it wasn't – it was little men running through with yokes, carrying things . . .

Over drinks in the mess, tales of tigers swimming the Straits of Johore, straight from the deep jungles of Malaya, tempted Marjorie Eavis (Mrs McCandlish) to explore. She had joined the PMs in 1943, during the Blitz, had been in India during partition and later in a troubled Aden. Following quieter sojourns at hospitals in England and Germany, she came to Changi in 1956. Marjorie had won her parachutist wings in the late forties, and this qualification persuaded the authorities to allow her to go into the jungle, where Malay troops commanded by British or Commonwealth officers were still hunting Communist bandits.

The vibrant, flower-bright jungle, filled with monkeys and birds, swept by below as the small 'pioneer plane' flew to land in a tiny clearing. Marjorie was 'immediately surrounded by half-clad Kemar belles who had never seen a woman before. I was in great danger of having my jungle kit of shirt, trousers, and tightly laced boots removed so that they could have a better look at me!' The plane had gone on to take supplies to other jungle outposts, but Marjorie was allowed to join the ground patrol, slithering silently through dank gloom, over lichen-covered tree trunks poised high above jungle streams, with deadly phosphorescent plants glimmering and on every leaf leeches that were 'well aware of my AB Rhesus negative blood . . . I did not realise until the patrol returned what a ghastly mess I looked – not the neat white dressed and veiled hospital Sister, but a creature crawling with ants after the blood seeping through my jungle gear.' Leeches festooned her arms, and the backs of her legs resembled bunches of bloated grapes. She was ordered to undress and don a towel and, 'protected by a circle of Malays, was passed lighted cigarettes to burn them off . . . Suddenly I felt hot breath on my back. It was the Sakai headman removing some in inaccessible places with his "Baccy-spittle"!'

Afterwards she heard that the headman had requested her as his sixth wife – 'the greatest honour he could bestow. However, with humility I replied that PMs were not allowed husbands . . . Madam regrets, but thank you just the same!'

West Germany

In the aftermath of war, British army and air force bases which opened in north-west Germany included two RAF hospitals, at Rostrup and Rinteln.

RAFH Rostrup, in the Bremen area, was built soon after the war, amid a landscape of bomb craters. Nearly a decade later, Doreen Hunt (Mrs Tomlin) found that time and nature had worked their spell: the hospital now enjoyed beautiful views across Lake Zwischenahn. The PMs' quarters lay a short distance away, in a spacious, single-storey block flanked by tennis courts.

Rostrup provided medical cover for three nearby RAF flying stations. As more and more personnel acquired cars, it handled a good many road-accident cases too. But the most demanding period Doreen Hunt experienced was during an epidemic of Asian 'flu, when 'the English school of Prince Rupert Wilhelmshaven was admitted *en masse* . . . We ran out of steam – everything that made steam was used, but it was not enough.' The RAF flew in with oxygen tents and other equipment, but despite all efforts a small boy and a young pilot died. 'Even the young National Service orderlies who would be counting the days to demob were magnificent. Their usual moans would be, "I didn't ask to work in a hospital, or join up." That was all forgotten and at last they became "one of us".'

In 1958, when many British troops left Germany, Rostrup gradually discharged its patients and staff went home. Joy Harris and two other sisters were posted a few miles north, to RAF Jever, where they opened a small maternity unit – and found themselves the only females in the officers' mess. Meanwhile Doreen Hunt was one of four PMs who attended Rostrup's final parade. Since they had not been certain of their final leaving date, they had not been able to send luggage ahead; the four sisters travelled with twenty-eight pieces of luggage, which did not amuse the customs officer who, at Parkeston Quay, asked what they had to declare.

When Doreen said 'a wire bust' his face fell and 'he insisted on my opening the container. He looked quite bemused – it was my dressmaker's wire bust frame. They didn't ask us to open anything else . . .'

The RAF hospital at Rinteln, near Hanover, had an even shorter history. Once an SS barracks, it was taken over by the wartime No. 8 RAFH in 1945 and was staffed by the RAF with some army personnel. The sisters' mess, built as part of the war reparations and intended to become a hotel at some later date, was suitably spacious and well-appointed, with a terrace where PMs could sit and chat while admiring the surrounding countryside. They did so until 1953, when the RAF handed over to the army and Rinteln became a British military hospital. It functioned in this capacity until 1996.

In its brief few RAF years, Rinteln provided a busy posting for PMs such as Susan Armistead (Mrs Sutcliffe). She enjoyed a lively MFH exercise dubbed 'Operation Pinnacle', and when the commander-in-chief's wife fell ill with an ulcer Susan escorted her home on casevac – and was rewarded by an invitation to lunch with the C-in-C himself.

Two tanks of the 11th Armoured Division collided and burst into flames at the end of an exercise. Alan Rosser was one of the survivors of the crash and the fire: 'After what seemed an interminable passage of time waiting for, and then travelling in, the ambulance, we arrived at Rinteln. By this time my burns had swollen and I was unable to see.' He remembers only 'a firm but caring voice which assured me I was all right now and that I would be "cleaned up" and given something to help me sleep'. He later discovered that the voice belonged to Sister Grace Haydock. But, blind as he was for several weeks, he couldn't see her. He came to know 'her voice, her step'.

I knew the instant she arrived at the entrance to the ward. The hum of activity was hushed when she set foot in her domain. She was the personification of the benign despot . . . her rule was absolute [but] she inspired confidence and calm . . . I believe I owe her my life . . .

I was flown back to hospital in Aldershot in due course, but by this time Sister had taken her leave. So . . . I never did see Sister Haydock.

When the RAF handed over the premises at Rinteln to the army, the sisters made sure they removed all mess property, including the red entrance carpet – 'I remember the looks of horror on the QAs' faces,' writes Muriel Dunn, who was about to leave with the Rinteln matron, Wing Officer 'Gertie' Grierson, in her red MG. They were moving on to a new, purpose-built RAF hospital at Wegberg.

Early Wegberg

Wegberg lies just inside West Germany, close to the borders of Holland and Belgium. Its RAF hospital was designed and built within ten months: designed in January 1953, it admitted its first patients on 1 November that same year. It was of unique design, the main buildings forming two 'D' shapes, the smaller inside the larger, with very wide main corridors; subsidiary linking corridors connected the two 'D's like spokes of a wheel.

Squadron Officer Doris Trick helped to equip the place and prepare for the opening and, when the day came, Margaret 'Jane' Clews and nine other sisters were posted out from the UK. Others came from Rinteln and they, as Jane Clews recalls, 'were not over-joyed with the move. We newcomers never failed to hear about that marvellous place up north!'

Coming from that 'marvellous place', Muriel Dunn's first impression of Wegberg was of a dark and unwelcoming hospital set in flat, unattractive countryside. The wide corridors, designed to hold huge numbers of casualties if needed (the Cold War was deepening and nuclear war a constant peril), 'seemed endless and it was said to be a quarter mile to the maternity ward where I worked. I delivered the first baby to be born there . . . Not all the wards were open immediately and the general night sister had a good step in between them. At one time she used a cycle to make her rounds!'

That bitter winter, which froze the Wegberg lake and even saw huge blocks of ice floating down the Rhine, lack of lagging on water pipes made itself evident. 'The water came down the metal rods which held the electric lights and light bowls, breaking them and scattering water and glass . . . One burst over an off-duty sister sitting on her bed . . .' They had ample hot water but no cold, so if someone wanted a bath she had to run the water and wait for it to cool (and hope that no one else nipped in first). Even the loos had to be flushed with hot water!

For Thérèse Saunders (Mrs Ayres), a memory that haunts her is 'a dreadful outbreak of gastro-enteritis amongst children and babies in Wegberg, and so many died despite our desperate efforts to save them. All leave was cancelled and we worked flat out for what seemed a very long time.'

Princess Marina (late Duchess of Kent, mother of Princess Alexandra) paid a royal visit to Wegberg while Doris Stanford (Mrs Kent) was running the children's ward. 'I had to spruce them all up – you know what children are like.' It was all terribly formal, everyone at attention, no sitting on beds, counterpanes wrinkleless . . . Tension reigned as the royal entourage appeared. Then one of the small patients, who had the habit of removing his clothes, suddenly started throwing off his pyjamas and 'made everybody laugh – it was rather nice'.

When a convoy of patients, including a baby with a serious chest condition, had to be rushed back to London's Brompton Hospital, Doris Stanford went with them. They flew in a Dakota, 'it flew very low, and I was so ill. I was quite ashamed – I was supposed to be looking after the patients . . .' After her earlier bad experience flying to Habbaniya, and now the Dakota trip, she realized she probably wasn't suited to aerial nursing.

National Servicemen

Before conscription ended in 1960, many young men of eighteen or so were called up to serve their country for two years. Some came willingly, some less so. David Snell had imagined being aircrew, but, 'despite any amount of kicking and screaming on our part, a large proportion of us found that we were going to spend two years in the Medical Branch'.

Sisters hold fond memories of these 'national service boys', who in civilian life might be apprentice engineers, carpenters, coalmen, clerks, or ballet dancers; a few were trained laboratory technicians – at least they understood the rudiments of hospital life.

Joy Harris remembers how the boys pitched in when inspections were due.

[We had] this awful brown oil-cloth you had to see your face in. You'd bumper it with these heavy great bumpers, and then everybody had to walk around with bits of old blanket on their feet. We had an AOC's inspection coming up at Ely and . . . we got on duty at quarter to eight in the morning, to get the place ready for the AOC's inspection, and it was spotless! – the boys on night duty had got it up to inspection standard.

As might be expected, the 'boys' had their favourites, among both PMs and patients. Nursing orderly M.J. Joy recalls that his job varied from taking temperatures and pulses to giving out bedpans. 'It has been known that some orderlies, dealing with an awkward patient who demanded a bedpan immediately, gave them a stainless steel one which had been under the hot tap for a couple of minutes . . .'

Tony Bowdler started his regular air force career as a nursing attendant at Wegberg. He was nineteen years old and most of his 'other rank' colleagues were national service conscripts. They thought of the sisters as 'ancient (all of ten years older than us), very efficient and wise. Most of the orderlies, for we were still called that at the time, detested the PMs as we appeared to do the work and they appeared to get the fun and money . . . The resentment was short-lived for me, but I do remember some of the old sweats being less than complimentary about the PMs.'

From another posting, at Halton, Tony Bowdler recalls 'the dearest, most loveable PM . . . Sqn Off Irene Turner . . . she had been in the service for ever.' She was in her early forties at the time, while he was a mere stripling of twenty-one. He most remembers her for the note pinned to her desk, which said, 'Orderlies are instructed not to rummage in sister's drawers at any time'! Tony doesn't think she saw the *double entendre*. Oh, no?

Both sides could play that game. Sylvia Emery (Mrs Pounds) says that she and her contemporaries worked on the wards in pairs, or sometimes alone, assisted only by national servicemen 'in varying stages of training'. In order to help the boys widen their experience and perhaps gain promotion, sisters allowed them to do some of the extra routine tasks such as writing up reports. One chap noted that a patient 'took a little custard, and vomited a trifle'! He didn't know what he'd written, so Sister Emery believed.

Who was kidding whom?

Early dialysis

RAF interest in the renal dialysis field began during the Second World War, when doctors realized that many casualties died not from injuries but from kidney failure, a common factor in acute injury. As a result, the Renal Unit at PMRAFH Halton came into being, officially founded in 1956 by Air Vice Marshal Sir Ralph Jackson. It possessed one of the original Kolff twin-coil dialysis machines – of which only two existed in the world at the time. Initially the machine offered only temporary relief to kidney patients, but it led to developments which eventually allowed for the long-term treatment of chronic renal failure.

Jessie Higgins, by then a senior matron, arrived at Halton just as they were beginning to perfect the machine. 'It was like a huge great boiler! I was terrified of it!' Interest in the new machine grew swiftly, especially after Guy's Hospital became involved in the research work, and groups of doctors and nursing sisters were sent to Halton for training.

> We used to have them for two weeks – six working days each week. They hated it: 'Trained by the RAF?' . . . They thought we did just ingrowing toe-nails and things. Didn't realise we delivered a thousand babies a year, apart from anything else. I put them straight, I said, 'Now . . . you came here to learn about something. There isn't another place in the world . . .

One renal patient, Flying Officer (later Wing Commander) Clifford Blunt, says he developed an allergy and lost large patches of skin from the 'sweaty areas' of his body. Treatment consisted of frequent medicated baths, painting the affected areas with gentian violet and exposing them to the air – which in practice left him lying on his bed under a cage, with the sheet folded back and his nether regions in full view. 'When visitors came, screens were placed around my bed to hide the blue-bottomed baboon from sight!' The screens went up during a visit by Princess Marina, commandant-in-chief of the Red Cross. Matron endeavoured to distract Her Royal Highness, but the princess was determined to see the mysterious patient. 'She stood at the foot of my bed and took a great interest in my treatment.

Whether I was more violet or red I will never know – but I was certainly in glorious Technicolour.'

'Bull'

Official visits of all kinds caused a good deal of angst. On one occasion at Ely, when Mary Page (Mrs Payne) nervously escorted Princess Mary round the ward, in order to avoid embarrassment she 'changed the diagnosis' of patients recovering from circumcision.

Shelagh Glenn (Mrs Barber) recalls:

> I arrived at Halton the day before the Princess Royal was making a visit . . . Sister said, 'Now, we're not having flowers in all the rooms, we're having potted plants in wards 1 & 2, and when ward 1 has been visited those plants will go to ward 3 and when ward 2 has been visited, they'll go to ward 4 . . .' I could just imagine me, in the PMs for one day, coming down the corridor with a couple of potted plants and bumping straight into the royal party. Sister added, 'And if I introduce you to the Princess and call you Miss Smith, then you *are* Miss Smith.'

And then there was all the pre-visit 'bull' – scrubbing and Brassoing and whitewashing . . . Matron Jessie Higgins heartily disapproved of the bumpering of floors of hospital wards and corridors to a high and dangerously slippery shine. At Halton she had many an argument with the CO on this subject – *he* liked to see every inch of space gleaming; *she* kept her floors scrupulously clean but not polished, even when a visit from the air chief commandant of the PMRAFNS was imminent.

Her Royal Highness duly arrived and was officially greeted by Miss Higgins and others before being conducted round the wards. During the tour, the Princess Royal remarked what a relief it was to have unpolished floors on which she could walk naturally – usually on such visits she had to teeter around trying not to slip over, and in consequence spent the following day in agony with stiff and painful muscles. 'Ma'am,' said Higgie, 'would you mind repeating that to the CO?' Her Royal Highness obliged. One up to Matron Higgins!

St Clement Danes

As the fifties drew to a close, an historic and moving ceremony, attended by the Queen and other members of the Royal Family, took place. On 24 October 1958, the restored building of St Clement Danes, in the Strand, which had been badly damaged during the Blitz, was reconsecrated by the Bishop of London. It became the church of the RAF. Matron-in-Chief Dame Alice Mary Williamson represented the PMRAFNS, along with retired matron Miss M.B. Charlesworth and Miss G.M.I. Jenkins for the reserve. The Roll of Honour included the names of three PMs.

THREE

On a jet plane

Much of the aeromed work was, and still is, what one PM called 'hard slog' – long hours, difficult conditions and the sheer drag of routine, with little glamour about it. However, conditions vastly improved with the introduction of jet engines. Suddenly the Far East could be reached inside twenty-four hours, the Antipodes within two days. The first turbojet Comets joined Transport Command at RAF Lyneham in July 1956. In 1959 came the turboprop Britannia, and in the mid-sixties both the workhorse Hercules and the sleek, speedy VC10 joined the aerial fleet. These two last-named aircraft could take up to seventy stretchers at a time and – much to the relief of patients involved, not to mention personnel who had the job of loading and unloading – stretcher cases could remain on board during the brief refuelling stops the new planes required.

April Reed experienced what she calls 'this incredible change. After I'd done about a year at Wroughton, on the aeromeds on the Hastings, I went to Germany for a few years, and when I came back there was the Comet, and the VC10. Absolute luxury in comparison.'

Dinghy drill

The arrival of jet aircraft synchronized with a move to more intensive aeromed training, leading to a professional qualification. This began in 1959 when the RAF introduced an Aeromedical Course for both nursing officers of the PMRAFNS and non-commissioned personnel of the RAFMS. SRNs emerged from the course as qualified flight sisters or flight nurses while state enrolled nurses (SENs), medical assistants and administrators became air-ambulance attendants.

Once she had been in the Service for a year, a PM might volunteer to take this course, which took place initially at RAF Lyneham and later at RAF Brize Norton. At first, ground training lasted for three days (later it expanded to eight days), small groups of trainees working with skilled instructors. They began in the swimming pool where, wearing black gaberdine flying suits, they learned survival techniques – emergency escape from crashed aircraft, decompression in a pressure chamber, use of life-jackets and how to handle a huge and unwieldy rubber dinghy – righting it, if necessary, climbing into it from the water, and then hauling an injured patient after them. Back on dry land they studied the effects of altitude on both patients and equipment, became familiar with the various aircraft they might be using, and learned how to load patients correctly, fix stretcher harnesses and pack medical panniers; they studied the relation of Greenwich Mean Time to other time zones, so that drugs could be given at correct periods, and they were taught how to handle a polio patient in and out of an aircraft while he was in a Monaghan cuirass – the RAF's portable version of an iron lung.

After initial instruction, students flew three aeromeds assisting an experienced nurse, then one flight when they were in charge but under supervision; after that, fully qualified, they were on their own. Changing needs, improved equipment and more modern techniques were incorporated into the training as time went by, and eventually all PMs – including some rather senior ladies – were required to pass the aeromed course.

Joy Harris was one of those later students.

I had done aeromeds in the days before you had to be trained, out in the Far East . . . but we found ourselves on a course with two nurse tutors and two matrons, I think it was . . . We got into great trouble doing the dinghy drill, because the only way you can really get into a dinghy when you're in the water – when you've got your Mae West [lifebelt] on – is to be dunked down, then you'll shoot up and they can grab you and pull you over. We couldn't get in, we kept saying, 'For heaven's sake, *push us under*!'

However comprehensive, no course can hope to cover every eventuality: each aeromed flight produces its own unique problems and PMs have learned always to expect the unexpected.

Sidelights

White ward dresses buttoned to the waist until 1960, when a Defence Council Instruction ordered somewhat daringly that, 'in future, Nursing Officers will wear dresses unbuttoned all the way down the front'. Most PMs, highly amused, took the words 'which are capable of being' as implicit between 'dresses' and 'unbuttoned'.

As a junior sister in the early sixties, April Reed found tights a headache: 'You had to have three colours: white to go with white uniform on the wards; black to go with the blue outdoor uniform; brown for mufti.' As for undies . . . at Ely, one matron

> . . . had this thing that we all had to wear white underwear under our ward uniform. It was a time when underwear was all bright colours. When you did a round with her, she'd be looking at you . . . trying to catch you against the light, to see, and – she always called you by your surname, of course – she'd say, 'Reed, you've got a blue petticoat on!'

A new member from 1961, Zena Cheel says, 'When I first came into the PMs, any serviceman, on admission to hospital, had to come in in uniform . . . those that were up and about wore uniform until lunchtime and then they could change into mufti, but mufti had to be collar and tie and flannels, or cords or something . . .'

In order to join the PMRAFNS, one had to face a selection board. Elizabeth Sandison travelled to hers by train, overnight from Aberdeen to London, in 1964. Next morning, after a medical, she went for her interview and came out wondering if she really wanted to join this 'club' where all they seemed to want was tennis-playing midwives – she did not play tennis and had done only part one midwifery.

Valerie Hand, too, was asked if she played tennis. Yes, she did. 'But are you any good at it?' came the demand – they obviously had the Dame Joanna Cruickshank Tennis Tournament in mind! As for Sheila Power (Mrs Bellamy-Knights), she had been in the army nursing service for four years; when she attended her interview with the

PMRAFNS they asked her how long she planned to give to the air force before she joined the navy!

Memorable aeromeds

In September 1963 an aeromed team including Squadron Officer Molly McNair set off on another trail-blazing flight. The signal which scrambled them is unclassified but still reads like gobbledegook to the untrained eye: 'UNCLAS H166/MED 20 SEP HQ PACAF AND HQ AAC . . .' Three lines later, it gets a little more comprehensible with 'SUBJECT IS AEROMEDICAL EVACUATION OF SERIOUSLY ILL PATIENT CMM FLYING OFFICER NORTHMORE RAF CMM AT PRESENT IN TRIPLER ARMY GENERAL HOSPITAL . . .' To put it plainly, Flying Officer Anthony Northmore, a Transport Command pilot based at RAF Changi, had been employed in ferrying equipment between Honolulu and Christmas Island. While off duty, swimming in Honolulu in July 1963, he had broken his neck when he dived into shallow water. His injuries had left him tetraplegic. The USAF hospital at Tripler had looked after him but in September his doctors decided he was well enough to be flown home.

The team from Lyneham made news because of the route they took – it was the first time such a mercy flight had crossed the North Pole, via Greenland and Alaska. They returned the same way, bringing their patient back to Lyneham, from where a Whirlwind helicopter whisked him away to Stoke Mandeville Hospital.

Another experienced flight sister, R.A. 'Penny' Penrose, recalls that by the early sixties regular aeromed flights served Germany, the Middle East and the Far East. In between these scheduled, routine flights, 'specials' were called for, 'for patients with poliomyelitis, fractured spines, burns, gun shot wounds of chest, sick babies and once six Aylesbury ducks to be taken to the Governor of Hong Kong to adorn his lake'. But her own most memorable patients were both world famous. In 1962, Sir Winston Churchill, aged 87, was holidaying in Monaco when he slipped and fell in his hotel room, fracturing his left thigh. Monaco surgeons performed an emergency operation but, as Penny Penrose explains, it was decided that the great man should be returned to England.

For if his injury should prove fatal his demise should not be on foreign soil . . . Flying Officer Tilley and I were having tea prior to returning to duty at 1700 hrs at RAFH Wroughton. By 1900 hrs we were flying from Lyneham . . . an MO plus two SNCOs completing the medical team. We arrived at Nice at 2100 hrs. Everyone knew who we were and we were treated like heroes and thoroughly spoilt . . .

Next morning the two PMs waited at the airfield while the doctor and medics collected the stretcher-bound Sir Winston and took him on board the Comet, 'courtesy of a forklift'.

Fortunately I had the foresight, whilst waiting, to purchase all the English newspapers which were available. Sir Winston avidly read all the news about himself and discussed the tennis at Wimbledon and horse racing with his secretary, who was travelling with us. We arrived at the Middlesex Hospital in London, being escorted from the airport by six police outriders . . . we carved our way through the London traffic as a knife through butter. A second operation was then performed, the patient making very satisfactory progress, much to the relief of the world . . .

Her next VIP aeromed happened in 1965 when 'I was posted to RAF Hospital Changi and in October I flew in an RAF Argosy with an MO and SNCO to Tonga, to escort Queen Salote, aged 65 years, on her journey for medical treatment in New Zealand'. The Tongan queen had become a great favourite with British crowds when, during the Coronation Parade, she had ridden through the streets of London in an open carriage, waving and smiling despite the rain. Now, when she was ill, Queen Elizabeth herself had asked that the RAF should provide transport and medical care.

Being a small island, Tonga could only accommodate certain aircraft on its small airport. It was therefore decided that the Argosy with additional crew could be the most appropriate aircraft to take Queen Salote from Tonga and transfer her to an RAF Comet with a second medical team to fly her from Fiji to New Zealand . . . Queen Salote was very frail and a bed was loaded on board should she find it more comfortable for travelling.

From RAF Changi, it took the Argosy six days to reach Tonga, with overnight stays, refuelling stops and a rest day, flying via the Cocos Island, Australia (3 days to cross Australia), New Caledonia and Fiji. 'Although the flying time had made for long days, together with the noise of the engine, when one saw the runway at Nakualofe the choice of aircraft was all too apparent.' Penny Penrose stayed with the hospital matron, a remarkable New Zealander.

> Not only did she supervise the nursing of patients, she administered the hospital, trained and lectured her staff ... The financial budget was limited and at times illness of many babies caused acute anxiety with lack of antibiotics, penicillin etc. Fortunately, not quite knowing what to expect, we had included a considerable amount of medication to our routine supply, which we readily offloaded ...
>
> We were entertained to a sumptuous Tongan feast seated on cushions on the floor, a long strip of coconut matting in front of us laden with chickens, sucking pigs, fish, fruit, yams, etc. whilst we were served by staff from the Royal Household. We were also invited to tea served on the most delicate of porcelain ... seated on the verandah of the Royal Household and entertained by singing and dancing.
>
> The route to the airport was a mass of people watching their Queen depart. She was very frail but very upright and we remembered how she had endeared herself to everyone at the Queen's Coronation. Our flight to Fiji was uneventful. The Queen was then transferred to the RAF Comet for the remainder of her flight to New Zealand. Sadly, she died in hospital a few days later.

Penny Penrose concludes, 'My years as an aeromed sister were the most superb experience one could ever wish for ... Happy days indeed. Memorable years.'

PM 'Ronnie' Oxborough also relished aeromed duties, which for her began in 1970. They were 'a very exciting part of my career in the PMs ... some trips enjoyable, some frightening, some tragic'. Recalling one particular trip to Washington DC, she recounts how 'a big fellow in the Irish Guards' had broken his neck by jumping off the side of a boat and hitting his head on a coral reef. Paralysed from the neck down, on a respirator and strapped in a turning frame, he was being cared for in the Walter Reed Hospital in Washington when the aeromed team went out to collect him. They worked with him to wean him off the American respirator and onto theirs for the flight home, but the treatment involved frequent turning of the frame so that for some periods he hung face down – not a pleasant position for anyone. In order to reassure him, Ronnie Oxborough 'sat on the floor under the frame, talking to him. One morning into the room walked a huge coloured gent built like Tower Bridge. He took one look at me, lifted me clean off the floor, put me on a bed and was about to send for the doctor – he thought I had fallen and couldn't get up! No harm done. Our patient had a good journey home.'

Some of the most rewarding of aeromed duties, according to those who were privileged to be selected for them, were the two-yearly flights which brought holders of the Victoria Cross and the George Cross back to the UK to meet the Queen. Anne Taylor felt very lucky to be chosen to accompany these men and their wives. 'They were lovely people, with amazing stories to tell.' Liz Sandison agrees that meeting the war heroes was 'an amazing experience, never to be repeated or equalled'.

Gan

Just two miles long by one mile wide, the staging post of RAF Gan lay in the southernmost part of the Maldive Islands, in the Indian Ocean. The runway drew a broad line down the length of the island and in the lagoon lay remnants of broken concrete moorings, an air sea rescue launch and a rusting old ship, not to mention sharks, manta rays, turtles and Moray eels lurking among razor-sharp coral – plimsolls while paddling were a must.

When, in December 1961, Princess Alexandra had to make a night stop at Gan, Jane Stott was sent from RAFH Changi to look after Her Royal Highness, the only other woman on the island being a WVS welfare officer. Later, Jane was attached to the sick quarters at Gan for three months, to assess whether the presence of a nursing sister might be beneficial. She found it an unusual posting: 'The Maldivians came to work every day in their flotilla of single sail canoe type vessels from islands in the atoll, and left every evening at sundown. Sick Maldivians came to be treated, but only with permission from their headman . . . Any terminally ill person was removed from Sick Quarters as, if dead, they would not be accepted back to their island.'

Since it was found impractical to have a nursing officer permanently on the tiny island, Gan's sick quarters were left in capable male hands.

Cyprus

When British forces withdrew from Egypt they ensured a base in the Middle East by enlarging their presence in Cyprus. By the late fifties about 30,000 British servicemen were stationed on the island, many with families. The RAF hospital at Akrotiri opened in 1956, some of its first PMs being transferred from the closing Canal Zone hospital at Fayid.

Off duty, the island offers abundant pleasures, from skiing in the snow-clad mountains to basking on golden beaches or swimming in the blue-green Mediterranean. But strife between the resident Greek and Turkish communities has made Cyprus, on occasion, an uneasy place to be. The strong RAF presence has kept the hospital busy, and over forty years its non-service patients have included both Greek–Cypriot EOKA terrorists and their Turkish–Cypriot opposition.

Owing to its barren, rocky location, the first hospital was fondly known as 'Alcatraz'. It was sited on the southern tip of Cyprus (near salt flats where pink flamingos mass at migration time) and it comprised five single-storey prefabricated buildings (intended as married quarters) set either side of a road. Its early days were not auspicious. When the first PMs arrived, the nearby airfield was still under construction and, what with heavy rains and lack of proper roads, hospital staff clumped through the mud in permanent gumboots. Orderlies bringing the first surgical patient, unconscious on a stretcher, found the trolley too wide to go through the door of the converted sitting room which served as the surgical ward; they had to manhandle the stretcher through a window (and send for 'Works and Bricks' to widen the door).

What was more, with a road running between, trolley-bound patients being wheeled from ward to theatre and back often had to wait for a gap in the traffic!

It was said that EOKA terrorists had tried to raid the hospital to obtain insulin for their leader, George Grivas; so the *bundu* (the surrounding scrubland) was strung with trip-wires that occasionally set off rockets and startled everyone – especially at three in the morning. Security appeared to have forgotten that herds of wild donkeys roamed free around the camp.

By 1959, however, improvements had been made – several caravans acted as changing rooms, sluice and Red Cross library. But the PMs had discovered the delights of being so close to a warm blue sea and social life was excellent, with RAF Akrotiri becoming the largest flying station in the RAF at that time – it held 2,000 personnel, with squadrons of bombers and fighters. When the growth of new trees, shrubs and flowers began to soften the environs, the peninsula turned into a very pleasant place to be, except for the bed bugs – and the terrorists.

During the hostilities of 1957–9, RAF casualties were few but bloody, mostly caused by snipers' bullets – often in the back – and by bombs. David Snell, a national service medic, recalls two particular incidents, the first with a Greek motor cyclist carrying a bomb. 'There was no need for any medical assistance ... they were finding bits of motorcycle and Greek for some weeks. The second was far more serious in that they destroyed a hangar and over £3m worth of aircraft. Fortunately casualties were limited to three station firemen with minor to moderate burns.'

There were, besides, many traffic accidents, and numerous cases of serious sunburn among newcomers who ignored all the warnings; the maternity unit was busy, too, with so many wives accompanying their husbands; but the hospital's main enemy was dysentery – one of the medical wards was kept filled by such cases and, given the climate, it was impossible to prevent infection from spreading. 1958 saw an outbreak so bad that sick quarters, the NAAFI and empty billets had to be used as wards and operating theatres closed for all except emergency cases.

One of the inevitable flying accidents made Ethnea Hancock think twice about accepting an invitation to go gliding:

I worked chiefly as a midwife there, although I had done some theatre work before I joined the service. One weekend I was asked to stand in for the theatre sister. She said, 'Nothing ever happens, you'll be fine. Maybe an appendix, but you'll be fine . . .' And at two o'clock on the Saturday afternoon a glider pilot crashed and put the steering column through his chest. So we were doing chest surgery that afternoon. It wasn't something the surgeon was doing all the time, either . . . these small places were not that well geared up for that sort of thing. It put me off taking up the offer to go gliding!

Having no proper mess of their own, nursing sisters at Akrotiri had to travel some distance to the officers' mess for meals and social occasions, including film shows. Ann Golding can never see the film *Psycho* without remembering the first time she saw it, in Cyprus, when just at the most gripping moment the tannoy announced, 'Sisters' transport!' and they had to leave to catch the coach back to their living quarters.

Princess Mary at Akrotiri

A new hospital, at Cape Zevgari, three miles from the main RAF camp, began building in June 1961. The Princess Royal visited it during its final stages and when it was completely operational she came again, in November 1963, to open it officially and grant it the use of her name. Ethnea Hancock was 'amazed by her stamina. The flight would have been eight or more hours at that time . . . She went up to Air House (home of the commander-in-chief) first, but then plunged into a really daunting programme – a fifteen/sixteen hour day, exhausting . . . She must have been quite elderly then, I remember she seemed terribly old.' The princess was in her mid-sixties at the time.

When the island gained independence in 1960, exiled Archbishop Makarios returned as president, and three years later the Greeks tried to seize control. The Turks resisted. Britain tried to remain neutral. Margaret Kingston tells how a friend of hers invited a Cypriot bishop to dinner and nearly got court-martialled for it – the bishop was *persona non grata* owing to the troubles.

However, remaining aloof was difficult when battle casualties needed help. Over Christmas 1963, Iris Rawlings (Mrs Kerse) was at Akrotiri.

> Greek-Cypriots were attacking their neighbouring Turks, burning villages and destroying property. On Boxing morning, Matron came up to my room to ask if I would go up to Nicosia, and to be ready within an hour. Three of us were to go – a midwife, theatre sister and myself as aeromedical sister . . .
>
> A Hastings came down from Nicosia to collect us . . . the landscape seemed to be ablaze as we overflew the burning Turkish villages. Fighting was intense in Nicosia, the walled city being held by the Turks and constantly bombarded by the Greeks. Within the walls was a Turkish hospital where their wounded were being treated. Our first task was to go into the walled city and take them to the airport, from where they would be flown to Turkey.
>
> A time was chosen when there was a lapse in hostilities while the Greeks were burying one of their martyrs. We went in, in uniform, in ambulances, and coming up to the walls was very dramatic . . . Above the sandbags, armed men were aiming their weapons at us. The ambulance driver asked if I was frightened and I said, 'No, I'm wearing this,' pointing to my veil. How naive can you get! He thought I was terribly brave! . . . We managed to evacuate our patients before hostilities recommenced. It was a great feeling seeing them off on the aircraft.

El Adem

During tours of duty at Akrotiri, a succession of PMs went on short attachment to the tiny staging post of El Adem, 500 miles away in the Libyan desert. Captured from the Italians during the desert campaigns of the Second World War, Libya was administered first by Britain and then as an independent monarchy under King Idris. El Adem served initially as a refuelling base for short-range aircraft. From the time of the Suez crisis, its role as a staging post increased. Aeromed and transport flights paused overnight to rest and refuel; Comet crews arrived to practise 'circuits and bumps'; and a resident

RAF Regiment squadron, living in tents, helped to clear the mines that still lurked among the sand-dunes.

Most PMs stayed on the base for about six months, some stayed a year; Jane Stott reckoned her thirteen-and-a-half month attachment to be the record. She and two colleagues named Jess and Joan arrived in January 1957, in the rainy season – they were glad of their Cyprus wellingtons, and of the break from terrorists and restricted travel. Along with Joan Parsons, of the WVS, plus her dachshund, the three PMs 'lived in an Italian-built block of rooms round an open-centre square . . . Salt-water soap was most useful as all water came from Tobruk by pipeline and was extremely hard and impure . . . laundry "whites" turned out grey.' Tobruk, where the RAF families lived, was sixteen miles away, still in ruins but beginning to be rebuilt.

The sick quarters at El Adem demanded special organization: when surgical operations became necessary, the MO had to call in army doctors to make up the team; and when a woman went into labour two airmen of the same blood group would stand by in case she needed a transfusion. 'In hot weather an air cooling unit was transferred from the servicing flight, and the cool air was pumped into the theatre through a Dettol-soaked sheet . . .'

Two of the sisters owned a VW Beetle, so they were able to visit nearby towns, though they had to watch out for desert rats, baby tortoises and stray camels. In camp, the only source of milk was tins of Carnation, and scorpions presented a permanent hazard. But entertainers visited to put on shows for the troops and they even had dining-in nights, with snails and desert game birds on the menu.

Even so, Ethnea Hancock found her six months in El Adem 'a bit of an endurance test. You were sent as a midwife . . . but not many deliveries so not much to do. You were seventeen miles inland from Tobruk, fairly good road between but in all other directions nothing but *bundu* roads, pretty ropey, and only two vehicles on the station – SMO's and CO's jeeps. But we survived.'

Tragedy in the desert

News of her own posting to El Adem left Jean Brown with mixed feelings, but fortunately two other Scots were to be with her: Isobel McDonald and Marie Morrison. During their tenure, in October

1961, a Maltese regiment came to RAF El Adem on desert exercises. Training done, the soldiers set off home to Malta, but as their plane took off it crashed, engulfed by flames.

Jean, Marie and Isobel were relaxing in their sitting room when the call came. By the time they arrived at SSQ, casualties were being brought in, many of them screaming in pain. None of them spoke English, so the sisters had difficulty in calming them. But they had to cope until the two MOs could arrive – both had gone home to their married quarters in Tobruk. Fortunately, Jean Brown had checked the crash ward only the previous day and had made sure of a good supply of intravenous fluids. She wonders if premonition prompted her.

Some of the men had 90 per cent burns. They died within a couple of hours. The British Padre Hodgson gave the last rites, while ambulance boys and orderlies helped to set up intravenous drips – not having enough drip-stands, they improvised with broom handles, which the orderlies had to hold. Meanwhile the sisters administered morphine supplied by the pharmacist. Within half an hour the MOs arrived and soon the team had everyone sedated and assessed. But Jean will never forget the smell of burning flesh.

A couple of years later, on his way back to London after treating King Idris, the eminent London-based orthopaedic surgeon Sir Reginald Watson Jones accepted an invitation to dine with the CO and officers of El Adem. He sat next to a nursing sister to whom he 'recounted his horror at having to do an operation in the Palace, surrounded by the King's advisers and many flies! Even in 1963 this was not what he was used to.'

RAF El Adem closed in 1969 when King Idris was deposed and Colonel Mu'ammar al-Gaddafi came to power in Libya.

Khormaksar Beach, Aden

In 1962 British forces became embroiled in a struggle for the hinterland of Aden, a territory known as 'the Radfan'; the war continued until 1967, when British forces withdrew from Aden and the Marxists took over.

The RAF hospital at Steamer Point had been operating since 1928, with RAF Khormaksar Beach ten miles to the north, on sandy flats on the shore of the old harbour. Also at Khormaksar, a camp for the Aden Protectorate Levies (APLs) had its own sick quarters, with male wards staffed by male SRNs of the RAFMS and a women's/families' ward supervised by four part-time British-trained civilian nurses. The hospital also employed local auxiliaries and *ayahs*.

Barbara Millar (Mrs Wight) was one of the sisters from Steamer Point who visited the APL sick quarters 'once a week, to give treatment of various sorts to the Arab soldiers and their families'. Then in 1959 the Khormaksar Beach APL Hospital (known as KBH) became a regular posting for PMs. The first contingent of four nursing officers, including Shelagh Firth, went out from the UK; two more were posted from Steamer Point. They were supposed to live in a building converted from two flats, not far from the hospital, but, says Shelagh Firth, 'As might be expected, the conversion was not completed, so [we] were accommodated in the Rock Hotel . . .' This lay in the main shopping area of Aden, ten miles away at Steamer Point. When problems with distance and transport made life fraught, they 'were assigned to a room in the Commanding Officer's (Wing Commander Cooney's) house – rather cramped, and I dread to think how much we disrupted their life!'

A strike of the local auxiliaries exacerbated early difficulties but, despite problems of language, cultural differences and the auxiliaries' lack of medical knowledge, after a short time 'they became very reliable and supportive'. Shelagh Firth enjoyed the social life, too, exploring Aden, shopping in Steamer Point, visits up-country and leave spent in Kenya, picnics with the BP fraternity at Little Aden, camel racing, shark fishing . . .

Everyone who worked at Khormaksar Beach APL Hospital found it 'very different'. It consisted of verandahed huts set about by trees and connected by black sandy paths. The huts offered 163 beds for local levies and their dependants, who could be numerous – a man might have several wives, each with children, plus his parents, his unmarried sisters and his juvenile brothers, and staff suspected that friends sneaked in under guise of 'relatives' too – would could tell? Consequently, beds were kept full, and nurses busy. As a general rule, men nursed men and women nursed women, with female and children's wards well away from the rest because of purdah rules. Common illnesses included all tropical diseases such as malaria, leprosy and TB; more unusual cases included mycetoma (also known as Madura foot, a severe fungal infection peculiar to Arabia, which often calls for surgery to excise the affected area).

For Zena Cheel, Aden provided her first overseas tour. She spent seven months at Steamer Point, then was posted to KBH: 'Khormaksar Beach sounds romantic, but it wasn't. Black sand, and very near Khormaksar airport. We used to have terrible trouble with aircraft flying over, especially if they were practising for an open day . . .' Having been brought up in India, Zena was unfazed by the local smells and noises, but some things did present 'a bit of a culture shock'.

> For instance, the first day I was there . . . it got nearer and nearer to lunchtime and I thought, they don't seem to be doing anything, so I said to this other sister, 'What do we do about lunch, then?' and she said, 'Oh, you'll see in a minute!' and across the *bundu* came this little chap with two huge great buckets, one full of rice and one full of curry, and under each arm a loaf of bread, and two big ladles. The patients dived into their lockers and brought out these little things that looked as if they should be under the bed as opposed to eating out of them, and those that were up went out on to the verandah, and he went round and he dolloped a bit of rice, and a dollop of curry, hacked off a bit of bread – and that was lunch! In the evening, they invariably had chapatti with a hard boiled egg – that was their supper. We used to have to go afterwards and hose down the verandah, where they'd been eating, because whatever they didn't want they just spat out, or threw out.

When Zena became sister-in-charge:

> One evening I was sitting there writing my report and I thought, I can smell something cooking! . . . These ladies had got one of the dressing bowls and into it they'd put onions and tomatoes and all sorts, and they were boiling it all up in the sterilizer!
>
> But it was very interesting . . . I never thought in my life I'd look after lepers . . . and we had people with all these different diseases, like bilharzia, that you hear about . . . A lot of these people had never been out of their villages and quite often if

they became ill the first person they would go to would be the witch doctor, or whatever they called him . . . We had a young boy about fifteen brought in, with meningitis, but he also had this terrific wound in his head, where they had put this red-hot needle, almost like a poker, into his head, to get rid of the evil spirit, so not only was he delirious from the meningitis but also from a high fever from the infection . . .

In time, Khormaksar Beach Hospital benefited from the permanent presence of twelve PM sisters and twelve male SRNs, plus local male orderlies and Somali *ayahs*. To Kate Crompton (Mrs Wilmot), her posting came as a shock: 'I had heard stories about KBH and was very apprehensive.' Nevertheless she, too, found it a fascinating experience.

Many of the female patients brought their babies into hospital with them whilst they received treatment. They made little hammocks under their beds for the babies. Mealtimes were an eye-opener . . . The toddlers, and all the babies old enough to eat solids, had minced liver and rice at lunchtime. They would sit down in a semi-circle and an *ayah* would roll the rice in a little ball and pop one into each child's mouth. She repeated this using minced liver. All TB adults had chicken curry and everyone else had ordinary curry – I've no idea what was in that!

On night duty, one sister would be in charge of the whole hospital. Says Kate, 'It was very strange walking between the female and male sections with Arab male nurses asleep on their beds by the roadside.'

In Britain, a new Labour government, elected in October 1964, decided that its forces could no longer afford to act as policemen to the world. It began to close some overseas bases and over the next few years British troops withdrew from the Middle East. When Doreen Francis arrived in Aden to take up matron's duties at KBH, she was told that within two or three years the British would be leaving Aden; meantime, the new hospital being built for the local troops (who would become the Federal Regular Army) would be used for British patients. Over the next three years, the work of this European Wing at KBH proved to be almost exclusively surgical, operating on casualties shot and injured by Arab terrorists.

Doreen Francis comments, 'We had a secure ward for Arab dissidents, and a helicopter pad where casualties were landed, particularly at dawn. We had many army units posted in.' Some army lines lay just outside the fence which abutted the levies' TB ward; hand grenades would be lobbed over to explode in the British lines. Pilfering posed another problem – hospital equipment had to be watched closely and even pushchairs used to convey babies to X-ray were padlocked to the verandah, otherwise they 'walked'. 'After eighteen years spent mostly in operating theatres,' says Doreen, 'it was quite a change.'

One of her nursing sisters, Alma Barnard (Mrs Tyack) enjoyed nursing the children: 'They were very trusting . . . They loved having injections – they thought that was something special, real medicine.' But their names raised difficulties: 'They were all called Ali or Mohammed, so they were numbered as by beds, surgical or medical – SB1/2/3 or MB1/2/3 – we had to make sure they stayed in the same beds so they didn't get muddled.'

Liz Lown (Mrs Armstrong) noted that 'a very special relationship grew up between the *Sisters* and the Arab, Indian and Somali women (the *ayahs*) who provided the basic nursing on the Arab families' ward. *Ayahs* always threw a tea-party for a departing Sister. They were being trained by the PMs to take over nursing care when the British finally withdrew.'

Troubled finale at Aden

Terrorist activities also began to affect Steamer Point hospital, on its hill above the main harbour. Monica Fern says:

Once the fighting really got going in the Radfan, we used to have the helicopters bringing casualties down to the hospital – a bit like M.A.S.H. – if the telephone rang you automatically put your uniform on and went over to the hospital . . . I looked after a nineteen-year-old soldier who had both his hands blown off by a hand grenade which he held too long after pulling the pin . . . Another patient had the top of his

skull sliced off by shrapnel – he was flown back to England
and a plate put in, but you wonder what sort of life he had.

For security, all buildings had to be searched once the Arab
orderlies and bearers had gone home and on two separate nights
midwives found something that made them call the bomb disposal
squad. New mothers dressed in nighties and housecoats, with babes
in arms, trooped from their ward to wait nervously outside while
the lads disposed of, first, a wrapped loaf of bread and, second, a
tobacco pouch inadvertently left by one of the proud new fathers.
On another evening, Monica Fern heard a commotion in the labour
ward – one of the Arab guards had fallen through the ceiling while
checking the roof space.

The hospital itself remained secure, but outside the walls terror
reigned. Sisters were on the patio of their mess enjoying an evening
drink when a bomb went off at the Post Office just below. Monica
Fern, 'craned to see, and somebody yelled, "Get down!"' As she
ducked, machine-gun fire erupted.

Another lucky escape occurred at a dinner in the officers' mess
at Tarshine. PMs present included a theatre sister named Diane,
from Steamer Point. They had reached the soup course when a
hand grenade landed on the long table. Diane pushed her chair
back, flung up her hands to guard her face, and threw herself side-
ways. The explosion peppered her with shrapnel. Monica Fern
recounts the denouement: 'Diane was prepared to have the shrapnel removed from her arm and side, but drew the line at exposing
her backside to the medics with whom she worked every day. So
she got a mirror and a pair of tweezers and removed the bits
herself!'

Others were not so lucky. Following a Christmas dinner on 23
December, as Monica and her fellow PMs relaxed over drinks
with their guests, 'the telephone rang to tell us a bomb had been
thrown into a room where a teenage party was being held, children of senior-rank officers – the C-in-C's son, the PMO's daughter . . .' The girl was seventeen. A piece of shrapnel had sliced into
her neck. 'Wing Commander Wynne-Griffiths was a few doors
down and when he heard the explosion he charged down to the
house and sent for an ambulance. He apparently sat astride her
with his thumbs on her neck . . . but she was dead on arrival at the

hospital.' The C-in-C's son had a piece of shrapnel in his leg, 'just underneath the femoral artery. It rather ruined everyone's Christmas.'

By May 1967 Steamer Point was on the point of closing. All work transferred to Khormaksar Beach. Shelagh Glenn (Mrs Barber) was one of the last PMs to be posted in.

> We were very busy. Awful lot of casualties. One thing I remember, if we had a dissident in [for surgery], they had to have two soldiers in the theatre, guarding them with guns. One of the regiments was the Argyle and Sutherland Highlanders, and there'd be these great big huge brawny men, who'd come and say, 'Sister, I don't have to go into theatre, do I? Can we stand outside?' So we used to put theatre gowns on them and let them stand outside the door . . .

Aden itself became a war zone and RAF personnel were confined to base.

> They had one little shopping centre which was open for an hour every afternoon, when it was guarded. That was the only time we could get out, we were almost like prisoners in the mess. Some of the MOs used to go by car down to the BP place at Little Aden and I knew a couple of them, so they used to take me, but even they would carry guns . . . When we were working in theatre they kept their guns in the dangerous drugs cupboard, and I had the dangerous drugs in my pocket. Bizarre, yes.
>
> And then Sue Quinn (Morgan now) and I were told that when the British went out of Aden, when the hospital closed down, we were going out to work on HMS *Albion* for about two months, to take casualties. We were kitted out in new uniforms, because we'd be on the mess deck, climbing on bunks, so we wore trousers and jackets. The week before we were due to go over, I went over by helicopter every day to get the mess deck sorted out and get the theatre ready – there was a small theatre attached to it, which was quite amusing because it was absolutely full – jampacked! – with 2 mil. syringes . . .

All the other PMs left Aden, Liz Lown among them.

> The day we abandoned KBH to its fate will live in the memo-
> ries of the sisters involved till the end of our lives. All
> European patients had been casevaced out. Numbers of Arab
> patients had been reduced to an absolute minimum – the rest,
> those too ill to leave the hospital, we simply had to abandon.
> To us, Western-trained nurses, it was a traumatic experience.
> To the locals . . . a soldier summed it up: 'We managed before
> the British came, we'll manage when you've gone – *Allah
> karim* "Allah will provide".'

Shelagh Glenn and Sue Quinn were the only ones left in the sisters'
mess. Sue decided she couldn't bear to be alone and so moved in
with her friend; they put wardrobes against the windows as Shelagh
recalls.

> I don't know what we thought was going to happen, but we
> felt safer that way. We were just going to sleep when we heard
> these footsteps coming along the verandah, so she squeaked,
> 'Oh! It's happening! They're coming!' and this voice said, 'It's
> all right, sisters, it's corporal of the guard, we're just doing the
> rounds. I'll be coming round every hour to see you're all right.'

Next day, they moved to HMS *Albion*, at anchor in the bay, where
they lodged with the Royal Navy.

> It was a bit difficult at first, being the only females on board
> with all that lot. But I must say they were very nice. We'd got
> a very nice suite – actually, it was the marine commandoes'
> Colonel's quarters . . . Luckily, we didn't have too many casu-
> alties. Most of the operating we did, the surgeon-commander,
> every day, used to go round the fleet and see what he could
> find – hernias, appendix, things like that, so if we weren't kept
> busy we were at least kept working.

The press seemed excited by the presence of female officers aboard
a marine commando carrier (back in 1967 it was very daring!);
Shelagh and Sue were subjected to photo sessions.

The TV cameras came too, and while we were on deck having photographs taken all flying had to stop, so there were we walking up and down the deck and everyone staring, making rude comments . . . The whole session finished and one of the photographers – I think he was from the *Daily Mirror* – said, 'Oh, I haven't got a film in my camera!' so we did it all again.'

Now that they were removed from it, the war seemed distant. By night, sometimes, they saw flashes as bombs and guns went off, but gradually the trouble died down and though a few casualties arrived by helicopter, the prepared 'casualty ward' on the commandoes' mess deck was not needed. 'The idea was that if there'd been a lot of casualties we'd have gone on with the ship – round to Mogadishu, and everybody would have been flown off from there, but luckily that didn't happen. When we left the ship, we went on a Bristol freighter to Bahrain . . . and then we flew from Bahrain back to UK.'

Hospital patients from Aden also travelled via Bahrain, where they were prepared for aeromed back to the UK. The last of them flew home from RAF Muharraq cared for by a medical team which included Elizabeth Sandison. She recalls it as

. . . quite an event, a full patient load on a Britannia, diverted into Gatwick – you can imagine all the panic at that in those days! One of the patients . . . Foreign and Commonwealth Office, stretcher case, not allowed to get off the 'plane . . . Customs came to see him on board and said to this lovely, jovial-looking gentleman, 'Have you anything to declare, sir?' He opened his briefcase and here were two revolvers with I don't know how many rounds of ammunition . . . They quietly took it away from him. He must have had the guns all the time, in the hospital, during transit . . .

Duty done, Liz Sandison returned to her base – the newly-named Princess Alexandra's Royal Air force Hospital, Wroughton.

A new Royal Patron

Following the death of the Princess Royal in 1965, the Service obtained the Queen's consent to the appointment of Princess

Alexandra (the Hon. Mrs Angus Ogilvie, now the Hon. Lady Ogilvie) to the role of Patron and Air Chief Commandant of the PMRAFNS. The appointment could not have been more appropriate: Princess Alexandra is not only a niece of the PMs' first Royal Patron, she is also the only daughter of George, Duke of Kent, who died in a flying accident in 1942 while serving with the RAF. She has two brothers – the present Duke of Kent and Prince Michael of Kent.

Like her aunt before her, after completing her education Princess Alexandra took a nursing course at Great Ormond Street Hospital before assuming her official duties. In April 1963 she married Angus Ogilvie (he became Sir Angus in 1989), second son of the Earl of Airdrie. They have a son and a daughter and, at the time of writing, four grandchildren.

Since accepting the role of Air Chief Commandant of the PMRAFNS in 1966, Princess Alexandra has paid many visits to RAF hospitals, welcomed as a well-loved presence by all members of the Service.

In 1968 Her Royal Highness visited RAFH Wegberg, West Germany. As part of the preparations for the occasion, Sandra Cranswick (Mrs Philpott) was selected to accompany the princess to the ladies' room.

> I had to practise shaking hands and curtsying, and was instructed in the exact words I had to say to her! However, she will never know of the concern shown beforehand to ensure her privacy. She was to use the bathroom in the flat of the matron, Wing Officer McNeill. This had a glazed door, but it was decided that a new curtain should be added for extra privacy. A maintenance man and I were tasked to decide how many layers of net were necessary for complete privacy – he held the net to the door and I stood at the end of the corridor to see if I could see him through the glazed door and net! We finally arrived at 3 layers of net being necessary to secure her complete privacy ... However, on her arrival, she immediately put us at ease and my 'chore' became an enjoyable and memorable occasion.

Many such occasions have been enjoyed by numerous members of the PMRAFNS in the years which have followed.

FOUR

Students and pupils

The story of nurse-training within the RAF is complex. It started in 1951, when the General Nursing Council approved RAF hospitals Halton, Ely and Wroughton as nurse-training schools for recruits of the RAFMS. Students both male and female might qualify as state-registered, non-commissioned staff nurses, ready for duty in hospital wards and SSQs. In some places they worked alongside nursing officers of the PMRAFNS.

However, from October 1962 the RAF also introduced nurse-training within the PMRAFNS, for 'intelligent young women with four O-levels or the equivalent', who wished to attain SRN standard. Applicants, either direct entrants from civilian life or transferees from the WRAF, entered what was officially designated the PMRAFNS NCE (Non-Commissioned Element). The three-year training typically consisted of six weeks' basic instruction at Halton and the rest at Ely or Wroughton, with secondments to Wegberg and Uxbridge providing, respectively, maternity and oncology experience. In common with their colleagues in the RAFMS, these students graduated as staff nurse junior NCOs, with the chance to rise through senior NCO ranks to become warrant officers.

Six years on, in 1968, the service also began training to state-enrolled level for the non-commissioned element; then in 1969 a new scheme enabled SENs and Pupil Enrolled Nurses to enlist on 'local service' engagements, living at home while being employed at a nearby RAF station or hospital – the hospitals involved were Nocton Hall, Ely, Cosford, Halton and Wroughton. The first member of the PMRAFNS to train under this new scheme was also a married woman – Aircraftwoman Mrs Marian Potter, who lived in Swindon with her husband while completing her SEN training at Wroughton.

Qualified SRNs and SENs continued to be recruited though, as had always been the case, only female SRNs could apply for commissioned posts; state-registered male nurses and state-enrolled nurses of either sex were offered non-commissioned posts.

Student tales

These were the Sixties, the era of the Beatles and the Campaign for Nuclear Disarmament, also the time when young people began to question the authority and wisdom of their elders. Stories told by student nurses reflect this change in mood.

Anne Sumner (Mrs Wynne-Jones) was in the WRAF, training at Wroughton for her SRN, when news came that student nurses could join the PMs.

> . . . change uniform, have our own rooms, and our own cleaners, but not have quite the same pay structure . . . the thought of an end to 'bull nights' [when students had to stay in and polish their shoes, buttons, floors, windows and anything else that might take a shine] was amazing to me, so off I went . . . There was a bit of rivalry between us and those who elected to stay in the WRAF. They were right at the other end of camp, by the NAAFI, still in billets, while we were in the hospital itself, in our own rooms . . . but we were still training on the same course, and working side by side on the wards . . .
>
> We were the first PM student nurses at Wroughton. We had the white dress and the cape, and we had our cardigans taken off us, and hats – these were replaced by the standard 'bowlers'. [Only nursing officers wore the 'Dick Turpin'; students' 'best-blue' hats were standard WRAF-type, which at the time had high, rounded crowns.] We went to have our heads measured for these bowlers . . . It was at the time of the fancy hairstyles, the french-pleat and back-combing, so mine was stuck up there – I'd been to a dance the night before and it was still

back-combed up when we went into Stores to get measured. By the time the hat arrived the hairstyle had dropped, my head was about two sizes smaller! I ended up with this dubious-looking bowler hat that sort of rested round the top of my nose . . . I was very often sent back off parade. They'd look at me with my funny bowler, my skirt that seemed longer than anyone else's because my legs were so short, and they'd boot me off.

We had some interesting little 'run-ins'. First of all, I mentioned they took the cardigans off us because we had the cloaks, but it was freezing cold in winter. We had a big dust-up about keeping our cardigans. Also, they gave us white canvas shoes – whereas Sisters had nice soft white kid shoes, we had these really, really hard white canvas shoes, they were terrible, they rubbed our heels . . . I led this mini revolution, I said, 'Right, nobody's listening to us, so we'll all go and report sick.' So after about the third person had reported sick with blisters on their heels, the MO came out, said, 'All right, how many are here for problems with your feet?' so we all stood up . . . It was agreed that they'd give us a chitty, or some money or something, to buy softer white shoes, but by the time we got that the damage had been done, the shoes were broken in.

On the question of cardigans, minutes of a matrons' meeting of 1969 may reflect this minor revolt in the ranks: 'When the weather is very cold, white cardigans may be worn by students and pupils, WHEN IN SCHOOL, but on no other occasion.'

From civilian life, Linda Kendall (Mrs McKenzie) joined Course 3, a mix of direct entries and girls transferring from the WRAF in January 1964. She too writes of rivalry between the two elements, 'especially as we had done less basic training than the WRAFs'. But in many ways little had changed – students were still being asked to bend over to see whether their 'popliteal space' (backs of knees) showed. If it did, they had to let down the hems of their ward dresses.

Course 4 began in June 1964, graced by the presence of Nadine Gay, along with six other girls who first met at Halton and still remain close friends. Nadine well remembers their transfer to Ely.

A mass of girls in blue uniform, luggage everywhere ...
People stared in horror at the bevy of beauties, looking more
like the cast of *St Trinians* than student nurses ...

The first time we were ordered to get ready in best blue
uniform – to be interviewed by the matron, Wing Officer
Higgins, a formidable character – had us all rushing about,
pressing and polishing. I, too busy talking, accidentally
poured Brasso all down the front of my jacket. Nothing we
did could remove it! We went in one by one to see her [but]
she barely lifted her gaze on me and my jacket.

Later, Miss Higgins mistook student nurse Nadine Gay for student
nurse Gaynor Morris, and when Nadine pointed out the error, 'she
snorted and said, "It doesn't matter, you're all as bad as one
another."'

In their second year, students gained paediatric and maternity
experience during a twelve-week attachment to RAFH Wegberg,
West Germany, and in their third year a sojourn at Uxbridge's Cade
Unit provided sobering insights into the suffering wrought by
cancer. 'The permanent staff had seen more death than any of us,
but were mostly kind and optimistic, which these poor patients
needed. We will never forget one lovely RAF doctor in the final
stages of bladder carcinoma ...' But one of the RAF medics at
Uxbridge made the girls laugh. 'His life's ambition was to kill
Matron's bad-tempered Pekinese, who had savaged his ankles more
than once.'

Students dropped out of the course for a variety of reasons –
'failed exams, failed hopes, failed contraception ...' However,
Nadine adds, despite all the legends of free love and flower power,
'not all of us had wild sexual adventures in the swinging sixties'.
One of her friends dared to invite a boyfriend to have coffee in her
room, and 'a particularly nasty WRAF NCO, who despised PMs
and must have been tipped off, decided to do a spot check ...
Keith, hearing her coming, tried to hide in the wardrobe. This was
always full of clutter, even a budgie cage, so unfortunately he was
discovered.' The pair were ordered to report to the CO, who made
an example of them: Louise went to Guildford in Surrey for two
weeks' punishment; her boyfriend spent a month in Colchester
Military Prison, where 'he rubbed shoulders with the likes of

murderers and high-profile offenders. None of them believed he had been sent there for having a cup of coffee in a nurses' home!'

From Uxbridge days, Cynthia Mayfield (Mrs Brown) recalls 'the noise from other service activities near to our quarters ... the Central Band of the RAF rehearsing, the Queen's Colour Squadron of the RAF Regiment likewise practising their drill, planes from Northolt flying overhead ...' Sleeping during the day while doing a spell of night duty was not easy! Neither was learning to give injections: 'Oranges are one thing, real live people something else altogether. But gradually we built up our confidence, and our ability to be convincingly economical with the truth ... "Oh, yes," we would say in response to the occasional nervous enquiry, "I've done this HUNDREDS of times before"!'

For student Pat Maslen (Mrs Perry) her association with the PMs began years before. Her father was in the RAFMS, stationed in Ceylon accompanied by his family, when his wife fell ill and had to be aeromeded home – husband and children, including Pat, all flew with her. Pat later joined the PMRAFNS NCE, Nursing Course 5. The very first injection *she* gave proved fateful – three years later she married the patient involved.

Diaries kept by 'Beth' Smith (Mrs Hamson) reveal how much of her off-duty time a student spent on uniforms: ward dresses, returned daily by the laundry service, had to be damp-ironed to make them presentable, and caps had to be starched. Her first ward at Ely was a 'dirty surgery' ward known as 'bums and gums' – 'haemorrhoidectomies and dental surgery, plus infected wounds'. I was very naive but keen to learn and visiting X-ray one day I asked what the small blue radiation machines pinned to the X-ray personnel's coats were. A lovely man whose name I've forgotten told me, "They're virgin detectors." Beth remembers some eccentric PMs, too, especially the sister in the maternity ward at Wegberg, who 'decided that all baby boys under her care should be called Julian.'

The girls may be surprised to know that they were regarded by at least one of the young male nursing attendants as 'super confident bunches of goddesses ... in their spotless white uniforms'. Enrolled nurse Geoff Holliday was still in his teens, at the stage of peeling slivers of yellow soap into a large jug bubbling on the stove, making the 'goo' to clean the floor before he swung a heavy bumper 'recklessly to and fro to achieve a superlative but non-slip shine'.

Having survived the temptations of becoming top of the 'black list' of undesirables which Deputy Matron read to each new entry of female students – 'it always guaranteed an early assignation if you were in writing as "best to avoid" in the dating stakes' – Geoff before long developed 'aspirations, some would say delusions' to emulate the girl students, and set himself on the long road to passing the exams he needed to become a state registered nurse himself.

Because of general cutbacks and a reduced need for newly qualified staff nurses, SRN training ended in 1977. But not before a few changes had been made: minutes of matrons' meetings for 1975 report that 'Wroughton School of Nursing has been moved to a permanent site – in a Porta-Cabin'.

Nocton Hall

A hospital which provided a favourite posting for many PMs was Nocton Hall, secluded amid acres of rolling Lincolnshire farmland. It took over the work of RAFH Rauceby in June 1947. The Hall itself became the sisters' mess, while the wooden wards reposed in grounds noted for the scent of wild garlic and the dance of springtime daffodils. Starting with just four wards, by 1954 Nocton Hall offered most of the usual hospital facilities, both for service personnel from the many RAF stations in Lincolnshire and for local people from the Sleaford area. Further departments added over ensuing years widened its scope to include a maternity wing, twin operating theatres, a central sterile supply department and a neuropsychiatric centre.

Margaret Kingston, who knew Nocton in the early sixties, loved it.

> The hospital was nothing, just hutted, but it had a happy atmosphere . . . The first time I was posted there, I went for a walk in the woods and picked some white flowers, put them in a vase in my room. My batwoman said, 'Sister, d'you know what you've picked there?' I said, 'No, but they don't smell very nice.' She said, 'It's wild garlic!' . . . I remember she was a bit late one morning. Eventually, in she comes with my cup of tea, saying, 'Sister, I've had such a fright! I was cycling up the drive and a BLACK MAN was walking towards me. He'd

got white teeth, but . . . he was black!' . . . I explained he was one of our American patients and a lovely boy. But she was so frightened . . . lived in that village all her life, and Lincoln so far away . . .

In those days of few cars, eight miles could be a day's excursion.

Many PMs enjoyed joining in amateur dramatics, 'particularly when National Servicemen brought their many varied talents,' according to Marion Wood (Mrs Donaldson). Nocton Hall's drama group produced a plethora of plays and pantos and 1961 seems to have been especially prolific. That year Kathy Mogg (Mrs Ostler) took part in three productions. During rehearsals for *Waltz of the Toreadors* she was almost knocked unconscious when the chap playing her husband 'flung me down and tried to strangle me. There was an iron bedstead (Airmen for the use of) underneath the flounces and my head hit the bottom rail'. Later both she and Marion Wood had parts in *Babes in the Wood*, in which Kathy played Robin Hood, 'rigorously rehearsed in singing and dancing by a professional actor doing National Service who had written and directed the show. After the second performance all the PMs involved went to the officers' mess for a party and I'm afraid the shellfish got me – food poisoning. By the next afternoon I was admitted to Ward 9 and the search was on for a replacement.'

Plucked from the obscurity of the chorus to save the day, Marion Wood was 'given the afternoon off to learn lines, refusing an offered phenobarb to calm my nerves – thought I'd better have my wits about me'. Visitors to Kathy Mogg's sick bed assured her the show had gone on.

Uxbridge

The Cade Unit at Uxbridge dealt with over a thousand cancer patients a year; more than 800 of these received chemotherapy and others were referred to the Westminster (now Charing Cross) Hospital for radiotherapy. As a junior sister, having finished her initial six weeks' service at Halton, April Reed came to work there. She remembers the patients as 'nearly all senior officers. We had Lord Trenchard, who died. They were practising his funeral long before he was dead.' But she was particularly moved by the bravery of younger patients dying of the disease. Everyone who worked on the unit felt the same. When the hospital closed in 1972, the Cade continued its invaluable work from premises at Halton.

Today, RAF Uxbridge still serves as a parade-training base for personnel chosen to represent branches of the RAF at commemorative events in London. Over the years these have included the Coronation Parade of 1953 and many Festivals of Remembrance.

In 1967 RAF Sergeant Kenneth 'Tug' Wilson 'was to lead the RAF contingent down the steps at the Royal Albert Hall'.

> We trained at Uxbridge and on the Tuesday afternoon there was a roar from the Officer Commanding the Queen's Colour Squadron, 'Sergeant Wilson! Leave your squad and take these b— women, put 'em in proper shoes and teach 'em how to march up and down steps!' What a task for a drill sergeant! I was used to drilling male recruits, not nurses . . .
>
> I became very diplomatic, pointing out that high heels and court shoes were really not intended for marching in. Once they had changed into more suitable footwear, I very gentlemanly grabbed two sisters by their arms and with me in the middle marched them up and down the steps at the bottom of Uxbridge square . . . Talk about shift work – three pairs of sisters to take up and down steps all afternoon.

Marching might not have been a forte, but nursing sisters had their followers. Security-conscious RAF police wanted to put a ring of security lights around the sisters' mess at Uxbridge, but Matron Kennedy refused to allow it. Her reason? 'My girls should have privacy to bid goodnight to their friends.' What a treasure!

Halton House

Without doubt, Princess Mary's Royal Air Force Hospital Halton remains dearest to the hearts of most PMs. Halton was where many of them spent their first few weeks in the service, where the pulse of the PMRAFNS seemed always to beat strongest. Especially they relished the ambience of Halton House, then as now the officers' mess of RAF Halton, which still hosts balls and reunions and other glamorous occasions, as it has done since the days when Edward VII was a regular visitor and when (allegedly) Lily Langtry bathed in the champagne-filled swimming pool.

Kate Crompton (Mrs Wilmot) wrote:

> I particularly remember the balls at Halton House. The setting was superb, with an imposing staircase sweeping down to the main entrance hall. There was a minstrels' gallery and the north and south drawing rooms opened into the main hall. The bar was painted gold . . . I lived in the Sisters' Mess [but] when it was being enlarged and refurbished half the Sisters moved to Halton House. That was rather a quiet, sedate Mess with lots of senior officers [who] must have had quite a shock with the invasion of the PMs.

Isobel Hipkin (Mrs Bedford), who was part of that invasion, found Halton House 'very much a male domain, with just a few WRAF and Red Cross personnel . . . An influx of twenty Nursing Officers caused quite some disruption.' The PMs were assigned to shared rooms on the second floor, far from the bathrooms and poorly heated by coal stoves – which came hard on two sisters recently returned from steamy Aden. Because of varying duty hours, mealtimes in the officers' mess had to be adjusted. At breakfast the resident male officers 'normally had a quiet meal behind the daily paper. They took some time to get used to these female intruders who talked!'

But the glamour remained: 'A real highlight of our stay was the Summer Ball, with trumpeters on the main staircase,' says Isobel, while Judy Cooke (Mrs Owens) remembers 'being shown the big V-bombers while wearing a long, emerald-green evening dress'.

However, it was not all high-jinks and dancing. Kate Crompton worked long hours in the plastic surgery centre, whose senior surgeon had worked with the famous Archibald McIndoe during the war. Starting in 1963, Kate 'did night duty every five weeks . . . 8 p.m. until 8 a.m., we worked 14 nights non-stop, with a sleeping day and two days off . . . Shortly before my time, the girls used to work 3 weeks non-stop!' The weather added its own inconveniences – Kate arrived at Halton in February, when the weather was so atrocious that 'the laundry van couldn't get through and nursing officers had to wash their own uniforms'.

Changes at Changi

The building of a whole new unit to link the two separate hospital blocks made RAFH Changi, Singapore, an easier place in which to work. Margaret Kingston, who went out to open the new families' ward, found it a delightful posting, but some of the other girls became depressed, for which Margaret blames the climate.

> It was the same all the year, you didn't have seasons . . . we used to say, wouldn't it be lovely to wake up and see some clouds? . . . and orchids – I never wanted to see another orchid. Coming from this flower area [she is a native of Spalding in Lincolnshire] I used to say, 'I'd love to see a daffodil, or a tulip.'
>
> One Christmas, the whole place flooded. The monsoon drains couldn't cope with the water and it just poured everywhere. Nobody could visit the patients. Nobody could go anywhere. And the sisters on duty were crying and the sisters off-duty were crying, everybody was home-sick . . .

Judy Hopkins (Mrs Foote) and her colleagues dealt with the monsoon in a practical way: they went to work in flip-flops and changed into white shoes on the wards, leaving off stockings. The hospital became a refuge for residents of the local children's home, which regularly flooded with every monsoon. But the handicapped youngsters loved it – it was like having a party.

In the row of married quarters which acted as accommodation for Changi PMs, Margaret Kingston lived close to her friend Molly McNair, at a time when the Ministry of Defence (MOD) were 'trying out new mess kits for PMs. We'd had all sorts, and somebody had the brainwave to use natural tussore [coarse brown silk], of all things, to make a mess dress. It was all tucks – most elaborate. Well . . . I used to look out from my balcony, most evenings, and there was Molly, in this new mess kit, gardening! I thought "the heat has got her." ' After observing this performance for a few evenings, Margaret asked Molly why she was gardening in mess dress. ' "Oh," she said, "MOD want it testing in all different climates, so that's what I'm doing." But it was hopeless, they didn't have it for long.' Margaret Kingston adds ruefully. 'It used to cost us a fortune every time they changed the mess kit. I think I had three different sorts.'

Poliomyelitis was still rampant in the early sixties. April Reed nursed many very serious cases, 'with the iron lungs and things . . . A sister named Margaret Wood was specialist aeromed polio-trained.' And there were civilian patients, resident Singaporeans, such as 'a chap brought in one night who'd been carved up [literally] by the rest of his family'.

Shelagh Glenn (Mrs Barber) was a theatre sister on the case. 'We worked for hours just suturing him up, then he went back into the ward and eventually, after a few days, was transferred to the civilian hospital in Singapore. As he walked out after being discharged they got at him again and finished the job!'

Marion Wood (Mrs Donaldson) says, 'Weddings, christenings and, sadly, deaths, were part of life in Changi. Four sisters married in my two years there. We had the Hospital CO in after a severe heart attack, and one of our physicians with a young family was killed in a road accident on his way home to lunch . . .' The CO of RAF Changi was also taken ill and casevaced home, but died soon afterwards. A memorial service was held for him at Changi and Marion and her friend Jane Bullen (Mrs Selway) attended. Marion says, 'It was a solemn service, but my abiding memory is of having to tiptoe on PSP (pierced steel planking used on many airfields) in heeled court shoes which were part of our best outdoor tropical uniform (black court shoes, travel dress and white Dick).'

On a lighter note, she reveals that, in order to feed the four night-duty sisters, 'a basket of food was provided by the Sisters' Mess, the meal prepared by the WRAF Nursing Orderly, and eaten in 3rd floor Sister's office. We sometimes requested a cake mix in the basket, and if no one was in labour as we went on duty it was easy to whip up a sponge and pop it in the ward oven.' Friends (and their boyfriends) often popped in to join the sisters at coffee break; they too enjoyed the cakes – until one evening when one of the sisters happened to mention that 'it had been mixed in a delivery bowl (sterilised, of course!)'.

After one of these convivial midnight feasts, as Judy Cooke (Mrs Owens) recalls, one of the naval officers sent a telegram saying, 'Thanks for the coffee and cakes and love to Ann Marie . . .' Unfortunately the matron, Wing Officer Dickson, saw the telegram and hauled the PMs up for a 'severe telling off'. But the Navy laid on the charm and matron was 'invited to very many pukka cocktail parties on such ships as the *Ark Royal*, and after that called them "such dear boys"'.

Whilst romantic dallying on service premises was strictly forbidden, some matrons could blink when it suited them. Twenty-five-year-old Flying Officer David Dodds was 'seriously courting one of the girls', and he relates how Wing Officer Jessie Higgins lent tacit approval – she addressed him as 'David, dear', though the object of his affections, Flying Officer Eileen Smith, remained simply 'Smith'.

Deputy matrons also played Cupid at times, as Judy Cooke (Mrs Owens) explains.

> I think there were twelve midwives and thanks to our Squadron Officers we organized our working shifts according to which boyfriend's plane or ship was in . . . One of the midwives, Jane Bullen, had a notebook with all of the ship's numbers in. The maternity unit was right on the sea and the ships had to pass in front to go up to the Naval base so, busy as we were, if a ship passed we used to tip the louvred windows up and wave the nappies out of the window.

In the late sixties, Clare Woolley (Mrs Fowler), ran the children's ward. Among hospital personnel she found a talented amateur artist, who 'kindly painted Walt Disney characters over the cots and beds. Unfortunately, one child took great exception to having the bed "belonging" to Dopey!'

Hong Kong

By this time the only other Far Eastern post for PMs was in Hong Kong, at the sick quarters of RAF Kai Tak, whose resident squadron was cared for by a small medical team: two doctors, a dentist and one PM, assisted by local orderlies. April Reed was the last PM there in 1960, after which the Medical Branch took over all Hong Kong duties.

Fifteen years later, however, the authorities decided that it might be useful to have a qualified aeromed sister on hand at Kai Tak. Following total withdrawal from Singapore in 1975, they sent in

Valerie Hand, who had already done a year's duty at Changi. She thought Hong Kong 'an amazing place'.

> The airstrip went out into the sea, and when you flew in, low over the sea, there was this strip of runway stuck out . . . you had to cross this six-lane highway and go up the hill to the officers' mess, which was on the side of the hill. From the balconies of the rooms, you overlooked this highway and RAF Kai Tak, and then the main Kai Tak airport beyond it. It was absolutely fantastic, the view . . .
>
> I used to do the local casevac flights with 84 Helicopter Squadron. They and the local Royal Hong Kong Auxiliary helicopters took it in turns to be on call, and the two doctors and I also had a call rota. We'd get called out to all sorts of things, like some Chinese woman in labour having a problem out on Cheung Chau island, and we'd fly to pick her up and transfer her to one of the local hospitals . . . [Or we] had to rescue somebody from the hillsides . . . depended whether you were in a Wessex or with the Hong Kong Auxiliaries, who flew Alouettes. But it made a change from the daily grind. Hong Kong was an experience. I loved it.

Valerie Hand was followed at Kai Tak by Shelagh Utley, who stayed there for two years. In 1978, soon after Shelagh left, RAF Kai Tak itself closed down and the medical centre moved to Shek Kong (pronounced Sek Kong), out in the New Territories. Other PMs were to be posted there in their turn.

With the 'boat people' crisis at its height in 1979, refugees from Vietnam crowded into boats and sought safety in Hong Kong. The derelict sick quarters at RAF Kai Tak was opened again by the British Red Cross. One of the Red Cross workers who helped with the refugees until they could be resettled was Helen Cookson, a retired squadron officer of the PMRAFNS. For this work she was later awarded the Florence Nightingale Medal, the highest honour in nursing, regarded as the 'Nurses' VC'.

Decade of diversity – the Seventies

Change and unsettlement loomed as the seventies began. Reductions

in the overall commitment of the RAF saw the withdrawal of forces
from the Middle East and the closure of some overseas hospitals. Cuts
in manpower led to additional closures of smaller hospitals in the UK
– Uxbridge, Padgate, Weeton and Cosford. However, for the PMs it
was also a time of interest and diversity, including chances to work in
unusual places and with nursing services of other nations.

As a prelude to the decade, a poignant occasion took place in
1970 when a service in the Nurses' Chapel at Westminster Abbey,
attended by the Queen Mother, dedicated the gift of special seats
and kneelers made by skilled needlewomen of all three nursing
services. Wing Officer Jessie Higgins (who had retired in 1968),
being an expert tapestry-maker and member of the Royal College
of Embroidery, was asked to work a cushion with a design showing
the PMRAFNS medical badge. Using the best materials supplied by
the Royal College of Embroidery, she considered it a labour of love
and was very proud to have been chosen. So she was somewhat
upset when Matron-in-Chief, having been to see the work in an
exhibition, remarked in amazement that there wasn't a mistake in
it. 'As if there would be!' says Higgie indignantly.

Changing courses

The General Service Training (GST) course, held at RAF Henlow,
had by this time become a requirement for all nursing officers. It
evolved into the Professionally Qualified and Re-Entrant (PQRE)
course, which in turn later became the Specialist Entrant and Re-
Entrant (SERE) course, and moved to the RAF College, Cranwell.
The course is designed to turn professionally-qualified civilians into
physically fit and service-aware officers, ready to take up their first
posts with the Royal Air Force.

Miche Shaw, practising midwifery at Nocton Hall and longing
for a posting to the Far East, was summoned to Matron's office and
informed that she had been chosen to go to Henlow as flight
commander on the very first PQRE course. Although she had no
teaching experience and had never even seen a signal, much less
considered how to teach the subject, she accepted the challenge and
with a good deal of homework and application her initial six-month
posting turned into two years in the job. A PM is nothing if not
adaptable!

Journey to the past – Oman

The Gulf state of Muscat and Oman (now Oman) was an isolated Islamic society, riven by blood feuds and slavery and ruled by a despot who turned the revenues from his oil deposits into gold which he kept in his palace. In 1970 the Sultan was deposed by his son Qabus, who determined to introduce a better way of life for his people.

Seeing medical aid as a priority, Sultan Qabus asked the British government for help and an RAF medical team went out – surgeon, anaesthetist, nursing officer, two male registered general nurses, two female SENs, a sergeant operating theatre technician and 'a Cpl Med Sec with 20 minutes Radiography training' according to Connie Bull, the nursing officer involved. The six men, fresh from the UK, stayed at RAF Salalah, an all-male domain; the three women, from RAFH Muharraq, in Bahrain, had a flat in the Sultan's palace.

The former ruler had begun to build a hospital but abandoned the project. So the 'hospital' set up by the RAF medical team consisted mainly of two bungalows which had been intended as accommodation for the staff of the uncompleted facility. The local populace dwelt mostly in palm-frond huts, deprived of most modern benefits including running water and electricity. However, the bungalows – which served as wards, theatre and night-duty quarters – obtained power from a generator and 'water was pumped up to tanks in the roof, from a bowser filled two or three times a day from the supply at RAF Salalah, by one of our RGNs (misemployed!)'.

In the air-conditioned bedroom (the operating theatre) patients were anaesthetized on the table – women had to be undressed while comatose because they wouldn't knowingly let men touch them. In the lounge (the ward) eight beds and several mattresses held patients – since they were accompanied and fed by relatives, the crush and scramble the nurses faced while trying to tend their patients may be imagined.

Modern sanitary facilities in the bungalows puzzled the local people – normal practice was to visit the beach, dig a hole, perform the necessary function, bury the evidence, and clean themselves with sea water and rocks. They tried to do something similar in the hospital toilets, with messy consequences which Connie Bull and the two SENs had to clean up several times a day. Writing to a friend about it, she added, 'To get my women and local girl nurses (under training from us) to know how to use the toilet, I decided the only way was by demonstration!! If you could have seen me surrounded by Arabs I think you'd have been in hysterics.' Connie was horrified to learn that her letter describing these events to Matron in Muharraq (humorously intended) had been seen at the Air Ministry by Matron-in-Chief *et al.*

> Imagine my thoughts when anyone of higher rank years later said, 'I've heard of you!' I had also ended my letter (I was a Flight Officer at the time), 'yours sincerely, Connie Bull, Matron of Salalah, Consultant Obstetrician and Gynaecologist (true – Arab women would not let men touch them), Consultant Physician to Royalty (I attended the Sultan's mother and sister, and the harem of his father), Jack of all trades and glorified char!' I was convinced my career was definitely limited to 16 years and no promotion. [She was wrong – she spent twenty-four years in the PMs and retired as a wing commander.]

Despite inadequate facilities, equipment and drugs, plus the inconvenience of being separated from the doctors on camp by a mined 'no man's land', there being a war on locally, their work varied from delivering babies to treating TB, performing minor surgery and vaccinating the Salalah population against cholera. For this last, Connie set up her clinic 'on a tree stump, armed with 2 syringes and 4 metal needles (as in the old days) and a spirit lamp to "sterilize"'. She vaccinated about 500 people in one day.

Major surgery was impossible without laboratory backup, but they began with hernias and cysts and eventually undertook 'some rather drastic surgical action to relieve abhorrent medical conditions'.

> We drained a hydrocele of 6.8 litres of fluid – he'd carried his testes in a wheelbarrow (Arabs don't wear trousers). We also removed a fungating breast cancer, which relieved the smell and made a husband very happy, [and] we borrowed the local

carpenter's saw to amputate the leg of a 28-year-old. We then had to turn a broom upside down for a crutch . . . the 'boys' at RAF Salalah kindly made him a peg leg . . . I will not forget the faces of those – like the amputee – who although deformed by the surgery were so exhilarated by it, because of their freedom from pain.

Connie Bull was in Salalah from September to December 1970 and again during March and April the following year. 'We also "trained" 4 local Arab girls – who were not even used to running water – to scrub up, lay up for a dressing, do it and remove sutures in a sterile manner. Achieved in 6 weeks mainly by sign language. I often wonder if they are working at the hospital, so modern today, and what status they hold . . . It was an experience not to be missed.'

A PM in Texas

For Elizabeth Sandison, then a flight officer in the PMRAFNS, new challenges opened when she became the first PM to go on an exchange posting with the United States Air Force (USAF). Attached to their flight school, at Brooks Airfield, San Antonio, Texas, for six weeks, she went through a flight-nurse training course there before joining the 11th Aeromedical Airlift Squadron at Scott Air Force Base, Illinois. 'It was at the height of the Vietnam conflict, so the amount of internal transfer of patients was phenomenal. We criss-crossed Continental US and Alaska, and down as far as Puerto Rico. Thousands of patients were airlifted around San Francisco, then moved on to bases near their homes, or to more specialist facilities.' Liz was also involved with casualties after Hurricane Celia hit Texas and devastated 85 per cent of facilities, including the hospital, around Corpus Christi Naval Air Station. Flying aboard a C-9 Nightingale, she and her American colleagues airlifted out twenty-one stretcher patients and fifteen walking wounded.

Her US detachment over, Liz Sandison returned to aeromed duties at what was now the Princess Alexandra Hospital, RAF Wroughton. She flew with an aeromedical team on one particularly harrowing mission when a civilian VC10 crashed on take-off from Addis Ababa, with huge loss of life. Among the passengers were 'numerous Embassy children going back to school, there'd been many fatalities and the survivors were desperately burned'. The aeromed team, flying in an RAF VC10 from Lyneham, evacuated sixteen severely burned patients. They staged through Cyprus, where the aircraft refuelled and where medical teams from TPMRAFH Akrotiri assisted at the airhead, providing much-needed equipment. Most of the patients recovered, but one woman died as the plane made its descent to England and later two little girls and a man died in the burns and plastic surgery unit at Halton.

Radical changes at Akrotiri

In 1973 another terrible air crash, in the Kyrenia mountains on Cyprus, killed thirty-eight people, including Helen Deery and Sheila Noble, two off-duty PMs from Akrotiri.

The hospital itself remained extremely busy, a lively place where social life was good and nursing officers enjoyed their postings. On one occasion, for a royal visit by Princess Alexandra, patients on Ward 6 were decked in made-to-measure pyjamas with matching cravats!

However, problems were soon mounting: first Whitehall ordered cut-backs which affected British forces on the island; then in 1974 Turkish forces invaded and once again civil war broke out between Greek and Turkish factions. In response, the Akrotiri hospital was put on a war footing: staff did not return to their homes but slept 'on the job', working an eight-hour rota. Most of the casualties coming in were British expatriates caught in crossfire, or shot while refusing to leave their homes, but before long a nasty strain of diarrhoea began to spread across the island. As civilian hospitals overflowed, Akrotiri treated both local Cypriot home guard and a crew of Turkish sailors from a sunken destroyer. Lying sick alongside one another on the wards, the rival factions got along amicably enough.

From Britain, PMs Helen Tyler and Margaret Luck arrived to help care for Turkish refugees at RAF Episkopi. Prepared for uncomfortable living, possibly in tents, they brought their uniforms, thick sweaters, wellington boots and sleeping bags – and were startled to be asked if they had evening dresses for the Christmas and

New Year parties! Their main task was making up hundreds of four-hourly milk feeds for mothers and babies, a production line that flourished as trust and friendship grew and older Turkish girls helped out. Eventually when the trouble abated and the island was partitioned, the Turkish families moved north, hopefully to enjoy a more settled and peaceful life.

The trouble subsided and curfews ceased, but travel for British nationals was restricted to Greek Cypriot areas in the south and parts of Nicosia. Owing to the reduction in service personnel on the island, only three wards remained open at Akrotiri. Enrolled nurses continued to live in their billets in the main WRAF block, but the sisters' mess closed and remaining nursing officers shared the No. 1 Officers' Mess on the main base.

1976 saw Akrotiri reduced even further, to only two wards. Nevertheless, preparations began for a visit by Princess Margaret. The programme had to be rehearsed, with PM Ethnea Hancock chosen as stand-in for the royal visitor. She says it was 'the strangest thing I have ever been asked to do'.

It started with standing at the top of aircraft steps with no aircraft behind me! I then had to walk slowly down the steps to inspect a guard of honour before being driven to Air House at Episkopi with the Air Officer Commanding. Being a relatively junior officer at the time, this was all rather daunting. Later I had to walk round the Sergeants' Mess being introduced as if I were Her Royal Highness and having to respond with appropriate small talk before going to the Officers' Mess for a similar reception followed by a rehearsal lunch!'

Joy Harris, who was in Akrotiri in 1977 as senior matron, recalls being a passenger in a helicopter which disturbed the flamingos on the salt flats, causing them to rise in a cloud of pink wings – a magical sight.

But for the RAF the best days in Cyprus had ended. On closure of the British Military Hospital at Dhekelia, the RAF hospital at Akrotiri became bi-Service under RAF command, having three-fifths RAF and two-fifths army personnel. In its new role, caring for the tri-Service community on the island, it is known simply as The Princess Mary's Hospital (TPMH).

Philatelic flight

In 1973, half a century from its formal beginning, the PMRAFNS had over a thousand members, including non-commissioned and trainee nurses – the trainees earned as much in a month as had been paid annually to a qualified sister in 1923. Only seven RAF hospitals remained, but PMs on exchange duties could be found as far afield as Asia, Australia and the Americas.

To celebrate the fiftieth anniversary of the royal charter which officially launched the Princess Mary's Royal Air Force Nursing Service, a philatelic first-day cover was issued. The stamp showed a tiny 1923 Vickers Vernon air ambulance, contrasted with a 1973 VC10. It was designed by Squadron Officer Dorothy Hutchins (who had shared the Belize aeromed adventure after Hurricane Hattie in 1961). She flew to Akrotiri on a VC10 aeromed flight, taking with her 11,250 special envelopes, and in Cyprus she stuck commemorative stamps on them all and had the covers date-stamped before flying home again. Proceeds from the sale of the covers went to the RAF Museum at Hendon.

Imperial Iran

For a brief but memorable period in the seventies, PMs were stationed in Tehran, on loan to the Imperial Iranian Air Force, for whom they set up a school of nursing. Among the nursing officers involved was Liz Sandison. In a varied career she had just spent three enjoyable years with the Inspectorate of Recruiting, responsible for spreading the word of the PMRAFNS, via high schools and nursing courses, to 'young people who often had no idea what to do with their lives . . . I loved it, a wonderful job.' Now she found herself heading for Iran.

Dorothy Lane and Polly Perkins had already undertaken the daunting task of setting up a school of nursing, and Dorothy Reid (Mrs Westman) had joined them when the course was established. In 1977 Liz Sandison and Margaret Ross (Mrs Upfold) relieved that original team.

Liz recalls that the task of setting up British-style administration and introducing Nursing Council policies

> . . . was a most uphill job because of their attitudes and the way they conducted business . . . you'd spend two hours with

Princess Alexandra visits RAFH Nocton Hall, 1969
(© British Crown Copyright/MOD)

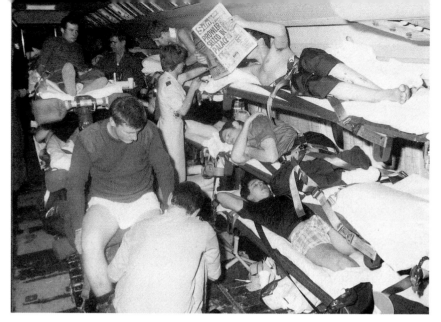

Medicine and dressings time for Falklands casualties flying home aboard a VC10 (© British Crown Copyright/MOD)

Princess Alexandra visits Wroughton during Falklands emergency, 1982. *Left to right:* Air Commodore Hurrell; Matron-in-Chief Air Commodore Joy Harris; Wing Commander Zena Cheel; HRH The Princess Alexandra; and a pupil nurse (© British Crown Copyright/MOD)

Wing Commander Anji Scofield (Matron, RAFWH Muharraq) giving a
daily briefing to her 'troops'

'Lady soldiers' with the Sheika's daughter in the palace, Bahrain, 1991

PMs make palm crosses for Palm Sunday – from their own trees!
Bahrain 1991

Transferring a casualty, Bosnia 1993, *centre:* Flight Lieutenant Lisa Bray
(© British Crown Copyright/MOD)

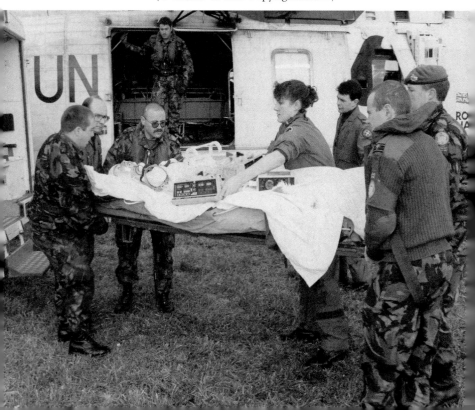

'the Generals', playing with a cup of coffee and a piece of sticky cake that you didn't really want, to get fifty pounds to replace a suction pump or other equipment for the school, whereas they would spend five thousand pounds on a silly piece of ornate nothing . . . [but] I would never leave without getting exactly what I wanted!

Although most Iranians considered nursing a very inferior occupation, some of the students came from very good backgrounds. Liz and her colleagues took them up to an Iranian air force holiday camp on the Caspian Sea. The girls had never had so much freedom before and they went mad painting their nails and plastering on make-up. Remembering those fashion-conscious, elegant girls that she knew, Liz finds it odd to see Iranian women now, on television, swathed to the eyes in black robes and veils. 'We left just as the Shah was about to be thrown out – the last few months were pretty tricky.'

Moving with the times

PM Susan Pound (Mrs Gray) made minor history in 1976. Her husband-to-be was based at RAF Stafford, with Susan at the closest RAFH at Cosford. However, 'Matron of Cosford Hospital, a rather formidable lady, would not consider me getting married and travelling from Stafford to Cosford.' Much paperwork later, Flight Officer Susan Pound/Gray became the first PM to be granted a married quarter in her own name. It was her husband who had to do the travelling!

However, Cosford itself was to close on 31 December 1977 after nearly forty years of service. It had been built in 1939 with the expectation of a useful life of ten years but, thanks to careful repair and renovation, the same buildings were in use thirty-seven years later. Cosford's last matron, Doreen Smedley, recalls the sadness of 'standing in the cold drizzly rain, six PMs with a lone RAF nurse' as the flag was hauled down for the last time.

Jubilees

As part of the celebrations for her Silver Jubilee, the Queen reviewed her Royal Air Force at Finningley on 29 July 1977 and, for the first time, a squadron of PMs was present on parade for the presentation of a new colour. Squadron Officer Judy Hopkins (Mrs Foote), chosen as officer commanding the squadron, says, 'To express fully in words how I felt is very difficult, but I was, and still am, extremely proud.' However, before the great day many hurdles had to be leapt, not least mastering the marching: 'Those few half-hours by the garages at Halton eleven years previously did not seem much help!'

The selected PMs went first to Uxbridge, to the Queen's Colour Squadron, for four days' intensive training to help them 'bond' and set them in the right direction. 'Drill sergeants have a reputation for a colourful turn of expression,' Judy Hopkins recalls ruefully. 'We were no exception in stimulating some memorable phrases. For years I had been led to believe that ladies should never shout and suddenly I was expected to have the voice of an RSM . . .' When Judy revealed that she was going on holiday to Wales, the drill sergeant suggested a good way to develop her voice would be to shout at the sheep!

Glossing over the nightly 'bulling' of shoes and worries over the fainting attacks that seemed to hit at random and deplete the squadron, Judy mainly recalls 'the sheer horror of arriving for the first rehearsal: there were all the other squadrons busy falling in, forming two ranks, then three, then turning about . . . and all the orders at true parade ground volume. No way were we going to do THAT in front of THEM.' However, they did do it, with a little help from the more-practised chaps (and trying to ignore the laughter in the ranks!). At last the great day came:

> I shall never forget marching on to the parade ground, with the music, the stands a sea of spectators – our backs were straighter and we marched so proudly – 850 men and women with the six Colours of the Royal Air Force, and 68 Squadron Standards on parade. I know I speak for all the PMs when I say that being on that special parade in the presence of the Queen was a very moving experience . . .

The PMs' own Diamond Jubilee, in 1978 (sixty years since the original 'temporary' Service was formed), was celebrated with a thanksgiving service in the central church of the RAF, St Clement Danes, London, followed by a reception at St James's Palace attended by HRH Princess Alexandra, Air Chief Commandant of the PMRAFNS.

This year also saw the very first issue of the *PMRAFNS Magazine*. Valerie Hand, who shared the editing with Sheila Joy, says it all began during a tri-Service middle-management course at Aldershot, when she and Sheila, faced with having to do a 'project', chose to test the feasibility of starting a PMs' magazine. Questionnaires sent out to retired members elicited a favourable response and when Matron-in-Chief Barbara Ducat-Amos heard about it she told them to get on and do it! Valerie enjoyed the challenge of 'getting it off the ground, finding material to put in it, deciding the format, going round publishers ... It started off with that nice blue cover, gold crest ...' Twenty-two years on, the annual magazine is packed with news and fascinating articles, all written by members of the Service past and present.

In her foreword to the first edition of 1978, Barbara Ducat-Amos told her members of cuts in the defence budget which, for the PMs, had meant closure of the hospitals at Changi, Cosford and Uxbridge. It had also caused Princess Alexandra's Hospital, Wroughton and The Princess Mary's Hospital, Akrotiri to drop the 'RAF' from their titles. Although still under air force command, at both locations RAF personnel now worked with army colleagues. Indeed, amalgamation of all three forces' nursing services was again under discussion – it had been a recurring background theme since 1918.

Aeromed advances

Although the closure of overseas stations had reduced the need for regular long-haul aeromedical flights, short-haul flights, plus worldwide emergency missions, remained an important duty for members of the PMRAFNS. For longer journeys, the VC10 was still in use; shorter aeromeds employed the more rugged Hercules aircraft and, increasingly, helicopters.

While Halton's renal unit continued to treat patients on its wards, the RAF's mobile dialysis teams – the only ones in the UK – were constantly on emergency call, often with two or three teams out at the same time on different missions. Advances in technology increasingly allowed their life-saving equipment to operate via aircraft power supplies.

In-flight nurse training is, of course, constantly updated, becoming ever more specialized. On long flights the change in time zones and the need to calculate the correct interval for giving drugs may entail wearing two watches; and, at altitude, changing air pressure may affect the drip rate of intravenous infusions. Particular injuries require patients to be placed in particular areas of the aircraft – those who need regular nursing attention must be easily accessible; others must lie where there's least vibration. And, if a patient's condition changes in mid-flight, with the nearest doctor perhaps hundreds of miles away, the nursing officer involved must know exactly how to phrase the questions which the aircraft captain will relay by radio. In such cases clarity is vital: even a small misunderstanding could be fatal.

On the subject of misunderstandings. . . .

Useful as they are for those in the know, jargon and acronyms can cause confusion. An example comes from Valerie Hand, the first PM to do the Basic Staff Officer course at Bracknell. This was, she says, 'for those who wanted to get on in the "big Air Force"', and a somewhat reluctant Valerie was persuaded to try it. The course covered service writing, operations, orders, court martials and public speaking, and included a variety of exercises and team projects. It was the exercise involving the acronym MSU that caused the problem – in that context MSU meant a major servicing unit, but when Valerie 'told the guys what it meant to me, they fell about laughing'. In nurse's jargon, MSU means a 'mid-stream sample of urine'.

'Anyway,' says Valerie, 'I passed the course.' And she did indeed 'get on in the big Air Force' – she was appointed Matron-in-Chief in 1994 and went on to become Director of Defence Nursing Services, retiring as Air Commodore in 1997.

PART V

Towards a New Millennium

ONE

The male element

In the light of demands for equal opportunities, it was inevitable that a purely female service such as PMRAFNS should succumb to the pressure for, in this case, 'men's lib', and allow professionally qualified male nurses to become PMs. Although state-registered senior NCOs of the Medical Service had had opportunities for commissions since 1976, these appointments had been in the Medical Technician Branch and applicants had had to complete full initial officer training; female SRNs were required only to complete the shorter 'special entrant' course before being commissioned into the PMRAFNS. However, on 1 April 1980, the Ministry of Defence inaugurated a unified nursing service, which made all suitably qualified SRNs, male or female, eligible for direct entry as commissioned officers of the PMRAFNS. Those with SEN qualifications became part of the non-commissioned element. On the same date, female nursing officers assumed the traditional male ranks of Flying Officer, Flight Lieutenant, Squadron Leader, Wing Commander, Group Captain and Air Commodore.

These changes did not occur without a few ripples: sisters at Wroughton caught hold of some of the 'boys', decked them in quatrecorn hats, handbags and capes, and made them walk through the mess. Gary Parkinson warns that someone may still have photos!

By this time, Geoff Holliday (who in the mid-sixties had dreamed of becoming an SRN) had passed his exams and been on several postings, including one to Muharraq in the Gulf. He was now a sergeant charge nurse at Ely, finding it 'more difficult, each passing week, to accept the anomaly which made my female colleagues commissioned and the men not.' He had mourned the fact that, as the service contracted, many fine NCOs of proven ability and with years of experience had been lost; so when the chance came to achieve a commission for himself he took it. 'It was a very proud me who went to the RAF College Cranwell . . . I was the first to do the Special Entrant and Re-Entrant four weeks Initial Officer Training, as a Flight Lieutenant in November 1980.'

Joy Harris was Matron at Halton 'when we started commissioning our NCOs. We had an establishment committee going on at the time, with a very old-school RAF officer – a Wing Commander – in charge of it, who wasn't keen on the idea at all: "You'll have a male Matron-in-Chief one of these days!" ' Fifteen years later, his prediction came true. Joy adds:

> But we did have trouble commissioning our boys. They used to put the male officers through Biggin Hill – and some of the most suitable chaps were getting turned down. Then one chap who we didn't think was suitable at all got through . . . When Matron-in-Chief of the time went into it, the thing they were failing them on was 'lack of aggression', and of course you don't want aggressive nurses!

In 1982, male and female PMs marching side by side represented the Service at the Royal Albert Hall Festival of Remembrance. Among them were a husband and wife, stationed at Nocton Hall.

Another aspect of this mingling of the genders is illustrated by a moment of revelation which came to Joy Harris later, while she was a resident of the officers' mess at Brampton. She had enjoyed the camaraderie of mess living for nearly thirty years but, with retirement looming, she realized she must soon think of finding a home of her own. 'The final push was, I think, the drying room on my floor of the mess. All the other members on that floor were men, so my undies hung to dry in the middle of their shreddies. Pride and vanity dictated that only my newest and best lingerie should be worn. It was time to seek another home!'

Not all of the ladies accepted the changes with such sanguinity: an ex-PM of the old school, hearing that the latest matron-in-chief was a male of the species, was heard to mutter darkly, 'They're getting in *everywhere*!'

Before long, however, this skirmish of the sexes was put into its proper perspective when British forces prepared again for war.

The Falklands Conflict

The Falkland Islands, remote amid the vastness of the South Atlantic Ocean, consist largely of bleak, treeless moorland exposed to rigorous sub-Arctic weather. Inhabited over the years by settlers from several European countries, they have been maintained as a British colony since 1833. The inhabitants consider themselves British, but being geographically close to Argentina they have also maintained links with that country. However, since the islands form part of the continental shelf of South America, Argentina considers 'Las Malvinas' an integral part of its territory – a claim more keenly pursued since rich deposits of oil were discovered off shore.

The first real signs of strife came in March 1982 when a party of Argentinians, arriving on the outlying island of South Georgia to dismantle a whaling station, raised the Argentine flag. On 2 April, Argentina invaded the main islands and in response the British gathered a force of ships which set sail to reclaim their sovereign territory. They recaptured South Georgia on 25 April, but the battle for the main islands continued through May and into June, when British forces proved superior. A cease-fire was declared on 14 June. Casualties continued to be flown home throughout the following two months.

Initially, planners had anticipated that casualties would be brought by sea from the South Atlantic to the nearest British base on Ascension Island (part of the British colony of St Helena), a voyage of ten to fourteen days aboard hospital ships before the men could be flown home. However, in the event, Uruguay offered hospital facilities at Montevideo, much closer to the Falklands.

Towards the end of April, RAF and army nurses at Princess Alexandra's Hospital, at RAF Wroughton, prepared to receive casualties. They shut down two-thirds of their wards and admitted only the most urgent new cases, thus freeing both bed-spaces and staff for the task ahead. The RAF hospitals at Ely, Halton and Nocton Hall released aeromedically trained staff to join the 'Operation Corporate' team; their remaining colleagues willingly undertook extra duties, despite serious undermanning imposed by a recruiting embargo. At first a trickle of patients with everyday medical problems and injuries came in from Ascension Island, but as May progressed to June and the fighting grew more intense, the flow of casualties increased.

Those of us who, through the media, witnessed the consequences of that war will not need reminding of the terrible effects wrought by Exocet missiles and other weaponry. Memorials on the Falkland Islands attest to the fact that many men, on both sides, gave their lives in the cause. Of those who survived, more than half suffered gunshot wounds; one-fifth had burns; some were disfigured for life; some lost limbs or were blinded; many suffered the appalling pain of trench foot; many succumbed to the effects of the bitter cold; a few were psychologically devastated. All of them had to be cared for.

Good medical management of the wounded depended on several links of a chain, each one relying on the rest. It began at the heart of the battle, wherever casualties occurred – in ships or in the field. This vitally important early work was followed by treatment in the surgical unit at Ajax Bay and then a stabilizing phase aboard the 'hospital at sea', SS *Uganda*, where naval and army doctors and nurses tended the wounded in zero temperatures with decks lurching under them. From *Uganda*, both British and Argentinian casualties were evacuated by sea from the war zone to Montevideo, a four-day voyage during which ambulance ships HMS *Hydra, Hecla* and *Herald* battled gallantly through forty-foot waves. Despite atrocious weather, casualties swiftly found themselves transferred to the British Hospital in Montevideo where, once assessed and stabilized, those well enough to withstand the eighteen-hour flight home were taken to the waiting VC10s. Men on stretchers with broken and shredded limbs; blinded soldiers leaning on ragged, bandaged comrades; bullet and shrapnel injuries, burns ... It was the largest movement of casualties, by air, ever undertaken by British armed forces.

For the PMRAFNS, the major task was the air evacuation link of the chain. This entailed a flight of 7,000 miles, by VC10, from Montevideo to RAF Brize Norton, with a refuelling stop at Ascension or, occasionally, in West Africa. From Brize Norton, patients travelled by ambulance or coach to reception and assessment at Wroughton. Finally, they were transferred to appropriate specialist units, base hospitals, or, for the more fortunate, to their homes.

In all, twenty-nine flight nursing officers and seventeen flight nursing attendants took part in the Falkland aeromeds, working in rotation. During major airlifts, each team comprised two medical officers, six flight nursing officers and eight flight nursing attendants. Their aircraft could carry up to sixty-six patients, of whom one-third might be stretcher cases, all needing different types of medical care. When the aircraft paused on Ascension to refuel, part of the flight nursing team would remain on the island while the others continued to Montevideo. This pause was intended to allow half of the team to rest, but in the event they usually helped out at the medical centre on Ascension. In turn, the other half of the team continued to work throughout the return flight from Ascension to UK, during the transfer to road vehicles at Brize Norton, and finally on the journey to Wroughton. By the time they handed over to their hospital colleagues at Wroughton, the team had often been on duty non-stop for twenty-three hours.

At the peak of activity, Wroughton personnel assessed and catered for 120 patients within two hours, a hectic time with many elements to be juggled and efficiently set in place, not only the all-important medical aspect, but paperwork, bed allocation, catering, stores, transport, the press . . . Another vital consideration was the comforting, both physical and emotional, of anxious relatives who waited in welfare rooms being fed and cared for by a squadron of Red Cross and St John Ambulance volunteers. These relatives were taken to meet the arriving patients amid tears – joy mingling with sorrow – and nurses stood by, their own eyes wet as they carried on with their work, matching lists of patients to available beds in wards. Within minutes, the patients were either tucked up in bed and being examined by doctors or, for the less seriously wounded, taken to places where they could rest and perhaps enjoy a beer and a cigarette. Cooks hurried to provide hot food; admin staff arranged onward movement to homes or hospitals; every spare member of staff turned to, bringing whatever comfort was needed – clothes, goodies, or perhaps only a smile and a friendly word. The returning men had lost close comrades, watched their ships go down in flames, struggled through moor and mud . . . endured all the horrors for which every fighting man prepares but which he hopes he will never see. Frequently, night-duty staff spent their time sitting on the grass outside the hutted wards, simply listening to wounded men recount their stories.

Many of the casualties had nothing left but what they were clad in – underwear and ruined uniform, if they were lucky; the rest had gone to the bottom of the South Atlantic, along with their ship. But stores and local people – often unasked – gave unstinting support.

For the staff of Wroughton hospital, and for their matron, Wing Commander Zena Cheel, it was a time they will never forget.

I didn't get home for six weeks during the Falklands War and, quite often, on a Sunday, one of the nurses would say, 'You're here *again* this weekend, Matron,' and I used to say, 'Yes, but so are *you*!' . . . And when they went off, they'd say, 'I live in block so-and-so, Matron, at Wroughton,' or, 'This is my address and telephone number, if you want any help please ring' . . . I remember the CO (Air Commodore Hurrell) taking a civilian surgeon round one weekend, and this chap said to the CO, 'You're very lucky to have so many staff, to be able to cope with all this,' and the CO said to him, 'You won't believe this, but half these people are off duty, and they don't get paid extra for it!' They'd be demanding overtime in the NHS, wouldn't they? So, it was simple – I tried to remember I was a nurse first and a matron second . . .

Let's face it, none of us thought that in our service time we'd be looking after war casualties. We thought there was never going to be another war – so the thing that really got to me was the stoicism of the nursing staff. These pupil nurses . . . young enough to be my grandchildren, some of them, but when we got the bad burns, and the amputations and all these things, they just got on as if they were looking after ordinary everyday patients . . .

We knew the Falklands War was on, we knew people were sailing out there . . . we knew there was going to come a time when our services would be called upon, but *how* we were going to be called upon we'd no idea . . . Apart from getting beds ready, we didn't even know what preparations to make . . . We had this Red Cross department that was part library, part occupational therapy, but also had things like toilet bags with a flannel, toothpaste, toothbrush and some soap, so on each bed table we put one of these bags, and some towels, pyjamas, and waited . . . In the meantime, the Royal Naval Association and the RAF somewhere nearby had heard that these people were coming to Wroughton, and we were inundated with cans of beer and we had to get extra fridges! . . .

All these men, when they arrived, looked as if they were in the Navy, all dressed in navy or bluish shirts, and navy trousers, all clutching these black plastic bags . . . the first few had trench foot and minor injuries. We welcomed them and then they were assessed by the medical officer . . . Depending on how well they were, they were given a can of beer . . . that was a very humble start really. What we didn't realize was that these bags that they had were their entire worldly possessions. As the weeks went by we learned . . .

After the first lot had gone, peeled off to their respective hospitals – the navy went to Haslar, the army went to Woolwich, and we kept the air force at Wroughton – the next day the nursing staff were making up the beds and Jo Boase [squadron leader in charge of the aeromedical ward] said to me, 'Matron, we're having great trouble with the linen store.' Unbeknown to us, the chaps had gone off with their towels, toothbrush and bits and bobs . . .

Stores were being difficult, fearing great loss of their equipment if this went on. So Matron Cheel appealed to the CO for some money out of the patients' 'comfort fund'.

If people wanted to donate money it went into this fund, basically for buying water jugs and vases, and little trays to put on people's lockers, that sort of thing, but I asked if I could have some money because, I said, 'I want to go down to Marks and Spencer's, in Swindon.' I went in my lunch hour, in my uniform, and I asked if I could speak to the manager and I explained who I was and said we were beginning to receive casualties from the Falklands War and I'd like to buy a hundred bath towels and a hundred hand towels, and maybe the odd flannels and things. I said, 'I've got an open cheque here and if you let me know how much it is the CO has said I can sign it,' and he said, 'Matron . . . we're going to give you half of everything.' So we got all these things. Some we paid for and others people *gave*. The shops in Wroughton . . . the little supermarket used to send pork pies and Dundee cake . . . the paper shop used to send all the newspapers that hadn't been sold . . . it all helped to make their lives that little bit nicer when they arrived.

Hospital staff eagerly watched the television, for news and to anticipate the kind of casualties they might expect. Then manifests began to come in, signals giving details of the wounded.

They tended quite often to come in in batches. We got a big batch of the burns after the *Galahad* went up . . . We knew we were going to have all these burns in and we knew there were very bad ones . . .

Anyway, we were looking this particular night on the telly and they were showing these people being transferred onto the hospital ships from Ascension Island, and we noticed they all had their hands in plastic bags . . . I did my plastics training in the air force, but when people had hands burned we used to wrap every individual finger, to stop them getting what they call the webbing . . . but evidently they found that if people put their hands in these plastic bags and they were occluded (so that no infection can get in), they can move their fingers, but all the exudate, which drips off their fingers, just collects in the bottom of the bag, but they can still use their hands within these bags . . . keeps them supple you see. So, once again, I went down to the local supermarket and I bought all the plastic bags that they had on their shelves. As I say, we learned . . .

One of the PMs at Wroughton was Squadron Leader Ann Golding, who recalls: 'When all the injured came back to Wroughton, it was horrific. All the relatives were waiting in the Red Cross room. They [the casualties] had to be seen by the doctors before they would release them to see their families. All the burns . . .'

Ann, too, remembers how kind people were in giving things.

It was fantastic . . . pyjamas, towels, toiletries . . . and television sets. It was a nightmare, because after they'd gone we'd got all these television sets. Did they give them to us, or loan them? And bowls . . . you see, everyone had a plastic bowl, to put their burned hands in, for treatment . . . Zena was overwhelmed by the number of fruit farmers in the area that were donating strawberries, really to go back out to the Falklands – all very well, but of course you haven't got space on the aircraft . . . I would ring up to get the numbers of things coming in, and all I could get was the number of these blooming strawberries, so I used to get really irate in the office – 'I don't want to know about the strawberries, I want to know about the patients!'

Matron-in-Chief Joy Harris happened to be on the airfield at Brize Norton as one of the VC10s brought home a plane-load of badly-burned Welsh Guardsmen, including Simon Weston. Joy found it 'horrifying'.

I'd just gone down to see an aeromed in and . . . I do believe it was Ishbel [McCabe (Mrs Bennet)] who brought him back, and left him in the ambulance, and she came out of it and . . . she was in tears, which she hadn't been able to give way to before, and at that point we saw his mother going into the ambulance . . .

I went to the NATO Women's Services Conference, either while the Falklands was on or shortly after. I managed to get Helen Renton, who was (D)WRAF, in tears on that conference . . . Just before I went, the Ministry gave me some photos to throw up and I gave a small talk on the people coming back from the Falklands, and the last photo that went up was a lad sitting in a pair of navy shorts and a shirt, sitting there looking so disconsolate . . . We'd spoken of how *cheerful* all the lads were, coming back, because they were all with their mates, and this boy . . . he looked disconsolate – it came out in the photo – I said, 'His friends have all gone off to different hospitals, or units, and so is he about to, and . . . what you see him sitting in is all he owns in the world at this moment' – and poor old Helen was quite upset. Well, rightly so!

Once settled in Wroughton hospital, the patients reacted in different ways, as Zena Cheel explains:

Some of them were terrible chatty and pleased to be home, but some of them were withdrawn . . . It was June, July sort of time, nice long evenings and the weather good. Some of them would just go and sit out on the grass, didn't want to be with anybody, others would sit and devour the papers because it was the only time they had got any news. Some learned for the first time how many of their mates had gone, or been injured . . .

But, we improved on the reception bit – we were able to get relatives down to greet them, and the people in Wroughton village were super because they put the relatives up. The CO's wife and the officers' and airmen's wives used to come over to the hospital and make tea and sandwiches and things. And we used to be swimming in beer . . . We had this huge great parcel arrive one day from Salisbury's, the people who make the hand-bags – they sent this HUGE great box, almost to the roof, full of bags, holdalls, overnight bags – a gift . . .

Once again, I went to Marks and Spencer's with the hospital Warrant Officer and we got 'on loan', for want of a better word, trousers of various sizes, shirts of various sizes, under-wear, socks and sandals . . . in one of the empty wards they set up this little 'tailor's shop' and after they [the wounded] had had a rest and had their treatments, they were kitted out, so they left us nicely dressed, usually with their relatives, their little holdall with a few goodies in it . . .

One week we had one flight in that was all amputees – some of them what they call 'hind-quarters' – really bad, hip and everything gone and I remember going round the ward one evening and chatting with them and saying I hoped they had a good night etc., and I said to one of these chaps, 'What are you going to do tonight?' and he said, 'Matron, I'm going to get legless!' Lovely sense of humour. And when they went out to the shower, the legless helped the armless and the armless helped the legless . . . with the shampoos and every-thing. The comradeship was incredible.

We continued to learn . . . I won't say we were perfect at the end of the war, but we did a bloody good job.

Then we had Princess Alexandra come down, which was lovely . . .

Staff and patients alike took heart from the informal visit which Her Royal Highness paid to 'her' hospital at the end of the emergency. She particularly wished to meet and thank members of the RAF, army and civilian medical teams who had helped to care for more than 600 casualties flown home from the South Atlantic. During the visit she also met the few casualties who then remained.

Nor was this the only royal interest, as Zena Cheel recounts:

One day I had a phone call to say the Duke of Edinburgh's chauffeur would be arriving and could I have somebody there to receive him . . . the Queen had sent these most beautiful flowers. There must have been at least a hundred boxes, all grown at Windsor Castle . . . So that was lovely, we spread them all around . . .

It was very nice to be able to get the families down to greet their men, so that they could see them from the word go. I remember Simon Weston's mother – she was a nurse herself – and I could hear him saying to her, 'Mother, at least I'm alive,' and she said to me later, 'He doesn't realize what he'll have to go through.' They'd been through so much, were so emotionally drained in many ways . . .

Among Helen Kell's many vivid memories of those days at Wroughton is an occasion when Matron Zena Cheel 'went ballistic' on discovering an ongoing problem caused by the khaki trousers issued for the patients. The trousers had rubber buttons which, says Helen, 'caused no end of problems with us trying to help with bodily functions!'

When the Wing Commander did her rounds and discovered this, an immediate signal was sent instructing stores to update and amend the style of trousers! Which occurred forthwith . . .

A lighter incident I recall, one Welsh Guardsman had a water-stained bottle of Chanel No 5 on his locker – to much teasing, he explained that he had purchased it, for his wife, outward bound on the *QE2*. When the *Sir Galahad* was hit he grabbed his perfume and reached safety. I said to him, 'If I was your wife, I'd never open it.' He replied. 'She b— better, after all my trouble in getting and keeping it for her!' The tenacity

of the Welsh Guards . . . a super bunch of men, and for a PM
a humbling experience.

Squadron Leader Josephine Boase comments:

> The staff throughout the entire hospital and supporting units
> were superb. Many of the flight nursing officers had only
> done their minimal basic training, but with assistance and
> initiative they learned – fast! Even the Head of Nurse
> Education (one of the many willing volunteers) was seen to
> administer care in the unique aeromed manner – pain-killers
> in one pocket, Y-fronts in another, lists in both hands and a
> pen clenched firmly between the teeth.

The man who became perhaps the best-known of the survivors –
Simon Weston – does not, of course, remember too much about his
stay in Wroughton. He was much too badly burned, facing years of
plastic surgery and physiotherapy. But his family will never forget. His
sister Pauline Hatfield wrote a long letter to Wing Commander Cheel,
particularly recalling 'the trays of sandwiches brought around for the
boys. Simon hadn't been eating since he was injured, due in part to
shock, and his mouth being burned. My mother persuaded him to try
a sandwich which she cut into pieces and fed to him. In all, he ate five
half sandwiches, which he thought was the most wonderful food he
had ever tasted.' The family are convinced that those few sandwiches
started Simon on the long and painful road to recovery.

Liz Kidman was in charge of nursing on the first Chinook helicopter that 'went from Wroughton and flew them up to London –
Woolwich, I think it would be, the burns unit. I shall never forget
that as long as I live. Twenty stretchers of burns patients, these lads
. . . so glad to be back . . .'

In her formal report on 'Operation Corporate', Matron-in-Chief
Joy Harris adds, 'The attitude and morale of the wounded was
tremendous. Nursing staff felt privileged to be able to help.'

The role of the rehab units

As always in the aftermath of war, rehabilitation played an enormous role for badly wounded servicemen from the Falklands. Some

of the disabled men went to what had become the Joint Services Rehabilitation Unit at Chessington, where 'Ronnie' Oxborough was a senior nursing officer. Most of her usual patients

> . . . were head injuries, both service and civilian personnel [but] after the Falklands War, I had the Welsh Guards on the unit for rehabilitation and treatment . . . Simon Weston eventually arrived at Chessington after many skin grafts and major surgery. He was my biggest challenge. He still required saline baths and many dressings which I'm sure caused him great pain and discomfort, but throughout all his treatment he still maintained a sense of humour. It was with great joy and delight – and tears – that we saw him and the other boys go home for the first time.
>
> The businessmen in Kingston-on-Thames decided they would like to entertain the Falkland boys – and the Northern Ireland boys – in some way, so they put on a dinner at the Seven Hills Golf Club in the company of Jim Davidson and Ed Stewart. It was a very funny and happy night out . . . Another proud moment came when I took my boys to Buckingham Palace to collect their Falkland medal from HRH Prince Charles.

Some of the staff from Wroughton also attended this moving ceremony, among them Matron Zena Cheel. She recalls that the event took place in the palace gardens, with medals presented to members of the various regiments by their royal colonels-in-chief.

> Prince of Wales for the Welsh Guards, Duke of Edinburgh for the Blues and Royals, Duke of Kent . . . I was lucky enough to be in the front row with my nursing staff and they came along and there was dear old Simon, at this stage with his face still terribly, terribly scarred. And along came this hoary old Warrant Officer and said to them, 'Remember, you don't have to stand up when the Prince of Wales comes to see you,' and one chap said, 'I *will*,' he said, 'he's my boss!'
>
> So . . . Prince Charles, Duke of Edinburgh, Duke of Kent, came along – and these people following with these trays of medals – and they had their medals pinned on . . . those in the

first rank then turned and pinned medals on colleagues standing behind them . . .

For Zena Cheel it was another emotion-charged moment, one of
many among her memories of those terrible months.

Chessington had for years been a medical rehabilitation unit
(MRU) for warrant officers, NCOs and other ranks, and latterly it
cared for army personnel as well as RAF. However, in July 1985 the
unit closed and its work transferred to Headley Court, formerly the
officers' MRU. A new remedial block was opened by the Duke of
Edinburgh that November, since when the unit has provided rehab
facilities not only for all ranks, serving and retired, of the armed
forces, but for members of the auxiliary services, civil servants from
the Ministry of Defence and, where appropriate, some civilians too.
Men hurt by the 'troubles' in Northern Ireland continued to come
in; others came from Cyprus, or from Germany, and road accidents
added to the list, as did orthopaedic injuries sustained while training or playing sport. While some problems, such as polio, have been
eliminated, others arise to take their place: today's young service
personnel are increasingly diagnosed with ankylosing spondylitis –
fusion of vertebrae in the spine.

Writing in 1987, Angela Scofield (who was to retire as Wing
Commander) explained that Headley Court's motto *Per mutua* ('by
mutual effort'), 'encapsulates the aim of medical rehabilitation . . .
It is the collective action of the team, each member making a unique
contribution, that makes rehabilitation effective . . . The patient's
day begins with the 15 minute warm up session, followed by ten 30
minute classes . . . this makes up a full working day . . .' It also
means that most of the wards are 'empty for most of the day. In
total contrast to a hospital ward, ours is busiest between 1630 hours
and 0830 hours. During the day the nurses are encouraged to visit
the departments to observe and assist the therapists . . . so that they
can carry techniques over into the ward situation . . . To watch a
patient struggle can be very frustrating for both of you, but it is the
only road to rehabilitation.'

It has been argued by some that rehabilitation, which covers such
skills as 'mothering' and counselling, has no place in a nurse's role
and may even be a waste of her specialist nursing skills. Liz Kidman
would not agree.

Headley Court was probably where I learned the most of all. It was a humbling place. I learned there was a lot more to illness than just getting people better. It had a knock-on effect, not only on the person who was suffering but the families . . . Simon Weston . . . some that were paraplegic . . . they didn't give up, they went on to achieve an awful lot of good things that they might not have done if they'd remained SAC Bloggs or Private So-and-so.

Snippets from the Eighties

Musing on the whole question of reaching the upper echelons of the Service, Air Commodore Valerie Hand chooses her period as Matron of RAF Hospital Ely as the most enjoyable time of her whole career.

That year at Ely was the best. Ely Hospital had such a special place in the city of Ely. It had been given the freedom of the city in '78 and all the citizens thought the RAF hospital was their hospital . . . There was this mutual friendship. It was lovely. As Matron, you really felt quite important, included in everything . . . From that point of view I always think of it as the best posting. Everything after that was a bit of an anticlimax, really. You went up to MOD as a Group Captain and had to make your own tea, down to earth again . . .

At the other end of the spectrum, new recruits are constantly being sought. The nursing service liaison officer has the job of spreading the word and helping to ensure that the brightest and best candidates come forward. In the late eighties, Helen Kell had this job: 'I loved it – it was the most enjoyable I have ever had – the demand and diversity, the ability to respond and work independently . . . I felt part of the "big RAF" and not just the Branch . . . I averaged 50,000 miles a year, self-driven . . .' She did recruiting drives in Ireland where 'security was tight and prevented me from taking the staff car as I wished'; in Scotland, wishing to appear immaculate for each presentation at schools or shows, or at the local careers information office, she changed clothes *en route*: 'the Highland cows had a PM "full Monty" ', and one day she and the

schools liaison officer 'got lost and found ourselves at Glamis Castle
– despite its being closed, we were offered refreshments, and a
personal tour, by a member of Her Majesty's staff'. In England, she
was stopped by red traffic lights at Greenham Common, scene of the
camp-in by women protesting about the American nuclear presence,
and there her 'staff car was jostled and rocked by a small crowd of
women. I escaped, as did the car, unscathed, but slightly shaken . . .
the eighties were a time of much political and social change and being
in uniform one was at the centre of repressed anger, on occasions.'

By that time, the government's cuts in defence spending were
chewing away at every aspect of the PMRAFNS. They continued to
bite even more deeply in ensuing years. For Matron-in-Chief
Valerie Hand, 'it really was very dismal and a time that I would
much rather forget'.

However, despite gloom at the top, PMs continued to work hard
and play hard. Many good causes have benefited from their activities over the years. In 1983, Senior Aircraftman Martin Hadnett of
the PMRAFNS, serving at Wegberg, was one of a seven-strong RAF
team of runners who competed in the first open international spar-
tathlon. Their challenge was to run from Athens to Sparta, following in the footprints of legendary Pheidippedes, a distance of over
250 kilometres, crossing no less than five mountain ranges. This
continuous run had to be completed in under thirty-six hours.
Martin himself didn't quite make it, but he raised DM1,000
Deutschmarks for worthy causes.

In that same year, Flight Lieutenant Tim O'Leary, also of
Wegberg, rode a small fold-up shopping bike the 400 miles from
Wegberg to Wellington in Shropshire, where his son was at a school
for handicapped children, which badly needed a hydrotherapy
pool. Collecting more and more money along the way, by laughing
people who admired the courage of this 'crazy Englishman', and
pausing only to sleep (and catch a Channel ferry), he made it in four
days and raised a magnificent total of 30,000 Deutschmarks. Not
only did the school get its hydrotherapy pool but Wegberg hospital
had a TV and video cable system installed from the proceeds of
what Tim dubbed 'Operation Saddle Sore'.

And there's music . . . At Halton, PM Amanda Cross was hailed
as the first lady bagpiper in the RAF when she joined the Halton
Pipe Band. They led the VIP parade at the Burma Star reunion in

1983 and took part in the RAF pipe band championship. Another high point was when the band flew by Chinook to RAF Odiham and Amanda piped the way off the helicopter.

On a more serious note, NATO's 'Exercise Lionheart' in 1984 provided a test of western Europe's readiness in case of a war fought with all the horrors of modern weaponry, conventional and chemical. PMs under the leadership of Wing Commander Maggie Pedder were involved in setting up a war hospital and performing aeromedical duties. Ethnea Hancock (later Group Captain and Matron-in-Chief) speaks for most of them when she says:

> I had never dreamed, when I first joined the PMRAFNS, that one day I would be going to wear a combat suit and NBC [nuclear, biological and chemical] protective clothing (noddy suit) for days on end! Getting ready was an exercise in itself. Most of the nursing staff [were] unused to coping with camouflage suits, webbing, boots and NBC clothing, none actually designed with women in mind. Puttees [long strips of cloth wound round leg and ankle] are still used . . . in time of war they could be used as bandages, but . . . they are not an aid to fast dressing.

After an introductory session of written briefs, slides and lectures, the medical team flew out to Gutersloh, West Germany, and took over most of a two-storey building, which became their command post and hospital. They had expected to have three days of preparation but 'suddenly, less than 48 hours after our arrival, we were on GENERAL ALERT'. Combat suits, numerous pockets bulging with essentials, had become normal attire, but all at once personnel had to start carting around a bulky haversack containing their personal protective gear – suit, boots and helmet. In the six days of the exercise they 'treated' more than a thousand simulated gun-shot wounds, blast injuries and burns, a stern test of their stamina and adaptability, but an experience they all felt was well worthwhile.

Elsewhere, aeromedical flights continued. Most of them were routine. Others were less so. In Beirut, terrorists booby-trapped a lorry and rolled it down a hill. The explosion destroyed a barrack block full of American soldiers. On 23 October 1983, a medical team from Akrotiri, including PM Fran Wooldridge, flew by

Hercules to bring out the injured US Marines. As they assessed and gave initial treatment to the casualties, under the tailgate of the Hercules, two helicopter gunships gave aerial cover and, bizarrely, citizens of Beirut continued to sailboard merrily in the harbour.

Twenty-one wounded men were brought back to TPMH Akrotiri, where Rosie Partington was senior matron. 'It was nasty,' she says sadly. 'They were very distressed.' One of the casualties died; nineteen were airlifted to the USAF base at Weisbaden, West Germany; the other remained in intensive care until he was flown home to the USA a week later.

The Harrods bomb

Terrorist activity closer to home called Halton's mobile dialysis team into action when, on Saturday 17 December 1983, an IRA bomb exploded outside Harrods of Knightsbridge. Among the wounded, a thirty-year-old police dog-handler sustained massive multiple injuries so severe that he was not expected to survive the day. He was taken to the Westminster Hospital, where his kidneys began to malfunction, but he was too ill to be moved to a dialysis machine. From Halton, a team of doctors and seven PMs (five nursing officers, including Flight Lieutenant Terry Smith, and two senior aircraftwomen) raced to the Westminster Hospital escorted by police with screaming sirens and flashing blue lights. On arrival, they faced a battery of cameras and crowds of onlookers – no, not for them but for the Prince and Princess of Wales, who had arrived to visit the casualties of the bomb. Soon after the team had set up their equipment the royal visitors arrived in the intensive care unit and, as Terry Smith reported, 'it was evident that they felt great concern over the horrific incident which had occurred some 48 hours previously'.

The young constable was critically ill with injuries over every part of his limbs, head and body. One of his legs had been amputated at the upper thigh and a dozen other complications tested the skill of the doctors and nurses attending him. What was more, his wife was eight months pregnant with their second child.

Over a period of six weeks, as the patient began to show signs of recovery, the renal team from Halton were made to feel at home among their NHS colleagues. In the fifth week the patient's wife gave birth to a second healthy son, another aid to the man's recovery. Though he still had a long way to go, by the end of January his kidneys were functioning properly and he no longer needed dialysis; the Halton team packed up at the end of 'a very satisfactory tour of duty'.

A second renal team from Halton, detached on 23 December to the Central Middlesex Hospital to dialyse another victim of the bombing, had a less satisfactory outcome: their patient, a police inspector, died on Christmas Eve.

The 'bubble'

Perhaps the most unusual and, for the team involved, the most complex of the aeromed flights undertaken in this period occurred in 1985 and involved PM Helen Ryan. Out in Sierra Leone, Jill Sanderson, a civilian midwife working with Voluntary Service Overseas, became seriously ill after contracting deadly, and highly infectious, Lassa fever. She was being cared for in Panjume Mission Hospital, 200 miles from the nearest airport at Freetown, but she urgently needed to be brought home to the UK.

For some years the RAF had had its own mobile isolation unit – basically a stretcher and trolley covered in a sealed plastic 'bubble' whose air supply and lighting could be run from an external source such as an aircraft or ambulance. Two days after the call came, the RAF had assembled its specialist aeromed team – nineteen personnel, some of whom were to enjoy a rare opportunity to train in a real emergency. Their lessons started on the first leg of the journey, out to Ascension Island. From there they flew to West Africa.

On arrival at Freetown, they learned that the patient's condition was far worse than they had expected. Her planned transfer to Freetown, by road, was impossible; so the Sierra Leone authorities made available their only helicopter. Helen Ryan explains: 'We had brought with us a smaller Isolator for the transfer, but this would not fit into the helicopter, so the anaesthetist elected to travel with the patient using barrier nursing techniques of gown, gloves and mask.'

The heat was another problem for the team, who arrived in Freetown dressed in theatre blues, plastic suits, overshoes and gloves, and then spent an hour on the sun-baked runway while the patient was transferred from the helicopter to the isolator, which was then lifted back into the VC10. They drank gallons of squash to keep themselves hydrated while they tended the patient, sited an intravenous drip and decontaminated themselves before getting back aboard the plane. The isolator had become like a greenhouse, but ingenious medical technicians rigged up a connection with the plane's air conditioning system, so the patient at least was kept cool.

Hampered by their plastic suits, ill-fitting rubber gloves and slippery plastic boots – lethal on a metal floor sprinkled with talcum powder (from their gloves) – they took it in brief shifts to care for Jill Sanderson. She was confused and semi-conscious. Among other problems, the tracheostomy tube which was helping her to breathe required frequent suction. All of this, says Helen, 'might have taxed us on a ward, let alone at 30,000 feet, in 2 layers of plastic, wearing someone else's gloves!' The flight lasted seven and a half hours and they fought all the time to keep their patient alive. Five minutes before landing, the intravenous drip stopped working and the patient required sedation. 'In order to achieve this and relieve her distress, which was compounded by the necessity to secure her stretcher harness for the landing, most of the medical and nursing team were standing when we landed . . .'

Some of the team accompanied the patient on her final transfer, still in the isolator and aboard an RAF pantechnicon, to Ham Green Hospital's exotic diseases unit. Thanks to their efforts, she recovered fully.

And Helen Ryan moved on to Akrotiri . . .

Tragedy in Cyprus

Considering the hours they spend in the air, the safety record for aeromed flights is second to none. Nevertheless, rare accidents have occurred – all the more shocking and saddening when they involve people on mercy missions.

In 1986 about a dozen nursing officers at TPMH Akrotiri, Cyprus, shared an accommodation block which Helen Ryan says was 'fondly referred to as Tenko [i.e. like a Japanese prison camp], but I don't think it had quite as many home comforts. As a small group we knew each other extremely well and being a long way from home relied on each other very much for friendship and entertainment.' Among the group was Fiona Johnstone, 'a lively nurse who was the life and soul of most occasions'.

In the early hours of Wednesday, 5 November 1986, word came that an expectant mother on the army base at Dhekelia was having problems in labour. A Wessex Mk 5 helicopter from 84 Squadron RAF Akrotiri was scrambled to bring the woman back to TPMH. Aboard the aircraft, along with the pilot and the loadmaster, were the nursing team of Flight Lieutenant Fiona Johnstone and Corporal Martin Cook, both of the PMRAFNS.

'This was a very routine hop,' Helen Ryan comments, 'one which had been done many thousands of times before.' However, this time something went wrong. Shortly after take-off the helicopter crashed in Limassol Bay and swiftly sank into the deep waters. A full search and rescue operation was launched. Searchers rescued the pilot but had to report the other three missing, presumed drowned. Their bodies were never recovered. 'Those of us who were there at the time,' says Helen, 'were devastated.'

A memorial service was held at RAF Akrotiri, where Martin Cook had worked at the station medical centre; his wife and two small daughters had joined him in Cyprus earlier that year. Another service at RAF Stafford brought together Fiona Johnstone's family and friends in the UK. Group Captain Miche Shaw, Matron-in-Chief of the PMRAFNS, read the lesson.

TWO

The Defence Medical Service

Having been pruned to a minimum as part of the overall reduction of the armed forces, on 2 January 1985 the medical branches of the navy, army and air force became a tri-Service organization known as the Defence Medical Service. Nursing branches, including the PMRAFNS, while still retaining their single-Service identities, became the Defence Nursing Services. It was anticipated that better liaison would lead to an easier exchange of ideas and, in some cases, a further exchange of posts. Already, air force and army personnel worked alongside each other at the hospitals at Wroughton and Akrotiri; both the naval base at Gibraltar and the army hospital at Rinteln had PMs on their staff; and a naval nursing officer was stationed at RAFH Wegberg.

In her president's address for the magazine that year, Matron-in-Chief Air Commodore April Reed commented, 'It has been a difficult year for the Medical Services, with . . . some fairly swingeing changes hanging over our heads like the Sword of Damocles. In the event, the actual recommendations were less sweeping than anticipated . . . with no changes to hospitals and other medical units . . .' Not yet.

The long-established nomenclature of nursing was also in the process of change: SRN (state-registered nurse) became RGN (registered general nurse); SEN (state-enrolled nurse) was now EN(G) (enrolled nurse general). However, the 1980s saw a move towards a single level of trained nurse – RGN – and, as a result, in 1988 the RAF ended its programme of training for SEN/EN(G). Enrolled nurses could, if they wished, convert to registered general nurses by completing fifty-four weeks' further training and examinations – this 'conversion' training entered the PMRAFNS programme in March 1987. EN(G)s not wishing to convert to RGN could choose to continue as they were until the end of their engagement.

Digital posts

Despite the climate of radical change, day-to-day duties continued. In a few places across the world unusual postings called for the presence of just one nursing officer. Such 'digital posts' existed on the staff at RAF College, Cranwell; at the St John's Ophthalmic Hospital, Jerusalem; at the medical centre in Hong Kong; and at the British missions in Islamabad and Peking. In the eighties, these posts were filled by PMs.

Flight Lieutenant Wendy Williams found herself 'adapting to the navy way of life', when she worked as a midwife in Gibraltar. The hospital overlooked the bay, with southern Spain beyond, and the mess had views across the Straits of Gibraltar to the Atlas Mountains in Morocco. Wendy thoroughly enjoyed the social life, the sport, and the chance to see Spain, despite some ribbing about being in the 'junior service'.

> I had to learn the language to survive and within a few weeks I was calling my room my 'cabin', going to the 'galley' for food and going for 'runs offshore' most nights – not, I hasten to add, athletic runs! My off-duty was now 'the watch', my uniform 'rig', and all the abbreviations I had just learned regarding the RAF were no use to me at all.

In China, the digital post at the British Embassy in Peking had, until 1973, been filled by an army nursing sister, on a one-year detachment from British Military Hospital Hong Kong. After the PMRAFNS took over, each sister was employed at the embassy for a full two-year tour of duty. Having diplomatic status, she left her rank and uniform behind and became instead a second secretary of the embassy.

Ishbel McCabe (Mrs Bennet) was the fourth PM to take this post, beginning in March 1978, though she had had a brief taster earlier, when she stood in while her predecessor took a couple of months' leave. This period helped her to assess whether she really wanted to spend two years in China. Her response: 'It seemed too interesting an experience to miss!' However, having seen her predecessor off on the train to Hong Kong, she returned to the empty flat feeling 'as if a gate had clanged behind me'. There was no going back, no way out of China without an exit visa – the Communist regime controlled its borders and its people with an iron fist. Though Ishbel met many interesting people of many nationalities, her acquaintances did not include any Chinese nationals.

Her first impression of Peking was 'intense cold, a drab and colourless city and people ... The streets were very dimly lit and scruffy, but the most alarming part was to discover cars or bicycles did not use lights.' Ishbel herself used a bicycle to get around the embassy and the British compounds which she had to visit, and, off duty, 'cycling round the *hutungs* – little back streets – was a pleasant way to pass an afternoon'. Of course British personnel were monitored everywhere they went – 'it's very easy to pick out a "round eye" on a bicycle' – phones were obviously tapped and no foreigner went anywhere without his or her personal China Travel Service guide. However, during Ishbel's two years these restrictions did ease and she saw signs of changes – 'Mao's portraits and sayings no longer dominated the city ... goods like suitcases, woollens, watches and make-up were advertised ... young men were growing and styling their hair, young girls wearing brightly-coloured clothing, including skirts and dresses, a thing unknown a year previously.'

In the clinic, however, old ways still obtained. Ishbel was particularly struck by the intravenous infusion apparatus – rubber tubing with the fluid contained in an open flask that could be topped up. 'Disposable equipment simply hadn't arrived in China [and] blood transfusions were almost always direct. I never saw them take one unit, they withdrew what they felt was needed!'

Pakistan has provided another stimulating post for a senior nursing officer. Around 200 people are attached to the British High Commission in Islamabad, including children ranging from six months to fifteen years. By means of morning clinics and afternoon visits, the nursing officer is responsible for their health. Pat Surridge, working there in 1985, also held weekly antenatal and family planning clinics for the Sweeper (Untouchable) people, who live in mud huts without sanitation. For their welfare, tetanus vaccination was a priority.

In the British clinic, staff undertook only minor surgery. More serious cases, requiring general anaesthetic, were sent back to the UK by aeromed flight or, in an emergency, treated at the local hospital. However, 'because of inadequate facilities and poor standards of hygiene' such cases would be transferred as soon as possible back to the two-bed ward in the British clinic. Pat Surridge dealt with about 200 patients a month. 'The most usual symptom is dehydration caused by food poisoning or some form of amoebic dysentery.' Nurses who served in the east during the Second World War would have found it all very familiar.

Return to Singapore

Forty years after the ending of the war, the government agreed to sponsor a pilgrimage to the major British war cemeteries in the Far East. In earlier days the Royal British Legion had organized trips for widows and others to visit war graves in Europe, but now with the government's financial backing those who had lost relatives and friends in battles in India, Burma, Japan, Korea and China were finally given the opportunity to pay their last respects. In 1985, a party of 230 war widows, veterans and ex-prisoners of war – senior citizens all – were accompanied to the rim of the Pacific by a medical team which included four nursing sisters – one from the navy, one from the army, and two from the air force.

Liz Kidman felt privileged to be chosen as one of the PMs on that trip. She says that many of the elderly passengers 'had never flown before, so embarking on a seventeen and a half hour flight, halfway round the world, was quite an adventure'.

At Bangkok the party split up into different groups to visit their own most relevant memorials. Liz and her group went to Singapore, from where they visited the Krangi cemetery. 'Many of the widows had anticipated the visit with mixed feelings – 40 years had dulled some emotions but many painful memories were revived of loved ones and comrades lost so long ago but never forgotten.' For some, sightseeing tours included a visit to Changi prison, which evoked more harrowing memories; and on the Sunday a multinational and inter-religious remembrance service took place in the presence of the Duke of Kent and other dignitaries.

> Some of the widows revisited Krangi. This time it was a private occasion, wreaths were laid and tears shed without the world's press looking on ... Despite other marriages, children, all those years, some of those women had been unable to grieve because they hadn't seen a body or visited a grave ... It was, for me, the most moving part of the pilgrimage.

In 1987, Squadron Leader Annie Reid escorted another party of war widows to the Tychaun cemetery, Bangkok.

> As you can imagine, this was a very emotional trip ... we could only help the ladies find the correct grave, then we left them in quiet solitude. I cannot express in words how I felt during those first few minutes in that cemetery: the graves were kept in such an immaculate state that I am not ashamed to confess that I could not hold back my own tears. The journey back to the hotel started subdued, but the ladies, after they had expressed their feelings of sadness, soon began to feel that they had, finally, laid their husbands to rest.

Fun and dramas at Wegberg

In West Germany in 1982, Senior Matron Miche Shaw had to find some way of entertaining her matron-in-chief, Joy Harris, on her annual three-day visit to Wegberg. Hearing that there was an exercise on,

> ... somewhere in the wilderness of Germany, I got permission to go out and visit them with my boss. First I had to kit Joy out in combat gear, much to her surprise. Our driver was given a map reference and we managed to get into the area, where a patrolling Land-Rover came to our rescue and guided us to camp. We were met by a medical officer Joy knew, which was a good surprise. He gave us a drink – almost surely a G&T! – and we watched as the men crawled around on their

In-flight care, Bosnia 1993 (© British Crown Copyright/MOD)

Old and new mess dress, 1994 (© British Crown Copyright/MOD)

Inaugural golf champion, Sergeant T. Smith, receives his trophy from Matron-in-Chief Group Captain (later Air Commodore) Bob Williams, September 1997 (© British Crown Copyright/MOD)

Tri-service uniforms at the Royal Hospital, Haslar 1998 (© British Crown Copyright/MOD)

Flight Lieutenant Diane Lamb, flight nursing officer, Aeromedical
Evacuation Squadron, HQTMW RAF Lyneham, 2001
(© British Crown Copyright/MOD)

stomachs in the undergrowth! It was a day Joy never forgot – she really revelled in the experience.

Five years later, freezing temperatures caused havoc when (yet again!) pipes burst in several departments of the Wegberg hospital and the shattering of a high-pressure steam valve badly damaged test equipment in the laboratory. The following summer, staff might have wished the water back to quench the disastrous fire that broke out. It destroyed the roof of No. 2 Maternity Ward, causing damage estimated at a million Deutschmarks.

PM Richard Laurence was working in the operating theatre when fire broke out.

> It was frightening. I'd scrubbed up for an ENT case. The surgeon was very miffed that we had to stop the operation [but] we had to abandon shop and get outside quickly . . . I remember distinctly waking the patient up in the car park. And the very next week, to the day, we had a bomb scare, so I woke another patient up in the car park . . .

In the late eighties IRA terrorist bombers turned their attention to British personnel and property in West Germany, where Richard Laurence lived in married quarters with his family.

> It was quite a stressful time . . . They could hide bombs better than I could find them. You got in your car, turned the ignition, gritting teeth, wondering . . . We lived next door to Joint Headquarters where they put a big bomb, which blew our French windows out. All the curtains flew up and the doors flew open. All you could hear was breaking glass, tinkling, tinkling, and all the car alarms went off . . .
> The car with the bomb was a Volvo estate, which just disappeared – crater in the road about ten feet deep. Cars that were next to it were just in bits . . . It broke about 3000 windows, so the German glaziers were clapping their hands! No, it was nerve-wracking. My daughters can still remember it. Not the thing going off, but the next day – it took them about two hours to get to school. Very unpleasant . . .
> A few RAF people got shot, apart from the army people, in a few of our favourite shopping places . . . Some RAF

Regiment were in Roermond [Holland], sitting in a car that got machine-gunned. One survivor came into theatre – he was in ITU and still getting death-threats – Northern Ireland phone number, calling up, saying, 'We're going to finish the job . . .'

But most Wegberg personnel have very happy memories of their years in Germany. Off duty they had opportunities to play sport, and to travel around Europe; they held fund-raising activities, and enjoyed social occasions. At one summer ball the officers hired a bucking bronco which was set up outside the mess. A certain (male) nursing officer, full of bravado, climbed astride it and 'clung on for grim death despite his No. 5 trousers opening up from crotch to turnup . . . He just clung on, would not let go, his best mess dress flapping around like a pair of chaps . . . It was very funny . . .'

In September 1992, Wegberg became the first RAF hospital to welcome a male matron (i.e. officer commanding nursing wing), in the person of Wing Commander Bob Williams. Otherwise it was not a happy year: government economies decreed that the number of beds should be cut from 171 to 90; as a beginning the paediatric and special baby care units closed in December 1992. The following year saw the combination of the medical and surgical wards, and then the closure of maternity, which had been one of the busiest of units.

Undaunted, in 1993 RAF Wegberg celebrated its fortieth anniversary in fine style, with a station party – an annual fête which included a fancy-dress bed-push – followed by a sunset ceremony, with the evocative sound of a trumpet accompanying the lowering of the ensign. A poignant moment. At least, it was supposed to be . . .

PM Kevin Mackie, the chosen trumpet player, explains:

Everybody was in high spirits after the fête and the bed-push. I'd been in the Vicars and Tarts team, and I was still in my vicar's garb because we'd gone straight from the fête to do the sunset ceremony and everybody there had done the same – they were still in their civvies, apart from the Air Vice Marshal – he was in uniform and so was Wing Commander Williams . . . I stood behind this tree to do it because I didn't want anybody to get me confused with the real vicar – I'd actually borrowed garb from a real vicar, the padre, so I looked the part! And because I had to wait for the cue, and the only cue I was going to get was from the AVM, when he started to salute, I had to keep popping my head round ... Lots of people said all they could see was this vicar with the trumpet popping his head round this tree! People won't let me forget it.

'Skywards'

The first-ever performance of a new PMRAFNS march was rendered in 1989 at HQ Music Services, Uxbridge, by the Central Band of the Royal Air Force under the baton of composer David Barker, to a select audience which consisted of Matron-in-Chief Group Captain Liz Sandison and her staff officer Wing Commander Bob Williams. Squadron Leader Phil Bush, a medical secretarial officer, says that 'listening to this jolly and bouncy march played for the very first time was an emotional experience'. He himself, as an enthusiastic member of the RAF Voluntary Bands organization, had been in on initial discussions about the project with Liz Sandison and former MIC Miche Shaw; in fact, it had been Phil who suggested David Barker as composer. David greeted the prospect with enthusiasm and, having written the piece, 'made the most noble of gestures in that he would let the PMs choose a suitable title ... rumour has it that a meeting of the elders was called. Very few are ever privy to the deliberations of such an august body [but] eventually the apt and most appropriate title of "Skywards" was agreed ...' The march is now available on a CD recorded in 1994 by 'probably the finest military band in the world' (of course!), the Band of the RAF College, Cranwell.

'Devastating'

As the eighties drew to a close, only five hospitals remained to be staffed by air force nurses – Ely, Wroughton and Halton in the UK, and Wegberg and Akrotiri overseas. Nocton Hall hospital had closed in 1983, though a remnant 'forward outpatients department', linked with Ely, held clinics there for personnel stationed in

Lincolnshire. That too was to end in 1991, shortly before its foster-parent hospital became the latest victim of defence cuts.

On 4 October 1990, the city of Ely learned that its RAF hospital was to be axed. For fifty years RAFH Ely had cared for both service personnel and the surrounding community, who regarded it as 'their' hospital. Indeed, only three years previously, it had been renamed The Princess of Wales RAF Hospital, with celebrations attended in person by Princess Diana. The *Ely Standard* now commented, 'If Ely's RAF Hospital is closed, it will be a bitter blow, not only for the RAF, but also for local people . . . If one hospital has to go, years of experience tell us it should not be Ely. We don't believe there is a better one in the UK.'

Despite all protests, The Princess of Wales RAF Hospital Ely closed in 1992.

Nor was it to be the last. In 1989 the National Audit Office had recommended that, with the threat of global warfare diminished, the requirement for separate naval, army and air force hospitals should be reviewed. It was decided that only three service hospitals should remain in the UK, all jointly staffed by tri-Service personnel under the Defence Medical Service banner. Additional secondary care facilities, termed Ministry of Defence hospital units (MDHUs), would open in certain existing National Health Service hospitals under the newly formed Defence Secondary Care Agency. Finally, the new Defence Medical Training Organization would inaugurate a tri-Service medical college at HMS *Dolphin*, Portsmouth, and Keogh Barracks, Aldershot.

Surgeon General Vice-Admiral Tony Revell commented: 'Nobody likes change, and this is pretty devastating . . . but when the whole service is up and running . . . people [will] see the advantages.'

It is too soon to tell whether he was right. What is certain is that the subsequent closures of Wroughton, Halton and Wegberg brought a great outcry, not only from air force personnel of all ranks and trades but from the civilian communities to whom these hospitals had given such excellent care over many years.

Ironically, in the period before these fine hospitals discharged their last patients they were once again called to stand by to accept war casualties – from the Gulf and from the Balkans.

The Gulf War

In 1990 the RAF found itself at war with the country which, seventy years before, had hosted its first overseas hospitals. That August, Iraqi forces invaded the small independent Gulf state of Kuwait. The Kuwaiti ruler fled and Iraqi President Saddam Hussein – long a thorn in the side of western democracies – declared Kuwait a province of Iraq. Peace moves began, but behind them the West gathered a coalition force – 'Operation Desert Storm' – designed to restore Kuwait and its rich oil fields to its legal rulers.

Once again members of the PMRAFNS found themselves on standby, at RAF Brize Norton and at Akrotiri. Nearly eighty personnel were detached from RAFH Wegberg and other specialists stood ready if needed; the RAF hospital at Muharraq in Bahrain, closed since 1971, was reopened and staffed by PMs; other nurses, attached to mobile field hospitals and No. 1 Aeromedical Evacuation Squadron, went to prepare in Saudi Arabia and Bahrain. At home the three RAF hospitals organized themselves to receive casualties, and many ex-PMs volunteered their services if needed.

That September, PMs Lesley Chew and Gillian Reid were part of a seven-strong tri-Service team sent to work at the King Abdul Aziz Airbase Military Hospital in Dhahran, Saudi Arabia. As tension grew, politicians set a date by which Iraq must withdraw from Kuwaiti territory or risk the consequences; the two PMs redeployed to RAF War Hospital Muharraq, Bahrain, from where Lesley Chew reported, 'The RAF War Hospital is now a 100-bedded facility which can operate conventionally or as a chemically-protected hospital . . . Hostilities broke out in the early hours of January 17 [but] few casualties are expected until the land battle commences. Meanwhile we continue to train all grades of staff ranging from musicians to GPs . . .'

Squadron Leader Angela Scofield went out as nursing officer-in-charge at Muharraq. On her staff was Richard Laurence, who describes how the old RAF hospital lay waiting, as if caught in a time-warp:

The hospital was physically walled-off – half of it was still used by the local population as a maternity hospital, the rest had just been left since 1971 . . . One of the rooms was piled full of incubators and dressings trolleys that somebody had stuck in there. You could tell it was an air force hospital right away – the way all the corners, ceilings and floors were rounded off, for cleaning purposes . . . So we just washed it down and opened it up. Very strange.

We set up the hospital with the usual Resus, where I worked. Theatres, wards, that kind of area, triage . . . We set an equivalent of about 100 and something beds in the COLPRO (collective protection area, the nuclear, biological, chemical tents, with positive pressure) – a nightmare to work in, you have to do lots of zips, air-locks and things. The idea is that, inside, the air pressure's higher, so any contaminant gets blown out . . . the pressure keeps it all away from the patients.

We had no significant numbers of casualties, just the usual – army people, you know, shooting themselves in the foot, jumping off the side of tall buildings, as they do. We had the usual appendectomies and minor stuff. But that was the same for all the British hospitals. I know some of the army hospitals never even got unpacked, out in the desert.

No. 1 Air Evacuation Squadron had flown out to Saudi Arabia in November 1990. One flight stayed in Al Jubail while the second split into two sections, some personnel going to Dhahran, others to 'glorious Bahrain' where, says Rachel Johnson, they spent ten 'very enjoyable weeks', with only the ground handling of one aeromed a week, plus 'endless NBC drills', to keep them away from swimming, eating out and shopping. However, after Christmas they moved on, in convoy, to a spot forty miles from the Kuwaiti border.

Talk about a culture shock! I think our lives changed 180 degrees in the 300 miles we travelled . . . It poured with rain and the road was like a quagmire, especially when following huge tank transporters . . . We were cold, hungry, tired, wet and miserable when we arrived at our destination about 2 a.m. [and] took shelter in the mud on the floor of 32 Field Hospital's newly erected evacuation tent.

For days we worked like Navvies – digging trenches, filling sandbags, putting up tents and cookhouses. We thought we would never finish in time for the fast approaching ground

battle deadline . . . Nightly the Scuds flew over our heads and
we had to don our NBC kit, just in case!

The air battle began on 17 January 1991. When Saddam remained
defiant, the coalition's ground forces opened their offensive on 24
February. To Rachel Johnson, 'caring for our first group of war casualties felt very strange. It was difficult to believe that these young
British soldiers had actually been under real battlefire . . . Some were
very frightened and some just relieved to be going home . . .' It also
felt strange to be nursing British soldiers alongside Iraqi prisoners of
war who were 'so pathetic and ill . . . poorly nourished, filthy dirty
and dressed in rags. I felt such empathy for them . . .'

In Dhahran, Flight Lieutenant Colin McMillan was with Medical
Support Troop Alpha (MST 'A'), sited at the vast King Abdul Aziz
Airbase, which covers twenty square miles and has a runway six
miles long. Colin and his team were sited 'two miles from the flight-
line . . . between the tempting targets of the base power station and
the fuel dump!'

> The Saudis were very protective of their sand and considered
> it holy . . . all the sand used for sand-bags at MST 'A' was
> imported. Neither would they allow non-Muslims to be
> buried in Saudi Arabia, therefore plans were made to repatri-
> ate all British dead.
>
> One remembers the heat, the sand, the smells and the sounds.
> The high temperatures of August days filling sand-bags merge
> with the freezing cold of the February nights on guard. I remem-
> ber the 'buzz' I had, and the sense of freedom when I helped the
> Americans with some of their aeromed flights. The smells and
> sounds of the bazaars in Dhahran and Bahrain mix with memo-
> ries of the Scuds coming in and the replying Patriots. The bore-
> dom of waiting being combated by learning German, developing
> computer skills or by learning to drive. I designed and made a
> unit flag which eventually was shown to the Prime Minister John
> Major on his visit at the end of the war and which now lies in
> the RAMC museum at Keogh Barracks, Aldershot . . .

Aeromed teams in the UK waited to be called into action. Liz
Kidman remembers the unbearable tension.

That was an awful time, because nobody knew what to expect,
or the scale to expect ... We were all put in the Gateway
Hotel, the accommodation at Brize Norton. There were three
TriStar teams and about eight VC10 teams, all ready to go. I
was i/c a TriStar team and what they said, basically, was,
'Prepare this TriStar to bring back two hundred walking
wounded, but we don't know how they'll be wounded or ...'
How did we do this? ... It was difficult. Nobody knew what
might happen or what we might have to do, or even where
we'd be flying them back to – whichever Health Authority
would take them. Thank God nothing happened!

The ground war ended after one hundred hours; the air war lasted
six weeks. President Saddam withdrew his forces and most of the
'Desert Storm' troops, with their medical and nursing teams,
packed up and went home, only too thankful that casualties had
been so low. A few PMs remained deployed in the Gulf area as the
devastation, including appalling fires and oil slicks, was cleared
up.

As the RAF War Hospital's matron, Angela Scofield, remembers,
the Sheikha of Bahrain invited 'all the "lady soldiers" on the Island
to a Reception at her Palace, as a thank you. The Palace was magnificent, all marble, crystal and mirrors.' Each of the 'lady soldiers'
who attended the reception was presented with a leather box
containing a solid gold commemorative coin.

Later, back at home, more expressions of gratitude were demonstrated when on 7 May 1991 members of both the PMRAFNS and
QARNNS took tea at St James's Palace with Princess Alexandra,
Royal Patron to both Services. And on 21 June the City of London
hosted a welcome home parade, for which Angela Scofield was
selected to lead the female RAF flight. She also received an invitation from the Lord Mayor and the Corporation of London to
attend the ensuing reception at the Guildhall. Guests of honour
were Their Royal Highnesses The Prince and Princess of Wales.

I was put in charge of a group of airmen, none of whom I
knew, and after being presented myself to the Princess of
Wales I had to introduce my group. She was interested in my
'black Dick' and said they had been talking about it on the

balcony. When I explained that I was a PM, Princess Diana said she would tell Charles when they got home!

Reflecting much later on the PMs' role in 'Operation Desert Storm', Squadron Leader Richard Laurence remarked rather sadly: '[Muharraq] was probably the last ever RAF hospital to be set up. It probably won't happen again in the foreseeable future . . . Our role is aeromed now. We may provide staff for an army hospital, but . . . the other side of it we couldn't do, because we haven't got the medical staff any more.'

Akrotiri's role

During the Gulf War, TPMH Akrotiri became a secure area for returning PoWs and RAF aircrew, among them Flight Lieutenants John Nicol and John Peters, Tornado flyers who had been shot down and held briefly captive by Saddam Hussein's forces. In their book *Tornado Down*, they remember a nurse who was 'all kindness, starch and cleanliness'. Bruised and dishevelled as they were, they tried to charm her into bringing them a beer, but she sternly reminded them of hospital rules. However, a few minutes later she reappeared with a smile and a six-pack of the local brew, saying, 'Just don't tell anybody that I gave it to you.'

Later that year, former hostages John McCarthy, Jackie Mann and Terry Waite passed through Akrotiri after being released from their long incarceration in Beirut. They too received attention at TPMH before flying home to England escorted by PMs, and all of them were debriefed at RAF Lyneham, under the care of a nursing and psychiatric team from PARAFH Wroughton.

The royal yacht incident

At the conclusion of the Commonwealth Conference in October 1993, the Royal Yacht *Britannia* docked at Limassol, Cyprus. Her Majesty the Queen departed for home aboard a VC10, leaving the ship preparing to sail to Saudi Arabia to meet the Prince of Wales. However, that evening many junior ratings on the royal yacht went down with food poisoning, consequent to partaking of 'tartan cack-leberries' (Scotch eggs). Happily for the more elevated of the ship's company, the dish had been served only in the junior ratings' mess.

At TPMH Akrotiri it was Sunday morning, just before lunch, when a phone call announced imminent arrival of nineteen casualties from *Britannia* with severe diarrhoea and vomiting. Squadron Leader Jan Oakman 'jumped into uniform' and began organizing Ward 5 to receive patients. Everyone turned to helping in whatever way necessary, with bedpan washer and loos working overtime; a porter rushed about removing red bags of dirty linen and restocking the linen cupboard, and assorted ladies wheeled drinks trolleys, while the hospital kitchens 'did a roaring trade in sandwiches for everyone involved in the work (the patients, needless to say, weren't at all peckish)'.

Hospital staff later attended the first all-ranks cocktail party to be held aboard *Britannia*, while at the hospital the CO designated the men's toilet on Ward 5 'Britannia Ward' – a suitably inscribed sign was made and fixed. Despite fears of what his reaction might be, the admiral of the royal yacht found the sign highly amusing and ordered a royal yacht plaque to be sent to hang alongside it. As a thank you to the CO and staff, he also sent a larger royal yacht plaque, which now hangs in the hospital's reception area.

The PMRAFNS Association

One of the first editors of the PMs' magazine, Valerie Hand, became project officer for a proposed PMRAFNS Officers' Association. Open to all serving and retired officers of the Service, the Association was launched in 1992 and its membership continues to grow. Every member receives news of the annual reunion and other events, and those who cannot travel to gatherings may still remain in touch through the pages of the magazine, which includes personal stories of past adventures as well as features on current happenings. Its articles have provided a valuable source of additional information for this book.

Resuscitation training

Continuing, as ever, to move with the times, the PMRAFNS decided to move into the field of resuscitation training, to which end they appointed one of their members as resuscitation training officer for the RAF. Flight Lieutenant Kevin Mackie was the man involved.

I was sent on an Advanced Life-Saving (ALS) Course, and an Instructor Course and was posted to RAF Wroughton. Almost within a month it all happened, and I was this new beast that nobody had ever seen in the services before. There were very few Resuscitation Training Officers (RTOs) in civvy street in those days. London, Manchester and Brighton were the main three areas . . . we were finding our feet. There's now an Association of Resus Training Officers and we've got people on the Resus Council of the UK . . . I still class myself as an RTO at heart, but at Wroughton, certainly, it was a new departure. I was responsible for the basic and advanced resuscitation training for all the staff, both ancillary and professional – or medical/professional – and as the role developed I was asked to teach at more and more places abroad. I ended up running an ALS course in Cyprus, went to Moscow . . .

The trip to Moscow, in February 1995, 'broke new ground in international relations'. It came about after former RAF medical officer Garth Manning (a retired wing commander), working as a freelance consultant with the UN, was asked to assess the standard of in-flight care, within the former Soviet Union, for refugees under the aegis of the International Organization for Migration (IOM). He made thirty-six recommendations, possibly the most telling being the observation that during aeromedical flights the Russian doctors did not assess any of their patients but went to sleep in Club Class! When asked how the situation might be improved, he recommended that they should ask for help from the RAF aeromedical evacuation team, from whose personnel Cathy Henderson and Kevin Mackie were selected to fly out to Moscow. As part of their equipment they took 'Resusci Annie', the doll used to demonstrate resuscitation techniques.

At Sheremetyevo Airport they underwent a lengthy arrivals procedure, 'devised especially to annoy weary travellers! We then had to go through the red channel in customs and have all our luggage re-Xrayed, which caused quite a stir when my Resusci Annie torso appeared on the screen . . . Two hours later we eventually cleared customs . . .'

They spent their first full day meeting IOM people and setting up their course, then enjoyed a weekend playing tourist around

Moscow and even managed to get tickets for the Bolshoi Ballet. In the following four days they gave two training courses, each for an audience of twenty-five Russian doctors, covering aviation medicine, in-flight care, in-flight emergencies and the latest resuscitation techniques. Kevin says, 'Initial feedback from both courses was extremely encouraging and we felt that we had got the message across . . .'

Thirty years before, such a trip would have been unthinkable.

This project provided yet another breakthrough for the PMRAFNS. Membership numbers may be relatively low when compared to those recorded during the Second World War, but the scope of experience for air force nursing officers continues to expand.

For Jackie Gross, one special experience was being part of the integration that took place in South Africa following the elections of April 1994, when apartheid ended and Nelson Mandela took up the reins of government. Jackie was attached to the British military and advisory training team which helped to recruit former guerilla forces into the new National Defence Force. In this role she was 'required to attend placement boards to see fair play, and to adjudicate on decisions made if necessary . . . Almost without exception the recruits had been seriously disadvantaged by Apartheid . . . Some had returned from exile and others had been working "underground" whilst carrying on with their normal jobs . . . It was a fascinating experience and one which I shall never forget.' The process took longer than was envisaged and when Jackie's posting ended another PM was sent to replace her.

Handover in Hong Kong

In the Far East, meanwhile, Britain prepared to hand Hong Kong back to Chinese rule.

Since RAF Kai Tak had closed in 1978, the British Military Hospital in Kowloon had looked after the health of British forces in Hong Kong, with satellite medical centres out in the New Territories, where the Ghurkas were based. The largest of these medical centres, at Shek Kong, had provided a digital post for an air force nursing officer.

'I was on my own with not another PM in sight for thousands

of miles,' says Liz Kidman, stationed at Shek Kong in the mid-eighties.

But that also had its advantages and it was very good experience. There was one big Med Centre with seven little ones, all of which had Ghurka midwifery units ... Anyone who needed to be in hospital within a couple of hours was flown by helicopter to BMH Hong Kong (Kowloon). Either one of the doctors or myself was permanently on aeromed call.

One month in every two the RAF Squadron did Search and Rescue for the Hong Kong government. I was also on call for that ... One night, there'd been an accident on a ship, four thirty a.m. we flew out. The ship was just about on the flying limit of the helicopter ... Because they couldn't understand me with the normal aircrew throat mike, I'd got a boom mike like the pilot used and, because it was windy and I was hanging out of the helicopter, they switched me off, so I couldn't hear what was going on. We didn't find anybody, and after a while I gathered that we had turned back. The crewmen were busy, getting things out, looking hassled, looking at me ... They'd pointed to something outside but I couldn't see what it was and because they were busy I didn't ask. Anyway, we landed at Kai Tak, which was very unusual. One of the crewmen grabbed me and said, 'You smoke, Liz, don't you?' I said, 'Yes, but you don't.' He said, 'I do now,' and dragged me off somewhere safe where we could smoke. He said, 'You're very calm about all this ...'

Turned out that they had got lost. What they'd been pointing to was Chinese territory with gunships aiming at us because we were over Chinese water. And in fact we were out of fuel! All the comings and goings ... the pilot had been preparing to ditch, getting ready to throw the lifeboat out, put us into it and then ditch the helicopter – and I'd missed it! Fortunately another crew went out and found the ship.

I was working with two RAF doctors. The rest were army, and there was one civilian – a lady doctor, GP, married to a judge in Hong Kong. The orderlies were Ghurkas, Chinese ... We had a ward of about twelve beds for tropical diseases – things the Ghurkas picked up on Exercise. Ghurka-trained

midwives (they'd done a crash course in it) looked after the
Ghurka midwifery units. At the Med Centre I had some lovely
nurses: one Ghurkali speaking one, two Nepalese – they were
married to Sandhurst-trained Ghurkas who alternated in the
post out there; we had a Chinese speaker – she was British
trained but married to a Hong Kong Chinese. She left because
of the [coming] Chinese take-over. Her family had been in
Shanghai when that was taken over, so she got out ten years
before . . .

Over those ten years, as the date for the hand-over to China
approached, British forces elements in Hong Kong combined into
one unit, called Shek Kong Station. Its medical centre's work had
become more like that of a GP's surgery by the time PM Sharon
Smith (now Squadron Leader Callcott) arrived there in July 1994.
'Never having worked in a Med Centre before, I was somewhat
daunted by the prospect. I tried to reassure myself that I was a qualified nurse and that nursing was the same wherever it was
performed. I was in for a big shock!' Fortunately she had on hand
Miranda Wong, who had worked at the medical centre for twelve
years as a general and children's nurse and midwife. Miranda
helped to answer such questions as 'Is this a verruca?' Sharon had
never seen a verruca, and as for 'Do you think these are monsoon
blisters, sister?' . . . HELP!! Chicken pox she was more prepared
for, having found a copy of *The Woman's Weekly Guide to Spots
and Rashes for Anxious Parents*, but she called on Miranda for a
second opinion.

After six months in Hong Kong Sharon Smith felt more confident, but as 'draw-down' to hand-over continued the unit
contracted yet again when its Chinese medics departed; then when
the army hospital in Kowloon closed in June 1995, Shek Kong had
to upgrade to medical receiving station level to take on the extra
maternity work. But 48 Brigade of Ghurkas was being disbanded
and RAF and army messes amalgamated. By the end of 1996 Shek
Kong Station had closed and on 1 July 1997 the whole colony of
Hong Kong returned to Chinese sovereignty.

THREE

Bosnia

The death of Marshal Tito of Yugoslavia in 1987 provoked the outbreak of a bitter and bloody civil war among Muslim, Serb and Croat factions in Bosnia, divided by religion, pride and ancient hatreds. In order to protect the innocents caught in the middle, and to ensure the safe passage of aid, the United Nations decided it had to intervene. It gathered forces from many nations around the world, huge powers such as America and Europe joined by troops from small countries like Nepal and Bangladesh, all wearing the blue UN beret and designated UNPROFOR (United Nations Protection Forces). Among this force, members of the PMRAFNS formed part of the British Medical Squadron, based in an area known as Sector South-West. Regional aid posts offered primary care for incidents in their locality while two medical support teams stood by to offer further help. And twice each week, from the small but vital aeromedical evacuation cell based in Split, a VC10 or a Hercules lifted casualties to hospitals in Germany or the UK.

The war in Bosnia dragged on. Dreadful atrocities were committed by all factions, with UNPROFOR forces tied by political niceties to doing little but pick up the pieces, bring food and blankets to refugees, and help the wounded – of whatever side. More and more PMs experienced the waste and futility of this war and in 1995 it was Kevin Mackie, then based at PARAFH Wroughton, whose 'name came to the top of the pile for out-of-area operations'.

We went as part of the Rapid Reaction Force and we sat in a place called Ploce, which was actually in Croatia. I had twelve medics who were assigned to me, who flew around on aircraft. Basically, if there was a helicopter in the air – an RAF helicopter, not a teeny-weeny army thing – it had a medic on board. Which we really had to fight for, but it meant we had full in-theatre casevac capability. We flew with crews at night, doing their night-training – we used the infra-red night-vision goggles, used them in the back of a kite with the lights off and doing tactical flying. We got shot at – as you do! Whenever anybody got into the helicopter, they'd ask me why I hadn't got a flak jacket on and I'd say, 'I'm sitting on two,' because if you're going to be shot from the ground it's going to be coming up through the bottom, so I used to sit on two flak jackets.

The site at Ploce was far from ideal, being on 'reclaimed' land and below the water line.

One of the funniest things . . . well, it was funny at the time, but you've got to live with black humour . . . when we first went there we had very small 'dunnies' that were dug-out, and then we had these big effluent containers – chemical latrine tanks – sunk into the ground, and on top of them they just put a toilet seat – that's what field sanitation is like . . . But, because we were below the water level, we had some severe flooding one night and these tanks just floated out of the ground and tipped up. So there was human effluent running past your tent – it was really quite challenging. What could you do but laugh? Our kit was safe, because our kit was off the ground, but . . . it turned into a health and safety night-mare, so we evacuated the site, and set up in some sheds in a nearby area that had concrete ground.

But the work side of it was great. I managed quite a few hours in both Pumas and Chinooks, and we did more than fifty aeromeds and casevacs in the time, so that kept us quite busy . . . We had a young Croatian lad, he was run over, nasty RTA [road traffic accident] and I actually took him to a local Croatian hospital, as a good-will thing, in the back of a helicopter.

You don't expect in the field to look after children – and

that's a big thing the services have learned, from humanitarian aid, that midwives and paediatric nurses are as important as trauma people . . . You're not talking about bomb-blast victims, you're talking about people with barbed-wire lacerations, or dysentery . . . things which you and I present every day to the GP, just everyday incidents that happen . . . We've got to be able to treat them all. Certainly the first casevacs from Bosnia were all primary care cases – troops who were just poorly, or dentally [sic] unfit, and had to be sent back.

Just before her retirement, Air Commodore Valerie Hand, in her role as Matron-in-Chief of the PMRAFNS and Director of Nursing Services, went on a visit to Bosnia.

I wanted to see what was going on . . . I spent a week there, flew out to Split, and toured the air force set-up there. I went on a merchant ship – royal fleet auxiliary – absolutely incredible, the supplies they had in the hold, catering for months, stores for all the troops out in Bosnia, amazing, unbelievable! Some of the army personnel lived on that ship, it happened to be in the harbour . . .

I went up country to an army camp – they were mostly army, but because I was tri-Service I could get to see all these things . . . They'd taken over what had been a large knitwear factory – just an empty shell of a building – and they had set up their camp – their field hospital, tents, emergency operating theatres, clinics and things, inside this shell of a building. And they were having a ball because this was what they'd been trained to do, what they'd joined the army for – but they weren't very busy, they had just a trickle of patients, mostly local civilians, but they were practising on each other and doing Exercises up there.

I was taken round into the village, the local town, and up to the village next door. We drove up in a Land-Rover, so we went through all this ravaged countryside . . . I've never seen anything like it. You see those pictures on TV, burnt out houses and things, shells, and it was like that all the way, village . . . after village . . . after village . . . after village . . . miles and miles and miles. Every time you came to a village it was just a burnt-out shell. I found it very moving. Couldn't even bring myself to take pictures of it. It was just awful. Awful! If you relate it to your own area, imagine it being Northleach, Bibury . . . It's absolutely horrendous. I was glad that I'd been. And the people were glad to see me . . . I think they are quite pleased when you go and see what they're doing in these remote places.

Kevin Mackie returned to England at the end of his Bosnia tour, to be met by his wife and ten-week-old baby daughter: 'a very emotional thing, one of the high spots of my life,' he says adding drily, 'Of course, in my absence Wroughton had closed – couldn't manage without me.'

The axe falls

In 1995 members of the PMRAFNS welcomed the appointment of their first male matron-in-chief, Group Captain (now Air Commodore) Robert H. Williams.

Having joined the air force as a boy entrant at sixteen, Bob Williams started his adult career in 1962 as a senior aircraftman on the renal unit at Halton. He commenced his SRN training at Wegberg in 1965 and rose through the ranks of the Medical Branch to chief technician. He gained his Queen's commission in the Medical Technical Branch in 1976 before transferring to the PMRAFNS in 1980. As we have seen, he was the first man to be appointed matron of an RAF hospital on posting to Wegberg in 1992.

Sadly, for him, one of Bob Williams' first tasks as matron-in-chief was to confirm, in the foreword for the 1995 magazine, the impending demise of the three remaining RAF hospitals – Wegberg in Germany, Wroughton in Wiltshire, and Halton in Buckinghamshire, all to be closed in 1996. As a result, PMRAFNS strength of 170 officers and 300 other ranks would be reduced to 102 officers and 178 other ranks – a total complement of 280.

News of the Ministry of Defence's latest cost-cutting plans brought a renewed clamour of protest. Service hospitals had a reputation as centres of medical excellence; they had provided care for thousands of civilians as well as members of the armed forces; and they had helped to pioneer many medical advances over the years. The remaining RAF hospitals were cherished by all who had served on their staffs and by local communities who had come to rely on their presence.

RAFH Wegberg had served personnel stationed in West Germany for forty-three years, caring for the sick and injured from a wide area and seeing the birth of thousands of babies. It was also well known for its annual bed-push charity day, whose events over many years raised a considerable amount of money for good causes, as well as providing fun for everyone.

Wroughton had opened in 1941 to receive the wounded of the Second World War. In 1976 the big hospital near Swindon had become a combined service unit, staffed by RAF and army personnel. In 1992 it had proudly reverted to being Princess Alexandra's Royal Air Force Hospital. Since this renaming came about with much ceremony, after five years of refurbishment, expansion and modernization, at a cost of millions of pounds, observers could be forgiven for assuming that Wroughton's future must be fairly secure. It was an invaluable asset to the local community.

One of its grateful civilian patients, Mrs Jan Gibson, says that her most memorable stay in a service hospital happened at Wroughton in June 1993, when she needed intense physiotherapy to alleviate her arthritis. 'Being blind and having a guide dog, I was rather apprehensive . . . I thought there was no way they would allow me to take my dog with me . . . How wrong can you be! A side ward was arranged for me to occupy, with my dog . . .' Guide-dog Yana became a focus of attention for off-duty staff, including the station CO, and nurses vied for the chance to take her for walks. A special visitor was PM Pat Surridge, who knew the pair from their visits to the orthopaedic outpatients' department. Late at night and early every morning Pat would come to take Yana for exercise, beginning a friendship which continued long after Mrs Gibson and her dog left hospital. During her stay in Wroughton, says Mrs Gibson, 'that dog was pampered, even to being offered a nightcap of Horlicks and toast. I ended up borrowing one of the signs to hang on the radiator above her bed, to say "Nil by Mouth"!'

If it had ever been in doubt, the hospital's usefulness was further emphasized when, despite political turmoil and personal danger, an aeromed team from Wroughton flew out to Sarajevo to bring back twenty seriously ill Bosnian children. The young patients might well have died if they had not been swiftly spirited to the care available in UK hospitals. Nevertheless, closing their ears to the numerous voices that cried against it, the government ended the life of Princess Alexandra's Royal Air Force Hospital, Wroughton.

For sixty-nine years the home of Royal Air Force medicine and cradle of the PMRAFNS, even the Princess Mary's Royal Air Force Hospital Halton could not be spared. Richard Laurence, writing the hospital's epitaph in a brief history, details some of its specialities: 'Medicine, General Surgery, Orthopaedic Surgery, Anaesthesiology, Nephrology, Urology, Gynaecology and Obstetrics, Burns and Plastic Surgery, ENT, Ophthalmology, Neurology, Psychiatry, Oral Surgery, Dermatology, Paediatrics, Maxillo-facial Surgery, Radiology, Oncology, Aviation Medicine, Tropical Medicine . . .' It had been the home of the Cade Cancer Unit, the Institute of Pathology and Tropical Medicine, and the Renal Unit – including Britain's first mobile dialysis team.

These three great Royal Air Force hospitals, last of the many that had existed over almost eighty years, all closed on the same day, 31 March 1996.

Primary health care

While many of the original RAF nursing sisters of 1918 had worked in the hospitals, others went to look after service personnel reporting on sick parades at station sick quarters. After eighty-odd years these sisters have evolved into today's practice nurses. They offer primary care ('doctor's surgery' style) at modern station medical centres across the UK and overseas, with the main focus on health education and preventive medicine. At present these medical centres remain under single-service control, so that those at RAF stations are staffed and run by air force personnel and cater mainly for air force patients – aircrew, groundcrew or other support staff, plus entitled civilians such as air force wives and families. The centres each employ a nursing officer or an NCO of the PMRAFNS (a few larger stations have both), and the work is both demanding and varied.

The first practice nurse at RAF Lossiemouth, in Scotland, was Debbie Gurney (Mrs Jones) who says, 'After many years of working in hospitals as part of a large team with numerous resources, I found myself working alone, at what appeared to be the "end of the world", with the nearest Nursing Officer working 300 miles away at RAF Leeming.' But pretty soon she had things organized, mornings being taken up by routine appointments for blood tests, dressings and minor ailments, 'with the usual handful of accidents thrown in to keep me busy. I still find it amazing the number of people who "walk" into aircraft. During the afternoons, as well as preparing patients for their medicals, I ran a "Well Women's Clinic", immunization clinics, and assisted the "docs" with their minor op clinics.' One afternoon a week was set aside to catch up on paperwork.

In addition, Debbie found herself voted in as duty medic, providing mobile emergency cover during flying operations – which at front-line Lossiemouth meant twenty-four hours a day. Two emergencies stick out in her mind: 'a Nimrod which, due to double engine fire, ditched into the Moray Firth; and a Jaguar which sustained double engine failure after a massive birdstrike and crashed into the sea. Luckily in both cases there were no fatalities, but plenty of "tachycardias" in the Station Medical Centre.' She also spent some time training with Lossiemouth's Search and Rescue Squadron, assisting on one occasion in the rescue of a climber on Ben Nevis, and as duty medic she spent a week in the sun while a Tornado squadron from 'Lossie' did armament practice at RAF Deccimommanu, on Sardinia. On leaving Lossiemouth she became the first practice nurse at another fast jet operational station, RAF Bruggen in West Germany.

Recent figures show fifteen nursing officers and twenty-six NCOs in post at RAF station medical centres, from Lyneham to Lossiemouth in the UK, and as diverse as Brunei and Ascension Island overseas. Squadron Leader Sharon Callcott, in charge of primary health care, observes, 'With more posts becoming available on more stations, PMs are increasingly high-profile in the RAF – people no longer have to go to hospital to see one!'

Secondary care

That year of so many swingeing closures and changes, 1996, also affected Akrotiri. The hospital's RAF ensign was laid up in the hospital chapel on 23 August 1996, as The Princess Mary Hospital in Cyprus became part of the newly formed Defence Secondary Care Agency (DSCA). This agency combines the medical and nursing branches of all three services into a single entity, in the field of secondary (i.e. hospital) care.

TPMH has a capacity of fifty-five beds (this number can be tripled if necessary), with an establishment of 127 personnel in the ratio 60:40 RAF:army. It includes a general ward, a dedicated children's ward, and a busy maternity unit, delivering up to three hundred babies a year, plus a full supporting network of operating theatres. With all the facilities expected of any well-equipped modern hospital, it currently serves the large tri-Service community on the island's three sovereign bases.

In the UK, following the closure of all other service hospitals, secondary health care is provided at the Royal Hospital Haslar (Gosport); at MDHUS at Northallerton, Peterborough, Frimley Park (Aldershot) and Derriford (Plymouth); and at the Defence Services Medical Rehabilitation Unit at Headley Court (Epsom). At these units, service nurses run wards for both military and civilian patients; service doctors, nurses and paramedics are fully integrated with their colleagues in the National Health Service.

Despite the undeniable impact of the Defence Cost Study, with the loss of the RAF hospitals resulting in redundancy for some of his 'highly loyal and talented nurses', Air Commodore Bob Williams remains 'optimistic that the PMs will still have a major role to play . . . not only in Aeromedical Evacuation, for which we retain single service responsibility, but also in supporting our sister services in time of conflict, or in lending humanitarian support throughout the world as we do at present'. The humanitarian support continues, wherever it may be needed.

Recruiting and training

Today's members of the PMRAFNS fall into three categories: nursing officers, non-commissioned staff nurses, and student staff nurses. Nursing officers are commissioned RAF officers; to join the Service they need at least two years' post-registration experience, preferably a second professional qualification, and demonstrable leadership qualities. They act as team leaders and nursing managers.

Staff nurses are qualified general nurses and mental nurses (RGN and RMN) who provide nursing support. (From 1997, when mental nurses and auxiliary air force nurses were incorporated, all RAF nurses came under one banner, as members of the PMRAFNS.) Student staff nurses will become tomorrow's nursing officers and NCOs; they are recruited to one of the individual services and remain members of that service, wearing appropriate uniform when on official duty.

Squadron Leader Pippa Ward, in charge of recruiting, says that a general decrease in numbers of school leavers looking for a career in nursing means that the pool of possible candidates grows smaller while the target numbers, after a few years of drastic cut-backs, are once again increasing. As the generation that served during the Second World War fades away, so fewer of today's young people understand the service way of life. Consequently, they may harbour some strange ideas. Pippa says, 'I spend a lot of time at careers fairs answering questions like "Do you have to wear uniform all the time?" or "Do you get leave?" and "Can you go home?" ' (For anyone interested, the answers are No! Yes! and Of course!)

> Before taking this job, I thought that recruiting would be a nice way of earning a living! In hindsight I can honestly say I have never worked so hard in my eleven years in the PMRAFNS. It is a rewarding job and I enjoy the travelling (3000 miles a month!) and meeting nurses in the NHS system. However, I have a whole new view of the recruiting world and, although I would recommend the job, it is not for the faint-hearted!

Following basic recruit and medical training, students move on to beautiful Hampshire, where beside the Solent they undertake their professional nurse training at the tri-Service Health Studies Department of the Royal Defence Medical College at HMS *Dolphin* (now renamed Fort Blockhouse), in Gosport. Here, students and tutors from all three services work amicably together. Initially the PMRAFNS took up only two places on a course of thirty students, but this number has increased significantly over the past few years, resulting in an annual intake of thirty PMRAFNS students.

All graduates become registered nurses with a Diploma in Higher Education (DipHEd); PMRAFNS staff nurses graduate in the rank of acting corporal. Following two more years' service, all nurses have the opportunity to apply to be considered for a commission. The PMRAFNS still welcomes nurses who have already done their training in the NHS; however, by undertaking professional training within the service, under the guidance of some of the best nurse tutors in the world, young men and women enjoy the advantages of imbibing military know-how along with their nursing skills.

Whatever career path they may follow, successful recruits and students all become fully fledged PMs, with the accompanying benefits and opportunities – good pay, with uniform and accommodation provided; the camaraderie of a service environment; a wide range of work experience; chances to specialize professionally, to gain further educational qualifications, to climb the promotion ladder; terrific opportunities for travel and social life . . . With such prizes on offer, only the best of candidates win through.

'Students always make you laugh, they do some strange things . . .' says Squadron Leader Annie Warburton, head of nurse training since 1992.

> I've seen a pupil nurse collect up thermometers to clean, put them in a great big bowl and pour a kettle of boiling water over them. So we lost that lot! And I've actually witnessed a student nurse putting the one and only stainless steel bedpan in a papier mâché bedpan masher – which wrecked the machine and made a hell of a noise . . .

As for the tri-service environment, Annie has not found any real problems.

> In terms of nurse education, I think it was inevitable. The nurse-teachers were luckier than most because we, as groups of people, had worked together prior to this happening. We had RAF student nurses who were on the navy student nurse programme with the University of Portsmouth. I already had one teacher working on the Haslar site, even before the rest of us moved, so it wasn't as traumatic as, say, closing Wroughton and moving to Haslar was for clinical nurses, who

were coming to work with people who they didn't know, perhaps had never seen before.

The Royal Hospital Haslar

The Royal Naval Hospital at Haslar is one of the oldest of military hospitals – it accepted its first patients in 1753. In the climacteric year of 1996, it became a tri-service unit of the Defence Medical Service and was renamed The Royal Hospital Haslar. Since that time, PMs have worked there alongside their naval and army colleagues.

In a pleasing link with the past, Mrs Sybil Morgan writes of a time in June 1948 when as Aircraftwoman Unsted of the WRAF she was stationed at RAF Bicester. On her way back to the station after taking leave at home in Gosport, she was hit by a lorry and spent six weeks on the seriously ill list in RAF Hospital Halton, with terrible injuries which almost resulted in her losing her right foot. For her eventual recovery she thanks 'the wonderful care and attention of all the nurses and doctors – they even came to see me when they were off duty'. She spent eight months in hospital, having several operations in that time, being taken for walks in one of the wicker 'prams', and even having the chance to meet Princess Mary when RAFH Halton celebrated its twenty-first birthday.

Fifty years on, in 1998, she found herself again being tended by air force nurses after suffering a heart attack and being taken to the Royal Hospital Haslar. 'Several times I was under the care of the RAF and they were wonderful. I will always look upon RAF nurses as being special.'

In December 1998 the government announced its plan to close the Haslar Hospital. No firm date has yet been set, but several wards shut down in June 1999 as military personnel were detached to help in the aftermath of the Kosovo crisis. When Haslar eventually closes, it is intended that a new MDHU (see below) will be developed within the Portsmouth NHS Trust.

Ministry of Defence Hospital Units (MDHUs)

Wards manned by service personnel already exist within certain NHS trust hospitals. The MDHU at Peterborough employs sixty-five medical and nursing personnel of all ranks, air force and army. They run both a surgical recovery unit and an orthopaedic ward, and they also help to staff the intensive care unit, accident and emergency, operating theatres and outpatients departments. These Peterborough PMs are 'parented' by RAF Wittering, which gives them a base to live and a place to socialize in the air force environment which they cherish and enjoy.

It was in the outpatients department at Peterborough that Margaret Kingston, who retired as a Squadron Officer in 1971, recently encountered a young PM.

> I was rather pleased . . . I went to this clinic and this girl came, and she looked so smart, and when she turned round I could see she was a sergeant PM. Got a nice little cap on and her dress was absolutely immaculate, and her sergeant's stripes up, so I called her over and I said 'Excuse me, you're in the PMs, aren't you?' She looked at me, as much as to say, what's that old girl know about the PMs? So I told her I *was* a PM for twenty years. She was helping out at the Peterborough District Hospital – they've got a few wards there. And she looked so smart compared with the other girls . . .

The pride remains. Once a PM, always a PM!

There are, however, sadnesses. The Service is now so streamlined that most of its members know one another personally; they become very close, like members of a family. A well-liked and highly respected friend and fellow officer was lost when Squadron Leader Peter Pullen died in a road accident on 14 July 1998. He held a senior position in the Peterborough MDHU and, at the time of his death, was preparing to take his turn for a tour of duty in Bosnia.

Tactical Medical Wing (Aeromed)

The third main role for today's PMs is still their forte – the aeromedical or casualty evacuation flights in which they are so skilled. The Aeromedical Evacuation Squadron, once based at PARAFH Wroughton, is now at RAF Lyneham, an integral part of today's Tactical Medical Wing. There, thirteen members of the PMRAFNS – nursing officers and senior NCOs – are constantly on stand-by to repatriate sick and injured servicemen and their families from destinations world-wide. Routine aeromed flights visit Cyprus and Germany; they bring refugees back from the former Yugoslavia; they also fly to countries where RAF squadrons may be exercising, and special aeromed flights go, as needed, to Royal Navy ships wherever they may be, or to army units on exercise.

In-flight training is constantly updated to incorporate the latest in technique and technology, the better to care for patients while in the air; it covers the handling of all types of patient in all types of aircraft, from the huge and noisy Hercules to the sleek VC10 and on to the smallest helicopter.

Another medal winner

Today's PMs are still winning medals. For example, as a result of saving the life of a man who collapsed and stopped breathing while exercising in a gym, Barry Wroe (now a wing commander) won the Sir Andrew Humphrey Memorial medal for 1998. The medal is awarded annually to the RAF medical officer 'considered to have accomplished the most meritorious act or to have contributed the most significant advance in the preservation or saving of human life'. Though normally made to officers of the Medical Branch, in exceptional circumstances – as in this instance – the medal goes to nursing, dental or paramedical personnel.

In a varied career, Barry Wroe has, among other things, been an instructor (flight commander) at Cranwell, where a student on one of the SERE courses has an abiding memory of him: '. . . our flight commander was training for the London Marathon at the time, so when I now say to people how much running we did at Cranwell, they say, "We don't do that any more!" Whereas, when I was at Cranwell, Barry Wroe was training, so every single lunchtime we were out jogging, so that he could keep his fitness up!'

Barry has also worked at Permanent Joint Headquarters, Northwood, helping to provide medical advice to UK military commanders, which in practice covers anything from giving guidance on immunization and staffing the provision of field medical facilities to flying out to Antigua to spend a morning assessing the danger and devastation caused by an erupting volcano.

A PM's life is *not* one of dull routine!

Dedication and Remembrance

Two special church services marked high points for 1999. At the annual reunion, held at RAF Halton on 5 June, members attended a service in St George's Church. The PMRAFNS Book of Remembrance was ceremoniously carried to the altar during an act of worship to dedicate a new stained glass window commemorating the PMRAFNS.

On the following day – 6 June 1999, exactly fifty-five years after D-Day – PMs brought home their Book of Remembrance to the RAF's own 'parish' church, the Church of St Clement Danes, in London.

Looking to the future

As this book goes to press, the authorities appear to be rethinking their draconian cuts to the Defence Medical Service. Proposed changes may see an increase in the strength of the PMRAFNS. As always throughout its eighty-odd years existence, the Service remains flexible, adapting to the times, riding with the blows and standing ready to answer the call of those in pain and distress. Its work grows ever more varied and its personnel ever more skilled and specialized.

What the third millennium may hold, who can say?

Squadron Leader Pippa Ward came across some interesting clues to the future: it seems that boffins are inventing space-age protective clothing for nurses and patients. In America (where else?) something going by the tongue-twisting title of the Defence Advance Projects Research Agency has come up with a Star Trek-style tricorder to detect germs and viruses, and a 'blood-scrubbing agent' which, injected into the blood stream, will destroy harmful micro-organisms and thus save personnel from the inconvenience of wearing protective suits. How thoughtful! Other projects include a 'smart shirt' for fighting troops. This has 'fibre optic cable woven into the material, with sensors and a transmitter which can identify wounds . . . and alert medics to the soldier's position . . . using satellite technology'. Sensors can also track a bullet through a human body and even identify its calibre, though it puzzles Pippa that the scientists seem to assume that the injured person won't notice he (or she) has been shot. She adds, 'What is even more worrying is the presumption that medics can read maps! Although technology hopes to make life easier, is there really any substitute for a professional, human and caring member of the PMRAFNS? I think not!'

The story so far

Eighty years ago, members of the RAF Nursing Service were all qualified nurses and all female; they held officer status but remained civilians; they wore starched white veils and long skirts; they were not allowed to travel in aircraft while on duty and they were strictly non-combatant. Today, both men and women may join the PMRAFNS with equal rights and equal opportunities; they bear all ranks from NCO to air commodore; they work alongside colleagues of the navy and army; both sexes might wear trousers, or flying gear, or camouflage battledress and 'bone-dome'; they most definitely fly, in whatever type of aircraft suits their purpose and, what is more, when necessary they carry arms and know how to use them.

They are also members of the Royal Air Force, required to take part in a wide range of service activities, from the rigours of recruit camp to a survival weekend at RAF Cranwell; from duty medic to mess secretary and orderly officer. On the social side, there are dinners and balls, opportunities to take part in expedition training in the Cairngorms, or adventure training in Cyprus; and sport – the annual Dame Joanna Cruickshank Tennis Tournament (to find a PM champion) and the Inter-Nursing Service Tennis Tournament continue to provide happy summer events, recently joined by the PMs' own golf championship. A glance at the annual magazine reveals PMs revelling in activities such as sailing, free-fall parachuting, equestrian team riding, swimming, netball, hockey, mountaineering, deep-sea diving, gymnastics, cricket, squash, judo, kung fu, skiing . . . the list goes on. Enthusiastic PMs take part in charity fund-raising events – bed-pushes, cycle rides, and the Nijmegen marches; they may be chosen to march across the arena representing their Service at the Albert Hall during the Festival of Remembrance, and at the Cenotaph next day; or even to line the route on grand state occasions.

Whatever their experience may have been, in war or in peace, not one of them regrets a single moment of service life. The sentiment of all of them was aptly expressed by Gwen Butler, whose career in the PMs, begun in 1925, took her from early Halton to Palestine and Iraq. During the Second World War she was matron of RAFH Lagens in the Azores and, after becoming the first matron of Nocton Hall, she went on to become senior matron at Halton. On her retirement in 1952, she recalled her twenty-seven years with the Service, adding, 'If I had my time over again I would not change one second of it. I think this is the most wonderful nursing service in the world . . . I have been thrilled with every minute.'

This book is a resumé of the main events in the story. For reasons of space, many fascinating personal accounts have had to be omitted. The choice was not easy: some gems have been kept for the postscript that follows.

However, this is not the end. Continuing chapters in the history of the Princess Mary's Royal Air Force Nursing Service are still being written . . .

POSTSCRIPT:
REUNION EAVESDROPPINGS

In the stories that follow, some names have been altered to protect
the authors!

Matrons

Why do matrons have such a bad reputation? Whatever the answer,
matrons of the PMRAFNS have left their own legends, still being told.

Doves

A PM says: 'Most of the Matrons were very efficient, great orga-
nizers, and they cared about people. It might not always have
seemed that way to nurses working under them, but . . .'

From the thirties: 'The two outstanding matrons were Miss Oliver
and Miss Clubb. They were both so very human . . . When I
returned from Aden I was posted as Matron to Air Ministry in
1939. I have never met a Matron-in-Chief who considered her staff
as Dame Emily Blair did. She was most particular that each member
be placed in wards or SSQrts to which she was most suited.'

From a wartime WAAF: 'Having come under WAAF, RAF and
PMRAFNS scrutiny, I found Matron Hards at Ely was a welcome
breath of fresh air – far from stuffy, and companionable to a degree,
she was a delight to know'.

From the sixties:

> You didn't have chaps in your room. You could only entertain
> them in the ante room and they had to be out by eleven

o'clock . . . Matron used to go around the corridors making sure no one was having a little snog anywhere. This doctor was absolutely potty about a friend of mine . . . decided he was going to propose. He got hold of her, opened this door and pulled her in, thinking it was a room, but it was the linen cupboard – a boiling hot linen cupboard. Matron was going along knocking on doors making sure nobody was in there, got as far as the linen room and hears this voice saying, 'Will you marry me?' and the reply, 'I can't marry you – I'm going to faint in this heat!' Matron interrupted, 'Couldn't you find somewhere a bit more romantic than a linen cupboard?'

A senior matron:

By the time the hospital had run down to these few wards, we were all living down in the officers' mess. I remember the CO saying one day, 'Pity the sisters' mess isn't open, you'd have beautiful accommodation.' I said, 'Yes, and I'd live there in absolutely solitary state. Down in the main mess everybody talks to everyone. But in a nursing officers' mess no-one's very keen on talking to the matron!'

A card written and illustrated for Scots-born Matron Mary R. Gall, on her retirement in 1960:

Mary Gall – Greetings from the PMRAFNS

Last week to Honkers,
Next week to Malay,
Back to Episkopi,
Off the next day.
You flew down the Red Sea,
Called in at Bahrain,
Your visits to Stations
Were never in vain.
One week to Malta,
The next week to SHAPE,
You've kept our flag flying,
And cut down Red Tape.
Sometimes by staff car,

And often by air,
A year at White Waltham
And Tavistock Square.
From Cosford to Changi,
From Wales to Kowloon,
The girls are all hoping
We'll meet again soon.
Wherever you turn up,
You're welcome, Miss Gall,
And now you're for Edinburgh,
Best of them all.
You've flown with the air force,
Touched down at the 'drome.
Most kindly of Matrons,
At last you are home.

So some are human, after all. As for the rest . . .

Dragons

From J.G. Kingan, once CO of RAF Halton:

A nurse nick-named 'Tatty', after a character in the radio series ITMA, decided to grace the PMs with her presence, only to discover that, while WAAF officers of RAF Halton lived in the normal mess and mixed socially with male officers, nursing officers of the sisters' mess at PMRAFH Halton were more closely guarded than nuns in a convent. Not that this deterred Tatty. She was sent for by Matron, who observed disapprovingly, 'I hear you have been seen in the company of an officer from the main camp.' Tatty admitted to the relationship, adding that she and the gentleman in question were, in fact, engaged to be married. 'I'm pleased to hear there's nothing untoward in this relationship,' said Matron. 'Congratulations. You may go.' Next day, Tatty was ordered to report forthwith to Ely. But she had the last laugh – she married her officer and retired from the service.

The matron of wartime Rauceby Hospital, a big, blonde woman with a passion for bridge, wanted young Sister Sunshine to make up a four.

When Sunny said she was too stupid and would rather do embroidery, she was given the task of smocking a dress out of a piece of apple-green silk which Matron had brought back from the East. 'For my sins, I had to smock the front and back – and she was a HUGE woman!'

Then there was the PM who refused to hurry even when a German plane flew low over the country road where she was walking – 'Matron says we mustn't run while wearing uniform.'

From a male PM:

> Miss Mangleworzel, matron at Halton, was a very fearsome character – bite the head off a junior doctor fifty yards away . . . I worked one Christmas Day. The hospital was very quiet. I'd finished my shift and decided to dress up as one of the nurses – student nurse, SEN – hat and everything, dress, even a touch of lipstick. What I hadn't realised was that Matron was doing rounds. In she walks, with me in full drag. She stopped and looked at me, dead-pan, and I thought . . . I'm dead! But she burst out laughing! I got on well with her after that. I was her deputy matron on my next posting. She said, 'I used to think you were such a stuck-up boy in theatre . . .' But if she was in a bad mood you might as well jump out the window . . .

Sister Molly Moonlight was happy to be posted to Wegberg to escape the proximity of Senior Sister Gripe. But as luck would have it Gripe was also posted to Wegberg, on the very same day. She gave Molly the choice of travelling alone by train and ferry or going as a passenger in Gripe's car. Not wanting to cause offence, Molly chose the car. Unfortunately the vehicle demanded mechanical attention, which delayed them. The evening before they were due at Wegberg they drove full tilt down to Folkestone, with a stressed-out Molly frantically searching the timetables for a suitable ferry. She found one and they arrived in good time, only to see the ferry just putting out to sea – poor Molly had read the *summer* timetable, and the *winter* schedule had just started.

Gripe was *not* amused. 'So what are you going to do now?' she barked.

'Cry,' said Molly – and did.

Touché!

During some local riots and disturbances in Bahrain, a somewhat unpopular Muharraq matron, who was known to enjoy a drink, came in one day and announced in annoyance that she had been stoned. 'What, drunk again, Matron?' came the riposte.

A sixteen-year-old boy apprentice (now a senior officer) came under Matron's constant disapproval. 'I could never do anything right for her,' he recalls. One day when she was showing him how to wrap a bandage she ordered him to cut some tape to hold the bandage in place. 'How long do you want it, ma'am?' he asked politely. 'Too long, or too short?'

At an annual reunion

Primula: 'Princess Mary came to Cosford when I was there. They were really fussy – if the shade of paint in the decor wasn't right . . . The dining room at Cosford was painted twice, for instance, and the carpet was too long . . .'

Myrtle: 'Who was it at Cranwell missed church service because she had to deliver a baby in an airman's married quarter? The mother's main worry was the risk of mess on her carpet – all she could think about was having to face the Families' Officer!'

Primula: 'When we were at Ely, Danny Whosit and Imogen Cartilage . . . she was in charge of maternity and he was consultant obstetrician. They were both very keen on horse-racing bets. On a Saturday morning, or whatever, they'd hope we weren't busy so one of them could go down to the bookie in Ely . . .'

Myrtle: 'Wasn't it Imogen, at St Athan, she stood on a floor polisher and went zussing out, almost out through the door of one of the Nissen huts. She was quite a big girl, wasn't she? And Scottish.'

Primula: 'The patients used to help clean the wards in the old days. It was always cleaner when they did it. They'd say to each other "Don't throw that down there – I've just polished the floor!" . . . As a junior sister, you had to sweep half of the ward – throw tea-leaves down, I remember – do exactly half, and the ward maid did the other half.'

Myrtle: The wards were a damn sight cleaner than they are now, you had to do high dusting around the rails around the beds . . . Mind you, Matron Millipede . . . she used to have the officers doing it – she'd dump a tray of cutlery on them: 'Clean that!' she'd say, or 'You do this! – she's not still with us, is she? Don't print this if she is! I remember when I first went into the service, she said, 'Never, ever . . . neither lend nor borrow!' and she'd never lend anything to another ward, but if she wanted something it'd be, 'Nurse, go and get such-and-such from the other ward', but if anyone came to her ward on the cadge . . .

Primula: 'And you opened all the windows – put the patients in bed, under the blankets, and opened all the windows in the morning, to air the ward, while you were cleaning. Every morning. However cold. Oh – they were all covered up, though!'

Myrtle: What do you suppose happened about the brooch – the one Dame Joanna's family gave? You know! Copy of the medical badge, studded with diamonds and rubies. They'd given it to her as a birthday present and after she died they presented it . . . It was given to all Matrons-in-Chief when they took office, and on formal occasions, when they were in mufti, they would wear it. Now we've got a male MIC . . . I wonder what Bob does with it!

Primula: When I was at Brampton . . . we used to call them 'bean-stealers' – the married chaps who had their married quarters outside the mess but still came and ate our mess rations for nothing. Some of the younger officers – PAs to the big bods on Support Command staff, formed themselves into the SLIME Club – that's Single Living-in-Members' Executive – and they held gourmet dinners, but only members of the SLIME Club were invited. Some very high-ranking officers found themselves excluded, but . . . they invited *me* to join them!

Myrtle: In sisters' mess one breakfast-time, all the cutlery was missing. We were about to call the police when we realized all the cruets were still there – solid silver all of them, so maybe we hadn't been burgled. Then someone spotted the cutlery under the chairs in the maids' dining room. The officers had been in, playing pranks. So we plotted revenge . . . A gang of us sneaked into the dining room at the officers' mess and somehow managed to cart away two hefty twelve-seater dining tables. Put them in the solarium off the orthopaedic ward. They weren't discovered for three days! So then the officers came and pinched the loo seats out of the sisters' mess . . . At which point Matron and the CO hit the roof, but other hospitals got to hear about it, and they started . . . so it spread.

Primula: Did you hear that story about the Dame Joanna Tennis Tournament . . . Ely, I think, 1988 or thereabouts. Dear old 'Gloria' Swansong, who was theatre sister there – straight-faced, not much sense of humour – you must remember her! Well, she was organizing the tournament and she got into a bit of a state because the mess stewards had set out a place for Dame Joanna, with a name tag, and were a bit peeved when she didn't turn up – they didn't realize she'd have been a hundred and twelve!

Myrtle: I remember doing an aeromed to Cyprus. Sitting in the back of this Hercules. Very noisy, very loud – and very full! We were flying over Italy, just had breakfast, and suddenly we just . . . dropped. Out of the sky. I caught my breakfast on the way back up again as we levelled off. I was absolutely terrified. I remember looking at the air loadmaster, who was normally so cool and contained – he was white as a sheet! Anyway, we got to Cyprus and were on the beach later that day, when the captain – the Flight Lieutenant who'd been flying the aircraft – mentioned the bumpy ride, and I said, 'I'm not flying in a Hercules again, it was just dreadful.' With that, the loadie looked across and said, 'You don't know the half of it. We were actually hit by lightning – and the hold was full of high explosives.' No wonder he'd gone white!

Primula: Were you there at Wroughton, when Doris . . . This Indian pilot had been admitted. Crashed his plane and injured himself. Anyway, Doris was night sister and he asked her . . . he said could she find out who kept leaving religious tracts and Catholic pamphlets on his side table. Well, she knew the day sister was a devout Roman

Catholic so . . . after a few discreet enquiries she discovered . . . The pilot had been asked his religion and he'd said he was a Parsee – Zoroastrian, or something, isn't it? The wardmaster had got him down as 'RC'!

The princess and the parrot

In the early sixties, Princess Alexandra was staging through RAF Gan, a tiny island in the middle of the Indian Ocean. Gan being a men-only station, PM Jane Stott was seconded from Changi to escort Her Royal Highness while on the island. The princess was due to be shown around the camp and to meet everyone, as usual, but they decided that one place should remain out of bounds – the back of the sergeants' mess, where lived a pet parrot whose language was even more colourful than his plumage.

So, the day came, the princess did the rounds, and then said, 'Isn't there something I haven't seen?' She had heard about the parrot! Reluctantly, they took her to see it and crossed their fingers while she talked to it, 'Pretty Polly . . .'

'BUGGER OFF!' said the parrot.

A deathly hush . . .

'Good heavens!' said the princess. 'It speaks English!'

APPENDICES

I

SIGNIFICANT DATES FOR THE PMRAFNS

1918, 1 April: Royal Air Force officially formed.

1918, 1 June: Royal Air Force Nursing Service (RAFNS) created; nurses posted to units in UK. Miss Cruickshank MIC from November.

1919: Former medical school unit (wooden huts) becomes RAF Hospital Halton. Many other units close on ending of First World War.

1921, January: RAFNS established by Royal Charter as a permanent branch of the RAF.

1922: First PMs posted overseas, to Iraq.

1923, 14 June: HRH Princess Mary becomes first Royal Patron; service renamed Princess Mary's RAFNS.

1925: First air ambulance service in UK, based at RAF Halton.

1927, 31 October: Princess Mary gives her name to the new hospital at Halton.

1923–34: PMRAFNS strength around 100.

1930: Retirement of first MIC, Joanna M. Cruickshank (later Dame Joanna). She presents a cup for the winner of the annual PMRAFNS tennis tournament.

1937: Service has 134 regular sisters, but as war threatens qualified nurses join a new PMRAFNS Reserve.

1939: Service has 184 regular sisters and 69 reserves, plus pool of 200 VAD nurses. By September, 6,000 volunteers apply for 460 reserve vacancies.

1941, 25 April: Defence (Women's Forces) Regulations grant emergency commissions; PMs don officers' rank markings but are still addressed by professional titles. Nurses are allowed (for the duration) to remain in PMRAFNS even when married.

1942, January: New post of principal matron established, to work at Air Ministry.

1943: 1,126 PMRAFNS sisters staff 33 RAF hospitals and 71 SSQs; in addition, nursing sisters work in a welfare capacity at 47 RAF stations.

1944: MBEs awarded to two PMs, the first women to enter Normandy after D-Day. Largest annual number of airborne casevacs: 300,000.

1945: Steady demobilization of PMRAFNS reserves in Europe. No major war casualties among PMs, but many honours and awards.

1948: Brief period of parachute training for PMs.

1949, 1 February: Women's services fully integrated into RAF. PMs hold commissions and adopt female officer rank though professional titles continue to be used inside hospitals.

1950: King George V approves the appointment of the Princess Royal, Patron of PMRAFNS, as Air Chief Commandant.

1950–1: Korean War proves the advantages of evacuating casualties by air. PMs attend airborne patients for first time.

1951: RAF Hospitals Halton, Ely, Wroughton and Wegberg approved as training schools for members of the RAF Medical Service.

1950s: Heyday of sea-trooping and long-haul aeromeds.

1956: PM Daphne Budgen killed on casevac duty when Anson crashes in Germany.

1956–7: Suez crisis; closure of canal obliges troopships to go via South Africa.

1959: Formal flight-nurse training begins at Lyneham.

1962, October: SRN training introduced: students become staff nurses/NCOs of PMRAFNS NCE (non-commissioned element).

1965: Death of HRH Princess Mary, the Princess Royal, Air Chief Commandant PMRAFNS.

1966: Appointment of HRH Princess Alexandra as Royal Patron and Air Chief Commandant of PMRAFNS.

1967, March: Training for SENs offered by all UK RAF hospitals.

1967: Wroughton becomes Princess Alexandra's RAFH.

1969: SENs and pupil enrolled nurses allowed to enlist on local service engagements.

1968–77: Overall reduction in commitment of RAF; closure of most RAF hospitals overseas, and smaller ones at home. Wroughton and Akrotiri staffed jointly with army.

1977: Discontinuation of SRN training at RAF hospitals.

1978: First edition of the *PMRAFNS Magazine* published.

1980, 1 April: Unified nursing service: integration of male nurses into PMRAFNS. Women officers assume male rank titles.

1982: The Falklands War: many casualties brought home by air, tended by PMs; PARAFH Wroughton is initial reception hospital.

1985, 2 January: PMs become part of the tri-service Defence Nursing Services (DNS).

1986, 5 November: Helicopter crash in Limassol Bay kills three members of the four-man crew, including PMs Fiona Johnstone and Martin Cook.

1987, March: Start of conversion training for enrolled nurses who wish to qualify as registered general nurses. RAF Hospital Ely renamed The Princess of Wales RAF Hospital.

1988: SEN training discontinued.

1990–1: The Gulf War: PMs on standby at Brize Norton, Akrotiri, Muharraq, and in Saudi Arabia.

1992: First male matron, appointed at Wegberg. PMRAFNS Association launched. RAFH Ely closes.

1993: PMRAFNS Trust formed.

1995: First male MIC appointed. PMs again called into active service, in Bosnia.

1996, 31 March: Closure of Halton, Wroughton and Wegberg. TPMH Akrotiri becomes part of Defence Secondary Care Agency. Conversion training ended. RGN training recommenced on opening of tri-service Royal Defence Medical College, Gosport. Start of MDHUs.

1998: Closure announced of Royal Hospital Haslar (only military hospital remaining in UK).

1999: War in Kosovo involves PMs in humanitarian work and movement of personnel closes some wards at Haslar.

II

HOSPITALS AND OTHER MEDICAL UNITS OF THE RAF IN BRITAIN

Earliest Hospitals, from 1917

London Area (mostly temporary sites):
Hampstead, North London:
  RFC Hospital, Mount Vernon, opened October 1917
  RAF Central Hospital, Holly Hill, 1 April 1918–May 1919
  RAF (Voluntary) Hospital, 37 Bryanston Square, January–November 1919
  RAF (Voluntary) Hospital, 82 Eaton Square, January 1919–January 1920
  RAF Officers' Hospital, 22 Fitzjohn's Avenue, opened April 1919
  WRAF Hospitals: 53 Hollycroft Avenue; 13 Parsifal Road; 24 Chesterfield
    Gardens, November 1919–January 1920
Croydon, Surrey: Convalescent Hospital, Shirley Park, January–November
  1919
Finchley, Middx: RAF Central Hospital, 1919–25
  Officers' Convalescent Hospital, established in Avenue House, closed
    November 1919
  RAF Central Hospital, East End Road, July 1919–June 1925, transferred
    to Uxbridge
Blandford Camp, Dorset:
  RAF & WRAF Hospital, September 1918–early 1920
  RAF Auxiliary Hospital, October 1918–early 1919 (opened in old work-
    house, solely to cope with flu outbreak)
Bolton Percy, Yorks: RAF Convalescent Hospital, Nun Appleton Hall,
  January–November 1919
Calshot, Hants: SSQ at flying-boat base, First World War
Cranwell, Lincs:
  RNAS sick bay, 1916–18
  RAFSH, 1918–40
Halton, Bucks:
  RFC Training School, 1917–19
  RAF Medical School and Hospital, 1919–27
Hastings, Sussex: 'The Hermitage' Hospital, January–May 1919
Matlock, Derbys: RAF Convalescent Hospital, Oct 1918–April 1919
  (re-opened Second World War)
Old Sarum, Salisbury, Wilts: RAF/Army Hospital, December 1918–early 1920

Members of the early RAF Nursing Service served also, singly or in pairs, at First World War WRAF depots at: Middleton Steventon; Saltley College, Birmingham; NARD, Sheffield; Glasgow; Hansworth College, Birmingham; Uxbridge; Shorncliffe; No.5 TDS, Peterborough; Aldborough; Farnborough; and Salisbury.

1920–39

By August 1920 most of the above had ceased to function. The WRAF had been disbanded in April 1920 (it reformed, as the WAAF, in 1939). Only three RAF hospitals remained, the largest being Halton, with a main hospital and an isolation unit; next came Cranwell, and finally the Central RAF Hospital, Finchley. A few staff nurses worked at individual SSQs at Uxbridge, Middx; Henlow, Beds; Manston, Kent; Flowerdown, near Winchester, and Calshot, Hants.

In 1939, as Britain once again geared itself for war, new RAF stations sprang up, and with them large sick quarters and hospitals – and more hospitals.

1939–2000

Blackpool, Lancs:
   'Cleveleys' RAF Officers' Convalescent Hospital, June 1943–November 1945
   Airmen's Convalescent Depot, 1940–6
Bridgnorth, Salop: RAF Station Hospital, August 1939–November 1947
Castle Archdale, N. Ireland: SSQ in Necerne Castle, 1940s
Catterick, N. Yorkshire: Army hospital, became tri-service Duchess of Kent Military Hospital, unit of the Defence Medical Services; closed April 1999 on relocation to MDHU Northallerton. DMS psychiatric unit remains at Catterick *pro tem*
Chessington, Surrey: MRU for WOs, NCOs and airmen from June 1950; joint services rehabilitation unit from August 1968; closed 1985, when it combined with Headley Court
Church Village, Pontypridd, S. Wales: RAFGH, September 1942–April 1946
Collaton Cross: MRU, January 1946 (renamed Chessington, 1950)
Cosford, Salop: Large SSQ, September 1938, became RAFSH/RAFGH, 1939–77
Cranwell, Lincs: RAFSH, 1918–40
Down Ampney, Glos: SSQ at RAF Down Ampney was central air evacuation centre for D-Day casualties and PoWs, 1944–6
Ely, Cambs (with annexe at Littleport): RAFGH, 1938/9–1987; Princess of Wales Hospital, 1987–92
Evesham, Worcs: RAFGH, May 1940–March 1946
Halton, Bucks: RAFH, March 1919–27. New hospital, Princess Mary's RAFH, opened October 1927; closed March 1996
Haslar, Hants: One of the oldest military (Royal Navy) hospitals, became a tri-service unit of the Defence Medical Service in 1996, when it was renamed The Royal Hospital Haslar

Haverfordwest, Pembrokeshire, Wales: RAFSH, February 1945–April 1946
Headley Court, Surrey: Officers' MRU, 1949–85; DMS MRU, 1985 to present
Henlow, Beds: RAFSH, September 1939–1948
Hereford: RAFSH, June 1940–November 1947
Hoylake, Cheshire: MRU 1940–December 1945, moved to Collaton Cross
Innsworth, Glos: RAFSH, June 1940–September 1948
Kirkham, Lancs: RAFSH, June 1940–June 1948
Littleport, Cambs: Opened 1939; became annexe to Ely RAFGH, August 1940
Lochnaw, Dumfries: RAFSH, September 1942–October 1945
Locking, Somerset: RAFSH, 1939–49
Loughborough, Leics: MRU, 1942–7
Matlock, Derbys: RAF neurological hospital, October 1939–May 1945
Melksham, Wilts: RAFSH, July 1940–6
Mongewell Park: MRU, 1945–50
Morecambe, Lancs: RAFSH, February 1940–October 1944
Nocton Hall, Lincs: RAFGH, 1947–83; FOPD linked with Ely, 1983–91
Northallerton, N. Yorks:
    RAFGH, January 1943–November 1947
    MDHU within NHS Hospital, opened 1999
Padgate, Cheshire: Large SSQ, 1938; RAFSH, May 1939–57
Peterborough, Cambs: MDHU within NHS Hospital, February 1996 to present
Rauceby, Lincs: Annexe for Cranwell RAFGH from 1 April 1940; complete hospital function transferred from Cranwell, 1 June 1940; returned to civilian use, 1945
St Athan, Glamorgan: Large SSQ, 1938; RAFGH, July 1940–1949; RAFSH 1949–61
Torquay, Devon: Officers' Convalescent Hospital, September 1939–January 1943. (After damage during two bombing raids, its function transferred to Cleveleys, Blackpool)
Uxbridge, Middx: RAF Officers' Hospital, 1925; WAAF Hospital, February 1940; RAFSH from August 1941; closed 1972
Weeton, Lancs: RAFSH, June 1940–December 1959
West Kirby, Wirral: RAFSH, 1940–December 1957
Wick, Scotland: SSQ (special treatment centre) April 1941; operating theatre open 1943; RAFSH, 1944–5
Wilmslow, Cheshire: RAFSH, July 1940– December 1958
Wroughton, Wilts: RAFGH, July 1941–67; Princess Alexandra's RAFH, 1967–76; Princess Alexandra's Hospital (RAF/Army), 1976–92; Princess Alexandra's RAFH, 1992–6
Yatesbury, Wilts: RAFSH, February 1939–December 1947

PMs have also worked, and continue to work, at SSQs on certain RAF stations around the UK.

III

HOSPITALS AND OTHER MEDICAL UNITS OF THE RAF OVERSEAS

1922–38 *(in order of opening)*

The earliest RAF hospitals overseas lay in the Middle East. They were formed from existing military hospitals manned by the RAMC during and immediately after the First World War.

Iraq:
> Baghdad, Indian and Isolation Hospitals manned by RAFNS from October 1922
> Baghdad/Hinaidi, No.23 Combined Service (RAF/Army) Hospital from October 1922; moved early 1923 to a new site and became RAFBGH Hinaidi, Baghdad; moved again December 1937 to Dhibban/ Habbaniya
> Basra (Basrah), RAF Combined (British and Indian) Hospital opened 1923; reduced to SSQ 1925; closed March 1928 but reopened briefly 1930s to cope with cholera epidemic
> Dhibban/Habbaniya, RAFBH/GH moved to Dhibban from Baghdad in December 1937; renamed RAF Habbaniya, May 1938
> Karradah, Indian Hospital, opening date not known; closed 1926
> Ser Amadia, rest and leave centre for RAF (summers only), 1932–54. PMs from hospitals in Iraq were attached here for short periods.

Egypt:
> Aboukir, SSQ, 1924–5 (closed because of riots); opened again from 1928–31
> Cairo, British Stationary Hospital (RAF/Army), 1920s

Palestine:
> Ludd (Lydda/Sarafand), Palestine General Hospital (RAF), 1924–40

Aden:
> Steamer Point, army hospital taken over by the RAF, 1 April 1928

1939–2000

Aden:
> Khormaksar Beach, Aden Protectorate Levies' Hospital, staffed by PMs 1959–67

Sheikh 'Othman: PMs stationed here 1941

Steamer Point: No.7 RAFH during Second World War; then RAFGH, closed 1967

Algeria: Algiers, No.2 RAFGH, November 1943–6

Azores: Lagens, SSQ/RAFSH, December 1943–October 1946

Bahamas: Nassau, SSQ/RAFH, October 1942–February 1946

Bahrain: RAFH January 1959–January 1964; became RAFH Muharraq, closed December 1971; active again as RAF War Hospital, December 1990–March 1991 (Gulf War)

Belgium: Brussels, No.8 RAFGH, September 1944–5

Burma:
  Kyaukpyu, Ramree Island, No.67 MFH, 1945
  Rangoon, No.65 MFH, July–November 1945; became RAFH Mingaladon, closed 1946

Ceylon: Katunayake, Negombo, hospital at staging post, 1950–60

China: Peking, British Embassy, digital post (one sister only), filled by a PM from 1973

Cyprus:
  Akrotiri: Princess Mary's RAFH, 1956–77; renamed The Princess Mary's Hospital (TPMH) and jointly staffed RAF/Army, 1977 to present. (On 1 April 1996 it became a Defence Medical Services [DMS] Hospital, part of the Defence Secondary Care Agency) Regional medical centre, current
  Nicosia, SSQ, current
  Troodos, medical centre, current

Egypt:
  Cairo (Abbassia/Heliopolis), No.5 RAFGH, 1942–7
  Fayid, RAFGH with families' wing at Abyad, 1947–56

France: Fontainebleau, French civil and military hospital, British wing, 1950s

Germany:
  Hamburg, No.53 MFH, 1945–6; became BMH
  Rinteln, No.8 RAFH, 1945–53; BMH, 1953–96 with digital post filled by a PM 1990s
  Rostrup, RAFH, 1952–8
  Wegberg, RAFH, 16 November 1953–31 March 1996

Gold Coast (now Ghana): Takoradi, RAFH, January 1942–November 1947

Hong Kong:
  No.80 MFH, became Static Hospital, September 1945
  SSQ opened June 1946, closed same year
  Kai Tak, SSQ/medical centre, closed 1979
  Kowloon, BMH, 1945/6–95, PMs attached 1980s and 1990s
  Shek Kong, army medical centre, PMs attached from 1979; closed on hand-over to China 1997

Iceland: Reykjavik, RAFH, March 1942–May 1946

India:
  Allahabad, Uttar Pradesh, No.11 RAFGH, 1945–1946
  Calcutta, W. Bengal, No.9 RAFGH, 1 January 1945–6
  Cawnpore, Uttar Pradesh, No.64 MFH, became No.12 RAFGH 1945–6

Chittagong (now Bangladesh), No.61 MFH, December 1943–July 1945
Imphal, Assam, No.60 MFH, January 1944–1945
Karachi (now Pakistan), No.10 RAFGH, April 1945–January 1948
Mauripur (now Pakistan), SSQ on staging post opened January 1948
Worli, Bombay, Second World War transit camp. SSQ opened January 1946, PMs withdrawn July 1947
No.62 MFH moved around the Arakan (area between Calcutta and Burma) 1944–6. Locations included Cox's Bazaar, Shillong, Khumbirgram, Comilla, Imphal and Meiktila

Iraq:
Habbaniya, RAFGH, 1938–56; RAFSH 1956–8
Ser Amadia, rest and leave centre, closed 1954

Israel/West Bank: Jerusalem, St John Ophthalmic Hospital, digital post filled by a PM 1980s

Italy:
Foggia, Apulia, No.4 RAFGH, June 1944–1946
Torre del Greco, Naples, No.1 RAFGH, replaced No.25 MFH, December 1943–May 1946

Japan:
Iwakuni, Honshu Island, British Commonwealth Air (BCAir) Hospital, July 1946–March 1948; RAF base and hospital active again October 1951–March 1955
Miho, Honshu Island, SSQ at RAF base, 1946–8
Okinawa, Ryuku Island, USAF/RAAF base, staging post for RAF casevacs, 1946–8 and 1951–5

Libya:
Benghazi, No.4 RAFGH, March 1943–April 1944
El Adem, SSQ at staging post, 1942–69
Tripoli, No.3 RAFGH, August 1943–January 1944

Malta: Luqa, No.1 RAF Field Hospital, August 1943; SSQ from May 1946

Pakistan: Islamabad, British Embassy, digital post filled by a PM 1980s and 1990s

Palestine: Tel Litwinsky, Jaffa, No.3 RAFGH, February 1944–January 1948

Saudi Arabia:
Al Jubail, medical centre/32 Field Hospital, 1990–1
Dhahran, King Abdul Aziz Airbase Military Hospital; PMs deployed here 1990–1

Singapore:
Changi, RAFGH 1947–72/3; ANZUK Hospital, then UK Military Hospital, 1972/3–5
Seletar, No.81 MFH operated here 1945/6; later an SSQ opened at RAF Seletar

Tunisia: Carthage, No.1 RAFGH, July–September 1943; No.31 MFH, September 1943–5

Yugoslavia: No.31 MFH was here during the late stages of the Second World War

IV

ROYAL PATRONS AND MATRONS-IN-CHIEF

Air Chief Commandant

1923–65   HRH Princess Mary, the Princess Royal, CI GCVO CBE RRC
1966–   HRH Princess Alexandra, the Honourable Lady Ogilvy, GCVO

Matrons-in-Chief

June–October 1918 Miss L.E. Jolley (*temporary service only*)
1918–30   Dame Joanna M. Cruickshank, DBE RRC
1930–8   Dame Katherine Christie Watt, DBE RRC
1938–43   Dame Emily M. Blair, DBE RRC
1943–8   Dame Gladys Taylor, DBE RRC
1948–52   Air Commandant Dame Helen W. Cargill, DBE RRC QHNS
1952–6   Air Commandant Dame Roberta M. Whyte, DBE RRC QHNS
1956–9   Air Commandant Dame Alice Mary Williamson, DBE RRC QHNS
1959–63   Air Commandant Dame Alice Lowrey, DBE RRC QHNS
1963–6   Air Commandant Dame Veronica M. Ashworth, DBE RRC QHNS
1966–70   Air Commandant Dame Pauline Giles, DBE RRC QHNS
1970–2   Air Commandant Ann S. McDonald, CB RRC QHNS

Directors of RAF Nursing Services and Matrons-in-Chief

1972–8   Air Commandant Barbara M. Ducat-Amos, CB RRC QHNS
1978–81   Air Commandant/Air Commodore Joan Metcalfe, CB RRC QHNS
1981–4   Air Commodore I. Joy Harris, CB RRC QHNS
1984–5   Air Commodore April A. Reed, RRC QHNS
1985–8   Group Captain M.M. Shaw, RRC QHNS
1988–91   Group Captain Elizabeth A.I. Sandison, RRC QHNS
1991–4   Group Captain Ethnea M. Hancock, RRC QHNS
1994–5   Group Captain Valerie M. Hand, RRC QHNS/Air Commodore DDNS 1995–7
1995–2001 Air Commodore Robert H. Williams, RRC QHNS/DDNS from 1999
2001–   Group Captain R. Annie Reid, OBE ARRC

V
PMs QUOTED IN THIS BOOK

This list details only those members of the PMRAFNS whose words are quoted verbatim in the text. They are listed alphabetically by birth surname. Many others, not detailed here, are mentioned in the book.

Eileen Adams (Mrs Knapper) PMRAFNS 1951–4; correspondence with the author 1999

Evelyn Addison (Mrs Glen) PMRAFNS 1943–6; correspondence with the author 1999

Mary Allen, VAD attached PMRAFNS 1939–45; correspondence with the author 1999

Susan Armistead (Mrs Sutcliffe) (Sqn Off Rtd) PMRAFNS 1943–51; correspondence with the author 1999

Alma Barnard (Mrs Tyack) PMRAFNS 1963–7; in recorded conversation 1999

Rona Black (Mrs McAlpine) PMRAFNS 1941–7; correspondence with the author, and wartime letters to her mother

Valerie Blackwell (Mrs Cornford) PMRAFNS 1942–5; correspondence with the author 1999

Janice Blood (formerly Hutton, now Mrs Oakman) (Sqn Ldr Rtd) PMRAFNS 1978–96; PMs Magazine 1998

Josephine Boase (Sqn Ldr Rtd) PMRAFNS 1967–88; PMRAFNS archive

Joan Botting (Mrs Peake) PMRAFNS 1940–6; diary and interview transcribed by her son Andrew G. Peake, Imperial War Museum

Christine Bramley (Mrs Bull) PMRAFNS 1954–8; PMs Magazine 1999

Jean Brown (Sqn Ldr Rtd) PMRAFNS 1954–8, 1960–73; correspondence with the author 1999

Constance P.I. Bull (Wg Cdr Rtd) PMRAFNS 1966–90; correspondence with the author 1999

Kathleen M. Burrows (Mrs Bennett) PMRAFNS 1945–58; PMs Magazine 1999

Gwen Butler (Wg Off Rtd) PMRAFNS 1925–52; information from her cousin Mrs Denize

Anne Caird (Mrs Austin) PMRAFNS 1948–51, 1954–5; PMs Magazine 1997

Helen W. Cargill (Air Cdt Rtd) PMRAFNS 1923–52 (MIC 1948–52); account of her life and career by her sister Jean Macrae, Imperial War Museum

Beryl Chadney, PMRAFNS 1943–7; correspondence with the author 1999

Elizabeth F. Chalton (Mrs Walker) PMRAFNS 1955–6; documents lodged at Hendon RAF Museum

W. Charlesworth, Matron, PMRAFNS First World War; PMRAFNS archive

Zena Cheel (Wg Off Rtd) PMRAFNS 1961–84; in recorded conversation 1999

Lesley Chew (Wg Cdr) PMRAFNS joined 1978, currently serving; *PMs Magazine* 1991

Margaret 'Jane' Clews, PMRAFNS 1951–5; correspondence with the author 1999

Judy Cooke (Mrs Owens) PMRAFNS 1962–5; correspondence with the author 1999

Lesley Cornwall-Jones (Mrs Howat) PMRAFNS 1953–5; *PMs Magazine* 1989

Violet Craig (Mrs Gibbons) PMRAFNS 1940–9; *PMs Magazine* 1978

Kathleen W. Cranston (Mrs Slim) PMRAFNS 1938–40; correspondence with the author 1999

Sandra Cranswick (Mrs Philpott) PMRAFNS 1966–70; correspondence with the author 1999

Margaret Crombie (Mrs Price) PMRAFNS 1949–51; correspondence with the author 1999

Kate Crompton (Mrs Wilmot) PMRAFNS 1963–6; correspondence with the author 1999

Dame Joanna Margaret Cruickshank (1875–1958), Matron-in-Chief of PMRAFNS 1918–30; her own writings, including unpublished draft of PMRAFNS history written after the Second World War

Sally Donovan (Mrs Pullan) PMRAFNS 1952–6; in recorded conversation 1999

Mary Drew (Mrs Mitchell) PMRAFNS 1941–6; *PMs Magazine* 1994

Muriel K. Dunn (Sqn Off Rtd) PMRAFNS 1951–72; *PMs Magazine* 1997

Marjorie Eavis (Mrs McCandlish) PMRAFNS 1943–52; *PMs Magazine* 1980

Mary E.R. Edwards (Mrs Sellors) PMRAFNS 1920–42; unpublished reminiscences (1964), PMRAFNS archive

Marjorie Ells PMRAFNS service dates not known; *PMs Magazine* 1979

Doreen A. Elston (Mrs Curston) PMRAFNS 1955–9; *PMs Magazine* 1999

Sylvia Emery (Mrs Pounds) PMRAFNS 1951–7; correspondence with the author 1999

Monica Fern (Sqn Ldr Rtd) PMRAFNS 1963–80; in recorded conversation 1999

Shelagh Firth (Gp Capt Rtd) PMRAFNS 1957–87; correspondence with the author 1999

Dulcie Flower (Mrs Wright) PMRAFNS 1945–8; correspondence with the author 1999

Doreen Francis (Sqn Off Rtd) PMRAFNS 1945–70; correspondence with the author 1999

Marianne Galletly (Mrs Hollowell) PMRAFNS 1941–5; correspondence with the author 1999

Winifred Gardner (Mrs Penman) PMRAFNS 1945–8; articles lodged at

RAF Museum Hendon, correspondence with the author 1999
Nadine Gay PMRAFNS NCE 1964–7; correspondence with the author 1999
Shelagh Glenn (Mrs Barber) PMRAFNS 1960–8; in recorded conversation 1999
Ann Golding (Sqn Off Rtd) PMRAFNS 1960–89; in recorded conversation 1999
Jackie Gross (Wg Cdr) PMRAFNS joined 1984, currently serving; *PMs Magazine* 1996
Debbie Gurney (Mrs Jones) (Sqn Ldr) PMRAFNS joined 1994, currently serving; *PMs Magazine* 1997
Ethnea Hancock (Gp Cpt Rtd) PMRAFNS 1961–94, MIC 1991–4; in recorded conversation 1999
Valerie M. Hand (Air Cdre Rtd) PMRAFNS 1967–71, 1972–95, MIC 1994–5, DDNS 1995–7; in recorded conversation 1999
Louise Hardy PMRAFNS 1923–46; *PMs Magazine* 1978 and 1979
Joy Harris (Air Cdre Rtd) PMRAFNS 1950–84, MIC 1981–4 in recorded conversation 1999
Jessie M. Higgins (Wg Off Rtd) PMRAFNS 1939–68; *PMs Magazine* 1996 and in recorded conversation 1999
Isobel Hipkin (Mrs Bedford) PMRAFNS 1963–9; correspondence with the author 1999
Kathleen Hird (Mrs Bion) PMRAFNS 1948–51; correspondence with the author 1999
Geoff Holliday (Sqn Ldr Rtd) RAFMS/PMRAFNS 1966–96; *PMs Magazine* 1985
Judy Hopkins (Mrs Foote) (Sqn Ldr Rtd) PMRAFNS 1966–82; in recorded conversation 1999
Noelle Horrocks PMRAFNS 1941–4; *PMs Magazine* 1982
Dorothy Hutchins (Sqn Off Rtd) PMRAFNS 1957–75; correspondence with the author 1999
Doreen Hunt (Mrs Tomlin) PMRAFNS 1953–8; *PMs Magazine* 1998 and correspondence with the author 1999
Julia Inkpen (Mrs Jenkins) PMRAFNS 1950–4; correspondence with the author 1999
Iris M. Jarred (Mrs Bartram) PMRAFNS 1942–6; in recorded conversation 1999
'Jenny' Jenkins PMRAFNS joined 1939, retirement date not known; *PMs Magazine* 1978
Rachel Johnson PMRAFNS 1985–96; *PMs Magazine* 1992
L.E. Jolley (Temporary Principal Matron) PMRAFNS June–November 1918; PRO records
Iris 'Fluffy' Jones (Mrs Bower, formerly Mrs Ogilvie) PMRAFNS 1939–49; unpublished memoir 'Normandy to the Baltic' (*c.*1985) and in correspondence and conversation 1999
Frances M. Keech (Mrs Judson, formerly Mrs Warner) PMRAFNS 1943–6; correspondence with the author 1999
Helen E. Kell (Sqn Ldr Rtd) PMRAFNS 1971–87; correspondence with the author 1999

Joyce F. Kellow (Mrs Wyatt) PMRAFNS 1944–7; correspondence with the author 1999
Linda Kendall (Mrs McKenzie) PMRAFNS NCE 1964–8; correspondence with the author 1999
Elizabeth Kidman (Sqn Ldr Rtd) PMRAFNS 1974–92; in recorded conversation 1999
Jean King (Mrs Flower) PMRAFNS 1956–60; *PMs Magazine* 1998
Margaret Kingston (Sqn Off Rtd) PMRAFNS 1951–71; in recorded conversation 1999
Olive Kirkham (Sqn Off Rtd) PMRAFNS 1950–66; correspondence with the author 1999
Mrs Joy Knowles (maiden name not known) PMRAFNS 1940s; correspondence with the author 1999
Richard Laurence (Sqn Ldr Rtd) PMRAFNS 1983–2000; in recorded conversation 1999
Tessa Lawless PMRAFNS 1951–5; *PMs Magazine* 1994 and 1997; and correspondence with the author 1999
Pamela Love (Mrs Batchelar) PMRAFNS 1947–51; correspondence with the author 1999
Elizabeth Lown (Mrs Armstrong) PMRAFNS 1965–9; unpublished memoir lodged at Hendon RAF Museum
Eve Loxston (Mrs Hall) PMRAFNS 1942–6; *PMs Magazine* 1999
Maureen Lumley (Wg Off Rtd) PMRAFNS 1942–74; correspondence with the author 1999
Kevin C. Mackie (Sqn Ldr) PMRAFNS joined 1990, currently serving; in recorded conversation 1999
A. Elizabeth Mansell (Mrs Ogden) PMRAFNS 1943–5; correspondence with the author 1999
Patricia Maslen (Mrs Perry) PMRAFNS NCE 1964–7; correspondence with the author 1999
Cynthia Mayfield (Mrs Brown) PMRAFNS NCE 1966–9; correspondence with the author 1999
Ishbel McCabe (Mrs Bennet) (Sqn Ldr Rtd) PMRAFNS 1986–91; correspondence with the author 1999
Colin McMillan (Flt Lt Rtd) PMRAFNS 1986–94; *PMs Magazine* 1992
Joan Metcalfe (Air Cdre Rtd) PMRAFNS 1948–81, MIC 1978–81, died June 2000; in recorded conversation 1999
Barbara Millar (Mrs Wright) PMRAFNS 1950–4; correspondence with the author 1999
Kathy Mogg (Mrs Ostler) PMRAFNS 1959–63; *PMs Magazine* 1985 and 1998
Mary Moultrie (Mrs Nicholson) PMRAFNS 1941–5; *PMs Magazine* 1983
Kate New (1883–1984), RAFNS 1918–20; story told to the editor of the *PMs Magazine* 1981
C.V. 'Ronnie' Oxborough (Sqn Ldr Rtd) 1968–84; correspondence with the author 1999
Mary Page (Mrs Payne) PMRAFNS 1953–7; correspondence with the author 1999
Dilys Palmer (Mrs Bore) PMRAFNS 1940–6; *PMs Magazine* 1993

Rosemary Partington (Wg Cdr Rtd) PMRAFNS 1957–88; in recorded conversation 1999

R.A. 'Penny' Penrose (Wg Off Rtd) PMRAFNS 1950–80; correspondence with the author 1999

Jean Ponsford (Mrs Howell) PMRAFNS 1942–5; *PMs Magazine* 1994

Susan Pound (Mrs Gray) PMRAFNS 1975–8; correspondence with the author 1999

Sheila Power (Mrs Bellamy-Knights) PMRAFNS 1967–72; in recorded conversation 1999

Monica Railton Jones (Mrs Chandler) PMRAFNS 1943–52; correspondence with the author 1999

Barbara Rampton (Mrs White) PMRAFNS 1944–7; correspondence with the author 1999

Iris Rawlings (Mrs Kerse) PMRAFNS 1958–66; correspondence with the author 1999

April Reed (Air Cdre Rtd) PMRAFNS 1955–85, MIC 1984–5; in recorded conversation 1999

R. Annie Reid (Gp Cpt) PMRAFNS joined 1975, MIC from March 2001; *PMs Magazine* 1988

Helen Ryan (Flt Lt Rtd) PMRAFNS 1984–92; correspondence with the author 1999

Elizabeth E.I. Sandison (Gp Cpt Rtd) PMRAFNS 1964–91, MIC 1988–91; in recorded conversation 1999

E. Thérèse Saunders (Mrs Ayres) PMRAFNS 1952–6; correspondence with the author 1999

Angela Scofield (Wg Cdr Rtd) PMRAFNS 1980–98; in correspondence and conversation 1999

Mary Michal 'Miche' Shaw (Gp Cpt Rtd) PMRAFNS 1963–88, MIC 1985–8; correspondence with the author 1999

Elizabeth Smallwood (Mrs Andrews) PMRAFNS 1941–5; *PMs Magazine* 1993

Doreen Smedley (Wg Cdr Rtd) PMRAFNS 1955–83; in recorded conversation 1999

Janet Smith (Mrs Campbell) PMRAFNS 1956–60; correspondence with the author 1999

J.E. 'Beth' Smith (Mrs Hamson) PMRAFNS NCE 1967–8; correspondence with the author 1999

Sharon Smith (Mrs Callcott) (Sqn Ldr) PMRAFNS joined 1987, currently serving; *PMs Magazine* 1995 and correspondence with the author 1999

Terry A. Smith, RAFMS/PMRAFNS 1966–97; PMRAFNS archive

Doris Stanford (Mrs Kent) PMRAFNS 1947–60; *PMs Magazine* 1999 and in correspondence and conversation 1999

D.M. 'Jane' Stott (Sqn Off Rtd) PMRAFNS 1953–69; *PMs Magazine* 1997

Anne Sumner (Mrs Wynne-Jones) PMRAFNS NCE 1962–3; audio-tape sent to author 1999

Pat Surridge (Sqn Ldr Rtd) PMRAFNS 1966–94; *PMs Magazine* 1986

Anne M. Taylor (Sqn Off Rtd) PMRAFNS 1956–71; in recorded conversation 1999

Ann Tickle (Mrs Waters) PMRAFNS 1952–7; correspondence with the author 1999

Gwladys N. 'Tommy' Thomas (Mrs McGregor) PMRAFNS 1939–44; correspondence with the author 1999

Annie Warburton (Sqn Ldr) PMRAFNS joined 1984, currently serving; in recorded conversation 1999

Pippa Ward (Sqn Ldr) PMRAFNS joined 1988, currently serving; *PMs Magazine* and correspondence with the author 1999

Christina Watson (Mrs Hunter) PMRAFNS 1941–6; correspondence with the author 1997–9

Marion Welch (Mrs Lampard) PMRAFNS 1918–30; letters and reports, PMRAFNS archive

Joan K. White (Mrs Cool) PMRAFNS 1943–6; correspondence with the author 1999

Mary Williams (Mrs Hancock) PMRAFNS 1944–8; correspondence with the author 1999

Wendy Williams (Wg Cdr) PMRAFNS joined 1984, currently serving; *PMs Magazine* 1988

Robert H. Williams (Air Cdre Rtd) RAFMS 1962–76; Med Tech Branch 1976–80; PMRAFNS joined 1980, MIC 1995–2001, DDNS 1999–2001; in correspondence and conversation 1999–2000

Marion Wood (Mrs Donaldson) PMRAFNS 1961–7; in correspondence and conversation 1999

Clare Woolley (Mrs Fowler) PMRAFNS 1962–70; correspondence with the author 1999

VI

INITIALISMS AND ACRONYMS

AC	Aircraftman (lowest rank in the RAF)
AMA	Assistant Medical Administrator
AOC-in-C	Air Officer Commanding-in-Chief
ARRC	Associate of the Royal Red Cross
BCAir	British Commonwealth Air Forces in Japan 1946–8
BMH	British military hospital
CAS	Chief of the Air Staff
CB	Companion of the Bath
CBE	Commander of (the Order of) the British Empire
CCS	Casualty clearing station
CI	(Order of the) Crown of India
C-in-C	Commander-in-Chief
CO	Commanding officer
DBE	Dame Commander of (the Order of) the British Empire
DDNS	Director of Defence Nursing Services (from 1985)
DGMS	Director General of Medical Services (from 1938)
DMS	Director of Medical Services (1918–38)
DNS(RAF)	Director of Royal Air Force Nursing Services (from 1972)
(D)WRAF	Director of the Women's Royal Air Force
(D)WRNS	Director of the Women's Royal Naval Service
EN(G)	Enrolled nurse (General)
FOPD	Forward outpatients department
GCVO	Knight Grand Cross of the (Royal) Victorian Order
GS	General service
IPTM	Institute of Pathology and Tropical Medicine (at PMRAFH Halton)
ITW	Initial training wing
LAC	Leading aircraftman
MDHU	Ministry of Defence Hospital Unit
MIC	Matron-in-Chief
MFH	Mobile field hospital
MO	Medical Officer
MOD	Ministry of Defence
NBC	Nuclear, biological and chemical
NCE	Non-commissioned element (students/staff nurses, 1962–77)
NCO	Non-commissioned officer

NHS	National Health Service
OC	Officer commanding
PARAFH	Princess Alexandra's Royal Air Force Hospital
PMO	Principal medical officer
PMRAFH	Princess Mary's Royal Air Force Hospital
PMRAFNS	Princess Mary's Royal Air Force Nursing Service
PMs	Members of the PMRAFNS
PoW	Prisoner of war
PQRE	Professionally Qualified and Re-entrant (officers' training course)
QAIMNS	Queen Alexandra's Imperial Military Nursing Service (until 1949)
QARANC	Queen Alexandra's Royal Army Nursing Corps (from 1949)
QARNNS	Queen Alexandra's Royal Naval Nursing Service
QHNS	Queen's Honorary Nursing Sister
RAAF	Royal Australian Air Force
RAF	Royal Air Force
RAFBH	Royal Air Force British Hospital
RAFGH	Royal Air Force General Hospital
RAFH	Royal Air Force Hospital
RAFNS	Royal Air Force Nursing Service (1918–23)
RAFSH	Royal Air Force Station Hospital
RAMC	Royal Army Medical Corps
RFC	Royal Flying Corps
RGN	Registered general nurse
RMN	Registered mental nurse
RNAS	Royal Naval Air Service
RRC	(Holder of the) Royal Red Cross
SAC	Senior aircraftman
SEN	State-enrolled nurse
SERE	Specialist Entrant and Re-entrant (officers' training course)
SNCO	Senior non-commissioned officer
SSQ	Station sick quarters
SRN	State-registered nurse
TPMH	The Princess Mary's Hospital
UN	United Nations
UNPROFOR	United Nations Protection Force
u/s	Unserviceable
USAF	United States Air Force
VAD	(Nurse of the) Voluntary Aid Detachment
WAAF	Women's Auxiliary Air Force (1939–49)
WO	Warrant officer
WRAF	Women's Royal Air Force (1918–20; and from 1949)
WRNS	Women's Royal Naval Service
YMCA	Young Men's Christian Association
aeromed	aeromedical evacuation flight, bringing patients back to home hospital
casevac	a more urgent and immediate evacuation of seriously ill or battle-wounded casualties

BIBLIOGRAPHY

Published works

Arthur, Max, *There Shall be Wings: The RAF from 1918 to the Present*
(Hodder and Stoughton, 1993)
Beauman, Katherine Bentley, *Partners in Blue* (Hutchinson, 1971)
Bowyer, Chaz, *RAF Operations 1918–1938* (William Kimber, 1988)
Bushby, John R., *Air Defence of Great Britain* (Ian Allan, 1973)
Cormack, Andrew (Text), and Volstad, Ron (Colour plates), *The Royal Air
Force 1939–45 (Uniforms)*, Osprey Men-at-Arms Series (Osprey
Publishing, 1990)
Escott, Beryl E., *Women in Air Force Blue* (Patrick Stephens, 1989)
Fairbairn, Tony, *Action Stations Overseas* (Patrick Stephens, 1991)
Green, Peter, and Hodgson, Mike, *Cranwell: RNAS and RAF Photographs*
(Midland Publishing, 1993)
Harfield, Alan, *Blandford and the Military* (Dorset Publishing, 1984)
McBryde, Brenda, *Quiet Heroines* (Chatto and Windus, 1985)
MTE Journal, 1941–5
Otter, Patrick, *Lincolnshire Airfields in World War Two* (Countryside
Books, 1996)
Rexford-Welch, S.C. (Ed.), *The Royal Air Force Medical Services* (in 3
Volumes), part of *History of the Second World War/United Kingdom
Medical Series* (HMSO 1954)
Ross, Tony (Ed.), *75 Eventful Years: A Tribute to the Royal Air Force
1918–1993*. Section on PMRAFNS by Gp Capt E.M. Hancock
(Wingham Aviation Books, Canterbury, 1993)
Taylor, Eric, *Front-Line Nurse: British Nurses in World War II* (Robert
Hale, 1997)
Thetford, Owen, *Aircraft of the Royal Air Force since 1918* (Putnam,
1988)
Tunbridge, Paul, *History of RAF Halton* (Buckland, 1995)
Woodman, Richard, *The Arctic Convoys, 1939–45* (John Murray, 1994)

Other sources

Air Historical Branch, London
College Library, RAF Cranwell

Community Relations, RAF Coningsby
Imperial War Museum, London
Personnel Records, RAF Innsworth
PMRAFNS history files, Matron-in-Chief's Office
Public Record Office, Kew
RAF Museum, Hendon
Royal Signals Museum, Blandford, Dorset

INDEX